Philosophical Issues
in Psychiatry II

International Perspectives in Philosophy and Psychiatry

Series editors: Bill (K.W.M.) Fulford, Katherine Morris, John Z. Sadler, and Giovanni Stanghellini

Volumes in the series:

Portrait of the Psychiatrist as a Young Man: The Early Writing and Work of R.D. Laing, 1927–1960
Beveridge

Mind, Meaning, and Mental Disorder 2e
Bolton and Hill

What is Mental Disorder?
Bolton

Delusions and Other Irrational Beliefs
Bortolotti

Postpsychiatry
Bracken and Thomas

Philosophy, Psychoanalysis, and the A-Rational Mind
Brakel

Unconscious Knowing and Other Essays in Psycho-Philosophical Analysis
Brakel

Psychiatry as Cognitive Neuroscience
Broome and Bortolotti (eds.)

Free Will and Responsibility: A Guide for Practitioners
Callender

Reconceiving Schizophrenia
Chung, Fulford, and Graham (eds.)

Darwin and Psychiatry
De Block and Adriaens (eds.)

Nature and Narrative: An Introduction to the New Philosophy of Psychiatry
Fulford, Morris, Sadler, and Stanghellini (eds.)

Oxford Textbook of Philosophy and Psychiatry
Fulford, Thornton, and Graham

The Mind and its Discontents
Gillett

Thinking Through Dementia
Hughes

Dementia: Mind, Meaning, and the Person
Hughes, Louw, and Sabat (eds.)

Talking Cures and Placebo Effects
Jopling

Schizophrenia and the Fate of the Self
Lysaker and Lysaker

Responsibility and Psychopathy
Malatesti and McMillan

Body-Subjects and Disordered Minds
Matthews

Rationality and Compulsion: Applying action theory to psychiatry
Nordenfelt

Philosophical Perspectives on Technology and Psychiatry
Phillips (ed.)

The Metaphor of Mental Illness
Pickering

Mapping the Edges and the In-between
Potter

Trauma, Truth, and Reconciliation: Healing Damaged Relationships
Potter (ed.)

The Philosophy of Psychiatry: A Companion
Radden

The Virtuous Psychiatrist
Radden and Sadler

Feelings of Being
Ratcliffe

Values and Psychiatric Diagnosis
Sadler

Disembodied Spirits and Deanimated Bodies: The Psychopathology of Common Sense
Stanghellini

Essential Philosophy of Psychiatry
Thornton

Empirical Ethics in Psychiatry
Widdershoven, McMillan, Hope and Van der Scheer (eds.)

The Sublime Object of Psychiatry: Schizophrenia in Clinical and Cultural Theory
Woods

Philosophical Issues in Psychiatry II
Nosology

Edited by

Kenneth S. Kendler

Josef Parnas

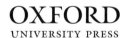

OXFORD
UNIVERSITY PRESS

OXFORD
UNIVERSITY PRESS

Great Clarendon Street, Oxford, OX2 6DP,
United Kingdom

Oxford University Press is a department of the University of Oxford.
It furthers the University's objective of excellence in research, scholarship,
and education by publishing worldwide. Oxford is a registered trade mark of
Oxford University Press in the UK and in certain other countries

© Oxford University Press, 2012

The moral rights of the authors have been asserted

First Edition published in 2012

Impression: 1

British Library Cataloguing in Publication Data

Data available

Library of Congress Cataloguing in Publication Data

Data available

ISBN 978-0-19-964220-5

Printed and bound by
CPI Group (UK) Ltd, Croydon, CR0 4YY

Preface

All the chapters of this book began as talks given at a conference held in Copenhagen, Denmark, on 14–16 November, 2010, sponsored by the National Danish Research Foundation's Center for Subjectivity Research and the Faculty of Health Sciences, University of Copenhagen. The conference was organized and chaired by the editors of this volume, Kenneth S. Kendler and Josef Parnas.

This conference had been initially scheduled for 21–23 April of that year. However, nature intervened. The eruption of the Icelandic volcano, Eyjafjallajökull, disrupted air traffic over much of northern Europe from 15–23 April. One of us (KSK) had made it to Amsterdam before the shutdown, while the other (JP) was safely ensconced in Copenhagen. After the initial eruption, for several days, there were anguished telephone calls each night trying to decide whether to proceed with the meeting or to cancel. Overnight, with no prior training, JP became an expert in volcanic ash and its distribution by wind currents. But finally, it became clear. We had no choice. We cancelled the conference expressing our regret to all of the participants and registrants and promising to find another date to try again.

The second time, the forces of nature were more cooperative. The conference went off without incident. We were very pleased that of the original invited speakers, all but one attended the rescheduled conference.

The conference itself was a highly stimulating 3-day experience. Each talk was followed by a formal commentary and then, an open give-and-take with the audience and other speakers, who were rarely shy about chipping in. So every speaker coming to the meeting was willing to present a paper of their own, comment formally on another, and agree to write them both up for publication. They were still willing to come despite these onerous responsibilities.

Like the first volume in this series (Kendler and Parnas 2008), we have tried to capture the interactive nature of the meeting through the organization of this volume. In addition to a general introduction to the volume and conclusion, written respectively by the two editors (KSK and JP), each individual paper has an introduction (written mostly by KSK or JP) and a discussion.

In working on a book like this, one naturally accumulates debts. Surely our deepest goes to the contributors to the volume. Their willingness to come back for a second try, to put up with all of our demands, and to (mostly) get their contributions in to us on time, all made the work on this volume much easier. The conference would not have been possible without the financial support of the National Danish Research Foundation. We also owe a debt of thanks to Jill Opalesky. She was involved, with her gentle manner and wonderful organizational skills, in all aspects of this project, from inviting the speakers, to setting up the schedule, to helping us keep straight all the submitted chapters and comments through their multiple revisions. We also want to acknowledge the steady efforts of Merete Lynnerup, who in her charming, no-drama manner, accomplished all local managerial and organizational tasks. We also thank Simon Höffding and Clarisse Sternberg for practical assistance during the conference.

We ended the preface to the first volume in this series with these words: "This project was, to use the philosophical term, emergent—in the end, the sum was much more than the individual parts." We are pleased to say that we also felt this way about the present volume and hope that you, the readers, will agree with us.

Kenneth S. Kendler

Reference

Kendler, K. S. and Parnas, J. (2008). *Philosophical Issues in Psychiatry: Explanation, Phenomenology and Nosology* (1st ed.). Baltimore, MD: Johns Hopkins University Press.

Contents

List of Contributors *xi*

Introduction *xiii*

Part I **The basics: the definition of psychiatric illness and rules for classification**

Chapter 1

Introduction *3*
Kenneth S. Kendler

Chapter: Classification and causal mechanisms: a deflationary approach to the classification problem *6*
Derek Bolton

Comments: The National Institute of Mental Health Research Domain Criteria (RDoC) project: moving towards a neuroscience-based diagnostic classification in psychiatry *12*
Michael B. First

Chapter 2

Introduction *19*
Kenneth S. Kendler

Chapter: Progress and the calibration of scientific constructs: the role of comparative validity *21*
Peter Zachar

Comments: Progress and the calibration of scientific constructs: a new look at validity *35*
Rachel Cooper

Chapter 3

Introduction *41*
Josef Parnas

Chapter: Taking disease seriously: beyond "pragmatic" nosology *42*
S. Nassir Ghaemi

Comments: What is psychiatric disease? A commentary on Dr Ghaemi's paper *54*
Derek Bolton

Chapter 4

Introduction *59*
Kenneth S. Kendler

Chapter: Is psychiatric classification a good thing? *61*
Rachel Cooper

Comments: Diagnoses as labels *71*
S. Nassir Ghaemi

Part II The historical development of modern psychiatric diagnoses

Chapter 5

Introduction *75*
Josef Parnas

Chapter: The nosological entity in psychiatry: a historical illusion or a moving target? *77*
Assen Jablensky

Comments: The Kraepelinian pipe organ model (for a more dimensional) DSM-5 classification *95*
Darrel A. Regier

Chapter 6

Introduction *99*
Kenneth S. Kendler

Chapter: The 19th-century nosology of alienism: history and epistemology *101*
German E. Berrios

Comments: The nature of the psychiatric object and classification *118*
Josef Parnas

Chapter 7

Introduction *125*
Kenneth S. Kendler

Chapter: The development of DSM-III from a historical/conceptual perspective *127*
Michael B. First

Comments: Evaluating DSM-III: structure, process and outcomes *141*
Harold Alan Pincus

Chapter 8

Introduction *143*
Kenneth S. Kendler

Chapter: DSM-IV: context, concepts and controversies *145*
Harold Alan Pincus

Comments: DSM-IV: some critical remarks *161*
Mario Maj

Part III **The problem of validity**

Chapter 9

Introduction *167*
Josef Parnas

Chapter: A philosophical overview of the
problems of validity for psychiatric disorders *169*
Kenneth F. Schaffner

Comments: Validity, utility and reality:
explicating Schaffner's pragmatism *190*
Peter Zachar

Chapter 10

Introduction *197*
Kenneth S. Kendler

Chapter: Structural validity and the classification
of mental disorders *199*
Robert F. Krueger and Nicholas R. Eaton

Comments: Seeing sense in psychiatric diagnoses *213*
Paul R. McHugh

Part IV **Application to major depression and schizophrenia**

Chapter 11

Introduction *219*
Josef Parnas

Chapter: When does depression become a mental disorder? *221*
Mario Maj

Comments: A sea of distress *229*
Josef Parnas

Chapter 12

Introduction *235*
Assen Jablensky

Chapter: DSM-IV and the founding prototype of schizophrenia: are we regressing to a pre-Kraepelinian nosology? *237*
Josef Parnas

Comments: Phenomenology, nosology and prototypes *260*
Kenneth S. Kendler

Part V The way(s) forward

Chapter 13

Introduction *267*
Josef Parnas

Chapter: Rendering mental disorders intelligible: addressing psychiatry's urgent challenge *269*
Paul R. McHugh

Comments: A search for coherence *280*
Assen Jablensky

Chapter 14

Introduction *283*
Kenneth S. Kendler

Chapter: Diagnostic threshold considerations for DSM-5 *285*
Darrel A. Regier

Comments: The tangible burden of mental disorder in the absence of mental disorder categories in nature: some reflections on Regier's contribution *298*
Robert F. Krueger

Chapter 15

Introduction *303*
Josef Parnas

Chapter: Epistemic iteration as a historical model for psychiatric nosology: promises and limitations *305*
Kenneth S. Kendler

Comments: Coherentist approaches to scientific progress in psychiatry: comments on Kendler *323*
Kenneth F. Schaffner

Index *331*

List of Contributors

Editors

Kenneth S. Kendler
Rachel Brown Banks Distinguished
Professor of Psychiatry
Professor of Human Genetics
Director, Psychiatric Genetics
Research Program
Director, Virginia Institute for
Psychiatric and Behavioral Genetics
Virginia Commonwealth University
Richmond VA, USA

Josef Parnas
Clinical Professor
University of Copenhagen
Psychiatric Center Hvidovre & Danish
National Research Foundation's Center
for Subjectivity Research
Njalsgade, Copenhagen, Denmark

Chapter Contributors

German E. Berrios
Chair in the Epistemology of Psychiatry
University of Cambridge, UK
Emeritus Consultant Neuropsychiatrist
& Head of the Department of
Neuropsychiatry
Addenbrooke's Hospital
Cambridge, UK

Derek Bolton
Professor of Philosophy &
Psychopathology,
Kings College London, Institute
of Psychiatry
Honorary Consultant Clinical
Psychologist
South London & Maudsley NHS Trust
Institute of Psychiatry
London, UK

Rachel Cooper
Senior Lecturer
Politics, Philosophy and Religion
Lancaster University
Lancaster, UK

Nicholas R. Eaton
Department of Psychology
University of Minnesota
Minneapolis, MN, USA

Michael B. First
Professor of Clinical Psychiatry
Columbia University
Research Psychiatrist
New York State Psychiatric Institute
Associate,
Forensic Panel
World Health Organization
New York, NY, USA

S. Nassir Ghaemi
Professor of Psychiatry and
Pharmacology
Tufts University School of Medicine,
Director, Mood Disorders Program,
Tufts Medical Center
Boston, MA, USA

Assen Jablensky
School of Psychiatry & Clinical
Neurosciences
The University of Western Australia
Centre for Clinical Research in
Neuropsychiatry (CCRN)
Graylands Hospital
Perth, Australia

Robert F. Krueger
Hathaway Distinguished Professor
Department of Psychology
University of Minnesota
Minneapolis, MN, USA

Mario Maj
Professor of Psychiatry
Director, Department of Psychiatry
University of Naples
President, World Psychiatric Association
Naples, Italy

Paul R. McHugh
Distinguished University Professor
Former Director Department of
Psychiatry and Behavioral Science
Johns Hopkins University
Baltimore, MD, USA

Harold Alan Pincus
Professor and Vice Chair of the
Department of Psychiatry
Co-Director, Irving Institute for Clinical
and Translational Research
Columbia University
Director of Quality and Outcomes
Research
New York-Presbyterian Hospital
Senior Scientist, RAND Corporation
New York, NY, USA

Darrel A. Regier
Executive Director
American Psychiatric Institute for
Research and Education
Director, Division of Research
American Psychiatric Association
Vice-Chair, DSM-5 Task Force
Arlington, VA, USA

Kenneth F. Schaffner
Distinguished University Professor
Department of History and Philosophy
of Science
University of Pittsburgh
Pittsburgh, PA, USA

Peter Zachar
Professor and Chair
Auburn University Montgomery
Department of Psychology
Montgomery, AL, USA

Introduction

Kenneth S. Kendler

The goal here is to introduce and briefly review some of the main themes you will confront in the rich series of chapters of this book, all prefaced by introductions and followed by comments.

Psychiatric nosology is a hybrid discipline. It is not science, but we all agree (I hope) that it should be scientifically informed. It is strongly pragmatic—having to serve the needs of clinicians, administrators and funders—but it should be more than that. It is influenced by a range of tensions. Here is a selected list on which we will briefly comment: clinician versus researcher, reliability versus validity, past versus future, psychiatry versus psychology, realism versus nominalism, descriptive versus etiologic models, and surface versus deeper phenomenological characterization of psychiatric symptoms and syndromes. Finally, we will talk about the problem of the governance of change in diagnostic systems. By what rules should this operate?

Nosologies have to serve at least two masters (not counting the administrative and insurance apparatus of health care)—researchers and clinicians. These needs are sometimes in conflict. Researchers want detailed, highly accurate diagnoses and typically ask more rather than fewer questions. Clinicians are always in a hurry and so for them the shorter and simpler the diagnostic criteria the better. The DSMs have tried to steer betwixt these two extremes, developing a single diagnostic manual for both communities. The ICD-10 took a different approach, producing two manuals—one for each.

Obtaining improved reliability was central to the development of operationalized diagnostic criteria and the rise of DSM-III. While subtle in its subforms (e.g., inter-rater, test–retest, etc.), it is nonetheless a far more straightforward concept than validity. Everyone wants a valid nosology, but there are many different possible meanings of that term. In its most simple form (at least as I see it—which requires that we reject some concepts such as "face" validity), validity from a diagnostic perspective means that the diagnosis does "some work in the world." That is, by knowing that a patient is in a diagnostic class we learn something of import.

One theme for DSM-5, especially during its early planning phases, was to try to move the central focus away from reliability and toward validity. One deep problem inherent in the goal to make psychiatric diagnoses more valid is that different kinds of validity might give us different answers. That is, the kind of criteria that might perform optimally to predict outcome or treatment might be different from those criteria which are best at predicting genetic risk factors. What do we do then?

Psychiatric nosology is historical-situated. It has a distinct past and now much debate about its future. The large majority of diagnoses in our manuals are clinical–historical concepts. Why are those particular diagnoses in our nosologies and not others? Why are certain historical figures so influential and others not? When we make changes, how much respect is due to the historical concepts and traditions? Under what circumstances should we chuck the whole thing out and start over?

The nature of what we should expect in the future is also a subject of debate. Are we in a "holding pattern" waiting for major breakthroughs that will thoroughly transform our diagnostic system? How much should we insist on a cumulative model for our diagnostic revisions? That is, are we trying to incrementally get better and better, thereby, trying to approach some external reality of "true" diagnoses? How much of a problem is historical instability in our diagnoses—making major shifts between versions?

In our diagnostic debates, we have to deal with two different historical traditions: the great clinicians of psychiatry, and the psychometrics of psychology. Until very recently, the former has been far and away the dominant paradigm. How should the well-developed tools of psychometrics (e.g., confirmatory factor analysis, item–response theory) be brought into the process of nosologic revision?

Questions about the nature of psychiatric disorders run through many chapters in this volume. That is, what kinds of things are they? Different terms can be used to describe this debate. On one side is realism: psychiatric disorders are clear and distinct, real things out there in the world for us to discover. On the other side is nominalism and social constructivism. Nominalism roughly suggests that categories like psychiatric disorders are not real, but rather, entirely human creations. Social constructivism is a bit more specific suggesting that these categories are, in the extreme, entirely the result of socio-cultural processes. They are not in any sense independent things that exist in nature. They are invented rather than discovered.

Realism can come in several flavors. At one extreme, we might expect psychiatric disorders to be nice, crisp universal categories like elements in the periodic table. Other softer versions might use more messy categories—like species—as a model for the kind of thing that psychiatric disorders are.

Realism and nominalism have very different predictions for the degree to which psychiatric disorders should or should not be stable over time and space. And there are hybrid positions that suggest psychiatric disorders are influenced by both real things in the world (e.g. features of the evolved human mind/brain system) and also by cultural, social and economic factors. Furthermore, for different disorders, the importance of these two classes of causes might vary.

For completeness, we would have to add the concept of essentialism, usually a version of realism (but there are also Platonic essences), that is, that psychiatric disorders—like elements of the periodic table—have crisp, clean essences, so that once you know the essence you know (just about) everything else you would want to know about a diagnosis.

A position between realism on the one hand and nominalism and/or social construction on the other is possible—pragmatism. Here the goal is to avoid metaphysical debates about the true nature of psychiatric illness and just get on with designing a system that best does what we want it to—predict course, relate to treatment response and/or reflect neurobiological or genetic risk factors.

Should psychiatric nosology, at its root, be descriptive or etiological? Put another way, should disorders be grouped together because they clinically resemble one another, or because they share key etiological features? DSM-III self-consciously eschewed etiological models, in part, to escape from the dominance of psychoanalytic theory. Since then, there has been an oft-expressed yearning for psychiatric diagnoses to be based on clean etiological models. Is this realistic?

From what we now know about psychiatric disorders, most of them are influenced by a wide array of risk factors spanning a number of levels (e.g., including molecular, neural, psychological, social, and cultural factors). Where will we chose the level of etiology on which to base our nosology? Only a minority of medical disorders—such as Mendelian genetic diseases—have simple crisp etiologies. No psychiatric disorder, at least given our current knowledge, comes close to having such a single clean etiology. If psychiatry moves toward etiological models, how will we determine the privileged level of explanation that will be used on which to base our nosology? Should it be the same across different groups of disorders (e.g., psychotic versus personality disorders)?

The symptoms of psychiatric illness can be understood at many levels. Some surface features, such as insomnia or weight gain, are relatively simple and usually easy to define and assess. Other constructs, like delusional percept, can be quite subtle. In the push to improve reliability of psychiatric diagnosis, DSM-III tended to include– for its operationalized criteria—symptoms and signs that were easy to define and rate. How much was lost in this effort?

It has been argued, with considerable force, that an unintended consequence of the popularity of the DSM has been the impoverishment of the psychopathological world of psychiatry. Here, some cultural factors are also at work. The major architects of the American DSM system had little knowledge of, or sympathy for, the phenomenological tradition that has so much influence on European psychiatry. They cited Kraepelin and may have read a bit of his work, but little more. Only at Johns Hopkins University was there a tradition of reading Jaspers and other classics of descriptive psychiatry from the European tradition.

Has the DSM, with its focus on reliability, sacrificed greater validity that would come with the use of subtler but critical psychopathological constructs? Or is it acceptable for diagnoses to focus on reliable surface features, with the understanding that arriving at a diagnosis should never constitute the sum and totality of a psychiatric evaluation?

Finally, the theme of the governance of nosologic change comes up at several points in this volume. Should we worry about "criteria for changing criteria"? Should we have a robust scientifically focused process, requiring strong empirical evidence to make changes? Or is informed opinion, that, for example, "DSM-IV was wrong and we can do better" sufficient to justify change? If we adopt the former, how do we deal with the very great differences in the quality of empirical evidence across different diagnostic categories? How could it be justified to require more rigorous rules for change in DSM-5 than were used to create DSM-III in the first place? Is there a risk of creating a catch-22 in which new diagnoses cannot be adopted if they have not yet been studied, but will not be studied before they are adopted?

These themes echo back to the questions about the nature of psychiatric disorders. Realists have an easy time of suggesting that psychiatric nosology should be cumulative.

They want to get closer and closer to the truth. Pragmatists, also, could easily imagine getting closer and closer to the practical goal they would set for a nosology. For social constructionists, by contrast, the very idea of a cumulative process makes no sense. There is no place toward which to accumulate.

So, we hope you find this book enjoyable and stimulating. The problems presented here will not likely go away anytime soon. We hope by providing the introductions, main chapters and comments, we have captured some of the excitement and interchange of the original conference on which these papers were based. Many of the tensions are likely inherent in the process of psychiatric nosology. We would be content with the hope that we have, in a small degree, illuminated these issues and clarified them, perhaps helping this critical process to move forward with greater deliberative wisdom.

Part I

The basics: the definition of psychiatric illness and rules for classification

Chapter 1

Introduction

Kenneth S. Kendler

In this succinct and rich essay, Derek Bolton sketches a recommended approach for psychiatry to the recurrent problems of its nosology. The particular question he wants to ponder is: how do we organize our broad diagnostic classes? In current DSM-5 parlance, this is the "meta-structure problem" (Andrews et al. 2009).

His message is largely a deflationary one. That is, "Don't get too hung up about it." His comments are a useful antidote to current preoccupation with nosology in psychiatry—fueled in part by our ritual practices, about every decade—of revising our two chief diagnostic systems: Diagnostic and Statistical Manual of Mental Disorders (DSM) and International Classification of Diseases (ICD). Our field is acting as if all depended upon getting this right. That may be a bit of an exaggeration.

However, he does not intend to be pessimistic about the prospects of classification per se. Rather, he suggests that the importance of getting classification "right" has probably been over-valued. After all, the main aim of the psychiatric science is not classification as an end in itself but rather identification of causes and interventions.

Bolton's underlying approach to psychiatric nosology is a pragmatic one. Diagnoses are good because they can do something useful in the world, like predict prognosis, functional magnetic resonance imaging (fMRI) results or, even better, treatment response. In this view, he shares much with Peter Zachar, another contributor to this volume, whose work on a "Practical Kinds" model for psychiatric illness could be profitably consulted (Zachar 2000, 2003). Furthermore, this approach is squarely within the instrumentalist tradition in the philosophy of science that our goal in science is to predict and, if possible, successfully manipulate the world, without getting hung up about the metaphysics, whether the constructs, which we construct to help us do so, are "real" or not.

In choosing particular diagnostic criteria, Bolton suggests that this too is a pragmatic decision. Subtype a disorder one way, he suggests, you might optimize predictive validity; and subtype another way, that might be best for treatment choice. In this, his views are very close to those I expressed some time ago about diagnostic validators (Kendler 1990). Once you chose what you want diagnoses to do, then you can go about selecting disorders empirically that perform best on those validators. But, the choice of validators reflects more a value judgment (what do we want most from our diagnoses?) than a scientific question.

In his emphasis on pragmatism in diagnosis, does this mean that Bolton gives up on the wish for nosology to reflect reality—or is there even a "there there" with respect to psychiatric disorders? This remains a controversial topic (see Kendler et al. (2010) for one recent review).

Very briefly, Bolton touches on the equally weighty issue of how we draw the line between psychiatric illness and the various forms of non-disordered suffering. Congruent with his thoughtfully argued book on this subject (Bolton 2008), he suggests that these questions do ". . .not primarily have to do with the sciences of causes, but which are rather to do with subjective and social phenomenology."

One of Bolton's main points, with which I have a great deal of sympathy (Kendler in press), is that the nature of psychiatric disorders do not yield up to a reductionist, "one-cause," etiological model which represents the ideal in medicine—what Bolton calls "the 19th/20th-century biomedical disease paradigm." While we might find this clear picture—where all roads lead to one essentialist cause—in Mendelian genetic disorders and some infectious diseases, it is really an exception even in medicine (where most morbid conditions in Western countries like hypertension and asthma are highly complex and multilevel) and probably out of the question for psychiatric disorders.

He also raises, in one of his rarer optimistic moments, the chance that, although at their most basic, psychiatric disorders will be highly etiologically heterogeneous; we might find a final common pathway through which these multiple causes act. He uses the term "biomarker" for such a common pathway. I might prefer the terms "emergent simplification" or "equifinality" but I think these are just different ways of framing the same possible process.

In closing, I cannot resist an anecdote about Carl Hempel. I have seen many references (mostly by philosophers) to Hempel's speech to the American Psychopathological Association in 1959 (Zubin 1961) in which he recommended the use of operationalized criteria that would one day give way to etiologic understanding. Typically, this reference is made with a sense of reverence for what was assumed to be a key historical event. I recently had an opportunity to ask both Dr Rodrigo Muñoz, the last living author of the famous and historically critical "Feighner Criteria" (Feighner et al. 1972), and Dr Robert Spitzer, who was key to the development of the Research Diagnostic Criteria (RDC) and then DSM-III (American Psychiatric Association 1980) and DSM-III-R (American Psychiatric Association 1987), about the importance of Hempel's talk. While both of them were aware of the talk, they both strongly denied that it had had any influence on the work that was done on the Feighner, RDC or DSM criteria!

Introduction References

American Psychiatric Association (1980). *Diagnostic and Statistical Manual of Mental Disorders, Third Edition*. Washington, DC: American Psychiatric Association.

American Psychiatric Association (1987). *Diagnostic and Statistical Manual of Mental Disorders, Revised Third Edition*. Washington, DC: American Psychiatric Association.

Andrews, G., Goldberg, D. P., Krueger, R. F. Carpenter, W. T., Hyman, S. E., Sachdev, P., *et al.* (2009). Exploring the feasibility of a meta-structure for DSM-5 and ICD-11: could it improve utility and validity? *Psychological Medicine*, **39**(12), 1993–2000.

Bolton, D. (2008). *What is Mental Disorder?: An essay in philosophy, science, and values (International Perspectives in Philosophy and Psychiatry)*. New York: Oxford University Press.

Feighner, J. P., Robins, E., Guze, S. B., Woodruff, R. A., Jr., Winokur, G. and Munoz, R. (1972). Diagnostic criteria for use in psychiatric research. *Archives of General Psychiatry,* **26**(1), 57–63.

Kendler, K. S. (1990). Toward a scientific psychiatric nosology. Strengths and limitations. *Archives of General Psychiatry,* **47**(10), 969–73.

Kendler, K. S. (2012). Levels of explanation in psychiatric and substance use disorders: Implications for the development of an etiologically based nosology. *Molecular Psychiatry,* **12**(1), 11–12.

Kendler, K. S., Zachar, P. and Craver, C. (2010). What kinds of things are psychiatric disorders? *Psychological Medicine,* 1–8.

Zachar, P. (2000). Psychiatric disorders are not natural kinds. *Philosophy, Psychology and Psychiatry,* **7**(3), 167–82.

Zachar, P. (2003). The practical kinds model as a pragmatist theory of classification. *Philosophy, Psychology and Psychiatry,* **9**(9), 219–27.

Zubin, J. (1961). *Field Studies in the Mental Disorders*. New York: Grune and Stratton.

Chapter 1

Classification and causal mechanisms: a deflationary approach to the classification problem

Derek Bolton

"Mental disorder" may be conceptualized in various ways, all controversial, none a clear winner, such as: conditions characterized by distress and disability, in or out of combination with deviation from population norms, from evolutionary design, or absence of understandability; and so forth (Bolton 2008). These conceptualizations of mental disorder are relevant to one prior classification question—is this condition before us in the class of mental disorders or not?—arising, for example, when considering whether to include or exclude a condition from the diagnostic manuals. A different classification problem concerns how to classify conditions within that class, once they are considered to be mental disorders. There are interactions between these two kinds of classification problem—but they usually not much discussed. I will consider briefly one aspect of this interaction at the end of the paper, but most of the paper is about the second kind of classification problem, the one usually called by that name: how to classify within the class of psychiatric conditions. I will consider the following issues and make the following points:

1. As is well-known, in 1959 Hempel recommended to the American Psychiatric Association that psychiatric conditions be classified by surface characteristics to begin with, to ensure reliability, and later, as the science matures, by etiology (Hempel 1965). Hempel's advice for the beginning stage was followed in the DSM-III on, and the question now arises after half a century of research, do we now know enough about etiology to classify according to it. In this context I will take the view that there is not much prospect that the science of the etiology of psychiatric conditions will deliver a single, optimal classification scheme—the reason being that the last few decades of research has uncovered systemic complexity, rather than reductionist simplicity.

2. Not to worry, however, because classification is not the main point of science, and psychiatry may be, for historical reasons, overoccupied with it. The main aims of science are rather *prediction*, refined by *causal explanatory models*, and, on that basis, if cause–effect relationships are sufficiently strong, making *technological*

applications including interventions. In brief, I will propose a deflationary approach to the classification problem: classification in itself is less important than often supposed to be, and less important than other tasks.

3. Regarding the prior procedure of classification, the one that picks out the mental disorders from normal, non-disordered conditions, I will suggest that this raises questions that are not primarily to do with the sciences of causes, but which are rather to do with subjective and social phenomenology.

Let me start then with an indication of the current state of the science. Much is known or reasonably hypothesized about causes of/risks for psychiatric conditions from research over the past 50 years, including: genetic risks, typically involving multiple (perhaps hundreds) of genes adding relatively small risk; pre-natal placental nutrient and hormonal environment affecting fetal programming; birth complications; early maternal and childhood rearing practices including neglect and abuse; life-stressors; maladaptive cognitive styles; social determinants such as social exclusion, poverty and wealth inequality; and so on and on; and all interacting, and all, presumably, affecting brain development and functioning in some way.

As to technological applications of these findings and hypotheses, in healthcare the primary tasks are treatment once someone is ill and, preferably, prevention before people get ill. Molecular psychiatric genetics may pave the way to psychopharmacogenetics. Psychological models of the maintenance of psychiatric problems may provide symptom relief, and preventative psychotherapy or other psychosocial intervention may be helpful in some conditions. Options of prevention by environmental intervention are apparently promising from the point of view of the science, since much is known about environmental risk factors, but many of the larger ones are social, and are problematic economically and politically. Achieving more mental health friendly parenting, relieving poverty, reducing wealth inequality—all such prospects apparently raise quite different viability issues than those the Victorians confronted in relation to cleaning water supplies and sewage-disposal. Nevertheless, these are the preventative interventions to which the science now points.

So—apart from all the sciences of causation, and all the problems of technological implementation in treatment and public health, while all this is being said and done— what is the role of the classification system? Is there any point in worrying much about its exact state?

There are familiar pragmatic considerations that can suggest improvements to existing classifications. It may be helpful to subtype a condition, for example, obsessive–compulsive disorder with or without comorbidity with tics, or conduct disorder with or without the trait of callousness. Whether this is helpful depends entirely, as is familiar, on what else of interest the differentiation predicts, e.g., developmental pathways to the condition, or treatment response. It is important to note that there is no a priori reason to suppose that subtyping according to any one kind of predictive validity, e.g., developmental pathway, will correspond to subtyping according to a different kind of predictive validity, e.g., treatment response. This is both because we are in the domain of multiple causes of small effect, but also because many kinds of "outcomes" interest us: there is much we have an interest in predicting; e.g., understanding of developmental pathway to a condition is critical for prevention strategies but is less important than knowledge of treatment responsiveness once the outcome has occurred. The main point for the present purpose is that the relation between cause and outcome is not one–one but many–many and in these circumstances there will be many differing subtypes each valid for its own purpose.

The position is the same in relation to the reverse possibility of enlarging diagnostic categories by joining two hitherto distinguished: we would want to gain more predictive scope and power than we lose, and because we are interesting in predicting many things that are not necessarily strongly correlated, there is unlikely to be a simple, single, absolute answer to this question whether or not the change of classification is an improvement.

The position in relation to classing individual symptoms into syndromes is also fundamentally the same: do we have more or less predictive power by including or excluding the one from the other? There is typically the same uncertainty as before— you gain some, you lose some—but in this case there is an overriding *pragmatic* consideration that stabilizes the classification system, namely, the need not to lose the previous 10 or 15 years of research into the condition as so far defined.

These considerations suggest that syndromes will tend to be left as they are, that different studies will suggest subtyping in various ways, not necessarily the same ways, and most of them are likely not to be sufficiently robust or large to make a difference to the classification system—though they may be of high value to the science and even to clinical practice—and finally, that we may move around syndromes within the system to different headings, e.g., obsessive–compulsive disorder may be classified with anxiety disorders, or on its own, without disturbing anything else.

The position suggested by these considerations is that classification is important but only up to a point. What is essential is to have a set of concepts, a language for communication, likely to be made more successful if it manages without controversial theoretical terms, as Hempel noted. This enables the science to get going, enables us to be confident enough about what we are studying, and that we are studying it again, a crucial condition of the scientific methodology of replication and the goal of generalizability. But so far this matter is pragmatic and pedestrian, hardly yet science at all, and after this point, what matters is prediction, explanation, and identifying mechanisms—and the classification system, the correctly called *system of nomenclature*, does not have to help with this, indeed the findings may be just that no classification system is likely to help with this, only insofar as it enables to research on mechanisms to proceed.

The line of thought I am pursuing here has to be understood by contrasting our current scientific paradigm with what went before it. Medicine has had great emphasis on classification. Why is that? To some extent classification in medicine is important for just the reasons, as sketched earlier, that some classing together is required to get the science off the ground at all—even to begin to ask a question about something, some kind of thing. But why in medicine has classification become as important as it is? Generally the point has to be: classification assumes fundamental importance if— and only if—it captures optimal predictive power, which in turn is likely to be derived from a model of causal mechanisms. This is why chemistry's periodic table of elements is the best classification of all: it is an optimal classification system *because* it captures a causal model that predicts all the phenomena of interest.

The critical point in the present context is that medicine between approximately the mid 19th century and mid 20th century managed this feat for some conditions. It constructed the notions of signs and symptoms, and of syndromes, taking into account course over time (a temporal, developmental, historical dimension), and then, in key breakthroughs in the new biomedicine, identified processes at the cellular level that causally explained those complex, variable surface features. Further, with the development of penicillin, treatment was developed too. Further, the understanding of causes and processes of transmitted diseases enabled prevention through public health interventions. Game, set and match to 19th/20th-century biomedicine and its disease theory. These discoveries of diseases changed public health and individual healthcare—*but* better classification was not in the least the main point, which was rather identification of associations, causal mechanisms, treatment and prevention.

The 19th/20th-century biomedical disease paradigm was taken into the new psychiatry at the turn of the century—along with, it should be added for completeness, quite distinctive paradigms from neurology and psychology. As is well known the biomedical paradigm had a stunning success early on with syphilis: it all worked in the new psychiatry too. Very diverse signs and symptoms at and over time were unified into a syndrome caused by a kind of bacterium, a spirochete, invading the central nervous system, and which was treatable by penicillin. This early game, set and match achievement of the biomedical model applied to psychiatry has not been repeated since, and there are, as is well-known, ample reasons from research in the past half century—as alluded to earlier—to cast doubt on whether it will ever be repeated, and indeed reason to believe that it will not be. As Professor Kendler put it in a recent paper on the philosophical framework for psychiatry: no more spirochete-like discoveries, but rather multiple causes at multiple levels (Kendler 2005).

The current science is complex and biopsychosocial, in the sense that it identifies multiple risks of mostly small effect that are biological, psychological and social—but it is indeed *complex*. Can it be simplified? Can we get *anything like* the 19th-century disease model back into the picture? As the disease model has been joined by others in general medicine (in fact, often sharing the same biopsychosocial complexity as for the psychiatric conditions), and has all but been given up in psychiatry, attention has turned to *biomarkers*, as an aid to more precise diagnosis of complex conditions, as well as utility in predicting, for example, treatment response. Then there arises the possibility that biomarkers may validate the classification system, by reducing the complex array of biopsychosocial causes to a single final common pathway, which is biological, underlying the thought referred to earlier, that all the distant (early) biopsychosocial causes and the current psychosocial causes must somehow be implemented in the brain.

This line of thought is a complex combination of philosophy of mind, especially post-dualist mind–brain identity theory, and the philosophy of explanation, especially the assumption that causes must be proximate to their effects, and theory of illness, especially the disease model.

The philosophy is plausible enough but the thinking that derives from the disease model in particular needs closer examination. One point is that it is an empirical matter, not an a priori one, whether or not there is a final common pathway leading from multiple pathways to a single clinical syndrome, especially when, as is often observed, the clinical syndrome is itself not an invariant (there are many symptoms/ combinations that can constitute e.g., major depressive disorder). To date, so far as I am aware, no or not many biomarkers of specific psychiatric syndromes have yet been found, despite looking. But further, and specifically relevant to the line of thought in this paper, even if and when a biomarker were found, the science of mechanisms, causes, treatment, prevention may well stay as it is. It depends on the extent and nature of the causal role of the biomarker. At one end of the spectrum, a biomarker may be just an (other) sign of the illness, *internal* (inside the skin) as opposed to external, but as yet hardly worth distinguishing from the *external* signs and symptoms of the illness, from the point of view of the etiological model, which, we may suppose, stays as highly complex and multifactorial as before. Or, at the other end of the spectrum, the biomarker may be something like a spirochete, in which case it has, let us suppose, a relatively simple mode of transmission into the body, in principle preventable, and a reliable response to treatment. But, as previously, it looks implausible now to continue supposing that there are spirochete-like discoveries still on offer in psychiatry—and in this case biomarkers, even if we find them, won't much change the current paradigms of complexity of etiology and features of the conditions that interest us.

A related point is that the differentiation between signs and symptoms is different in psychiatry compared with general medicine. In acute medical care the symptom of distress (physical or mental) is likely not to be the critical point, and may indeed in trauma be a good sign (of consciousness and life), the critical issue being more likely to be an inner, beneath the skin, sign of something potentially catastrophic. In psychiatry, by contrast, especially in distress-related conditions such as anxiety and depression, the symptoms of distress are more constitutive of the illness, and the opposed concept of sign has a much less critical role. To put the point another way, the mental phenomenology, and its immediate behavioral associations, and its interpretation in the social context, have a defining role in our concepts of mental illness, and it is likely that, whatever else we may want our diagnostic categories to capture, we want them to capture these phenomena. Disturbing states of mind and related behavior are, after all, what bring people to the clinic. In this sense what we see as fundamental to mental disorder, regardless what else it may be or how it is caused, will place some constraint on the content of the classification system, the terms in which it is written. In the great paradigm of illnesses as diseases, the classification of illnesses is the classification of diseases. In the current late 20th/early 21st-century paradigm of complexity and diversity, one (relatively) stable and causally important fact is that disturbing states of mind and related behavior are what bring people to the clinic, and capturing the surface phenomenology is likely to be expected from any psychiatric classification system, arguably as a primary adequacy criterion.

Chapter References

Bolton, D. (2008). *What is mental disorder? An essay in philosophy, science and values.* Oxford: Oxford University Press.

Hempel, C. G. (1965). Fundamentals of taxonomy. In *Aspects of scientific explanation. And other essays in the philosophy of science.* New York: Free Press, pp. 137–54.

Kendler, K. (2005). Toward a philosophical structure for psychiatry. *American Journal of Psychiatry*, **162**, 433–40.

Chapter 1: Comments

The National Institute of Mental Health Research Domain Criteria (RDoC) project: moving towards a neuroscience-based diagnostic classification in psychiatry

Michael B. First

There are a variety of goals of a classification of mental disorders for which the current DSM and ICD systems have had variable success in meeting. These include facilitating communication, improving diagnostic reliability, aiding the prediction of future course and treatment response, and facilitating research into the identification of underlying causal mechanisms of illness. Undoubtedly one of its most important goals is to facilitate communication among clinicians, researchers, administrators and patients regarding psychopathological presentations by establishing a common language. In this regard, both the DSM and ICD systems have been highly successful given that virtually all communications about mental disorders are expressed using terminology from the DSM and ICD which provide a convenient shorthand for describing clinical entities. Long gone are the days in which clinicians used idiosyncratic terminology or employed diagnostic terms that meant radically different things to different clinicians based on geographical location, training, and professional background. A second goal of a classification is to provide diagnostic definitions that can be applied reliably, so that different users of the system can arrive at the same diagnosis given the same clinical presentation. In this regard, the DSM and ICD have been moderately successful in that it has been demonstrated that good to excellent diagnostic reliability can be achieved by researchers using structured diagnostic interviews (e.g., (Zanarini and Frankenburg 2001)). However, the reliability of diagnostic definitions as applied by clinicians has been shown to be fair to good at best (Sartorius et al. 1993; Spitzer et al. 1979), an issue that will be further examined in the DSM-5 field trials (Kraemer et al. 2010).

With regard to the third goal, namely to facilitate the prediction of course and treatment response in order to improve clinical care, DSM and ICD have been only modestly successful. While some diagnostic distinctions have predictive value in terms of what treatments are more or less likely to be successful (for example, a diagnosis of bipolar disorder versus schizophrenia predicting greater likelihood to respond to mood stabilizers), the diagnostically non-specific nature of most psychiatric treatments renders these instances more the exception than the rule. With respect to the final goal, that is, facilitating the identification of the underlying causal mechanisms of illness, the current DSM and ICD systems have been spectacularly unsuccessful. Initially, as Bolton notes in his paper, there was the hope that the evolution of psychiatric nosology would mirror the developments of 19th-century medicine, in which syndromes were identified for which etiological processes at the cellular level would be discovered that causally explained the surface features. Unfortunately, besides the identification of the spirochete as the etiological factor underlying the psychotic disorder general paresis of the insane, the reductionistic 19th-century disease model has not been applicable to any other psychiatric syndrome. Indeed, despite 30 years of intensive effort, the field has been unable to find a single biological or genetic marker that is specifically associated with a DSM category (Charney et al. 2002).

Bolton begins his paper with the question of whether, given the vast body of psychiatric research over the past 50 years, there is enough known about the etiology of mental disorders to move beyond a descriptive nosology to one based on the pathophysiology of mental disorders. He answers this question by suggesting that "there is not much prospect that the science of the etiology of psychiatric conditions will deliver a single optimal classification scheme, the reason being that the last few decades have uncovered a systemic complexity, rather than reductionist simplicity." Bolton then proposes what he describes as a "deflationary approach" to psychiatric classification which de-emphasizes the importance of classification, noting that "psychiatry may be, for historical reasons, overoccupied with it." Bolton notes that "classification is important but only up to a certain point," and that "what is essential is to have a set of concepts, a language for communication" that "enables the science to get going so we can be confident about what we are studying." His "deflationary perspective" calls for the field accepting the fact that the DSM and ICD are unable to help with prediction, explanation and identifying mechanisms, but as long as these systems enable research into the underlying mechanisms to proceed, the "primary adequacy criterion" should be that they be able to describe the "disturbing states of mind and related behavior" that bring people to the psychiatric clinic.

One question that immediately arises is whether Bolton's claim that our current classification systems are in fact enabling research into the discovery of the mechanism underlying mental disorders is in fact the case. The diagnostic paradigm that has framed research efforts for the past 30 years is based on the assumption that the best approach for defining mental disorders is in terms of syndromes, i.e., groups of symptoms that covary together. In 1972, the first set of operationally defined syndromes, "Feighner criteria," were developed for 15 conditions via a group consensus process by researchers at Washington University in St. Louis (Feighner et al. 1972). Subsequent research criteria sets (e.g., RDC (Spitzer et al. 1978) and the various editions of the DSM from DSM-III onward) were all built on the foundation of the Feighner criteria, with the goal that these criteria sets would be continually refined and validated, ultimately leading to discovery of the "diseases" underlying the disorders. Unfortunately, using diagnostic categories based on clinical syndromes as temporary "stand-ins" for phenotypes has led to a dead-end in terms of providing a framework for conducting research into the etiology and pathophysiology of mental disorders.

Not only has the syndromal approach embodied by the DSM *not* been helpful in facilitating research efforts to understand the mechanisms underlying mental disorders, but some have suggested that this approach may be holding the field back. Hyman (2003) cautions that "scientists attempting to discover genetic or neural underpinnings of disease have all too often reified the disorders listed in DSM-IV-TR as 'natural kinds.'. . . When investigators perform an imaging experiment, they recruit only patients with DSM-IV-TR schizophrenia or major depression. . . In reifying DSM-IV-TR diagnoses, one increases the risk that science will get stuck, and the very studies that are needed to define phenotypes are held back (p. xix)." Similar concerns have been raised by the authors of the neuroscience white paper (Charney et al. 2002) that was part of the Research Agenda for DSM-5:

> The over-reification of the DSM categories has led to a form of closed-mindedness on the part of researchers and funding sources. For example, researchers involved in new drug development tend to focus their efforts on treatment of DSM-IV-defined categories, despite widespread evidence that pharmacologic treatments tend to be effective in treating a relatively wide range of DSM disorders. Furthermore, the erroneous notion that the DSM categories can double as phenotypes may be partly responsible for the lack of success in discovering robust genetic markers (p. 34).

In a recent review paper, Hyman (2010) summarized his position regarding DSM-IV reification problem as follows:

> [DSM-IV] created an unintended epistemic prison that was palpably impeding scientific progress. Outside of their ongoing research projects, most investigators understood that DSM-IV was a heuristic, pending the advance of science. In practice, however, DSM-IV diagnoses controlled the research questions they could ask, and perhaps, even imagine (p. 157).

What then can be done to help researchers break out from the diagnostic shackles imposed by the reification of the DSM-IV system? A major challenge posed by the DSM and ICD systems is that they are being used simultaneously by clinicians, researchers, educators and administrators to serve very different purposes. Given that the primary goal of the DSM and ICD systems is to be clinically useful (First et al. 2004), there is a limit to how far the system can be stretched in order to accommodate the needs of researchers who are exploring the underlying pathophysiology and genetics of mental disorders without compromising the needs of clinicians. One approach, suggested by both Hyman (Hyman 2007) and First (First 2006) is to broaden the DSM research appendix to include experimental diagnostic constructs for research purposes that would supplement and "shadow" the existing DSM classification which could be updated by appropriately constituted committees as new information emerges from neuroscience and genetics. A disadvantage of this approach is the tendency for the research classification to be framed using the same diagnostic paradigm that applies to the main classification. For example, virtually all of the entities included in the DSM-IV research appendix are framed in terms of diagnostic categories defined by patterns of descriptive symptoms. Furthermore, based on prior experience with the

DSM-IV appendix for "criteria sets and axes provided for further study," it is unlikely that researchers will make much use of such a research appendix. In the 17 years since publication of DSM-IV, with the exception of the experimental criteria for binge eating disorder and premenstrual dysphoric disorder which been cited in hundreds of studies, the remaining 21 criteria sets and two axes have received very little attention from researchers. While the basis for their lack of usage has not been empirically examined, likely reasons include the lack of involvement of the wider research community in the development of these research criteria sets and perhaps most importantly the lack of incentives for researchers to adopt these particular criteria sets in their studies.

An alternative approach for breaking free of DSM/ICD diagnostic constraints is to completely rethink the diagnostic system from scratch and to develop a new diagnostic framework rooted entirely in neuroscience and genetics. Such a system would function as a modern day neuroscience-based "Feighner criteria." The Research Domain Criteria (RDoC) project, developed by the National Institute of Mental Health in the United States, is intended to establish "a framework for creating research classifications that reflect functional dimensions stemming from translational research on genes, circuits, and behavior." (Insel and Cuthbert 2009, p. 989). The RDoC project is a direct consequence of one of the aims of the NIMH 2008 strategic plan, namely, to "develop, for research purposes, new ways of classifying mental disorders based on dimensions of observable behavior and neurobiological measures." (National Institute of Mental Health 2008). The goal of RDoC is to shift researchers away from focusing on the traditional diagnostic categories as an organizing principle for selecting study populations towards a focus on dysregulated neurobiological systems. The initial stages of the RDoC project are devoted to specifying those basic dimensions of psychological functioning and their corresponding brain circuits that have been the focus of neuroscience research over the past several decades. In deciding which of the many domains of functioning should be included in the RDoC framework, priority is being given to those domains that can be related to problem behaviors found in the symptom lists of conventional disorder categories (Sanislow et al. 2010).

It is important to understand that the RDoC project is not intended to function as a diagnostic classification system in the way that the DSM and ICD do. Unlike the DSM, ICD and other medical classifications which are designed to exhaustively describe and delineate the different ways that psychiatric patients might present symptomatically in terms of conceptually high-level concepts such as disease or disorder, the RDoC project is primarily a research framework to assist researchers in relating the fundamental domains of behavioral functioning to their underlying neurobiological components.

There are several a priori assumptions that inform the design and implementation of the RDoC project (Insel et al. 2010). The first is that at some fundamental level, mental disorders can be conceptualized as disorders in brain circuitry (in contrast to neurological disorders that are defined in terms of identifiable lesions in the nervous system). Secondly, these dysfunctions in neural circuits can be identified using the tools of clinical neuroscience, such as electrophysiology, functional neuroimaging and new methods for quantifying connections *in vivo*. Thus, the central organizing elements of the RDoCs system are brain circuits.

The current draft of the RDoC framework has identified five major domains of functioning as its central organizational elements, each containing multiple, more specific constructs. The Negative Valence Systems domain includes constructs for active threat ("fear"), potential threat ("anxiety"), sustained threat, loss, and frustrative nonreward; the Positive Valence Systems domain includes constructs for approach motivation, initial responsiveness to reward, sustained responsiveness to reward, reward learning, and habit formation; the Cognitive Systems domain includes constructs for attention, perception, working memory, declarative memory, language behavior and cognitive control; the Systems for Social Processes domain includes constructs for imitation/theory of mind, social dominance, facial expression identification, attachment/separation fear, and self-representation; and the Arousal/Regulatory Systems domain include systems involved in sleep and wakefulness. For each of these constructs, the RDoC framework will list the current state-of-the-art measurements/elements at several different units of analysis, including genes, molecules, cells, circuits, physiology, behavior and self-reports. (Cuthbert and Insel 2010). Thus, in concrete terms, the "product" of the RDoC effort is a matrix, where the constructs form the rows and the various units of analysis forming the columns (see Table 1.1). In order to fill in the various cells in the matrix, NIMH is in the process of convening a series of conferences involving experts from each of the domain areas for the purpose of refining the list of domains and constructs; this includes providing working definitions, as well as compiling for each unit of analysis a listing of the measures and components that contemporary research has identified as pertaining to a particular construct. These meetings will result in the production of an annotated listing of the state-of-the-art measurements/elements at each level of analysis, which will be published on the NIMH web site for a period of continuing commentary, with final specifications of the framework available on the NIMH website for free downloading (Cuthbert and Insel 2010). The ultimate intent is that researchers would be guided to the most advanced measures in various areas, and could use these measures for selection of both independent and dependent variables in their grant submissions to the NIMH. For example, under the current system, researchers often select study participants based on their having a DSM diagnosis in common (e.g., social phobia). Under the RDoC framework, a researcher interested in fear circuitry might recruit all patients presenting to an anxiety clinic, with an independent variable of fear potentiated startle and dependent variables comprising scores on fear, distress and symptom measures (Insel et al. 2010).

The RDoC approach represents a true paradigm shift in the classification of mental disorders, moving away from defining disorders based on descriptive phenomenology and instead focusing on disruptions in neural circuitry as the fundamental classificatory principle (Kendler and First 2010). Whether RDoC ultimately has an impact on future clinical classifications of psychiatry will depend on how well this new approach performs for research, i.e., how well the new molecular and neurobiological parameters included in the framework end up predicting prognosis and treatment response (Insel et al. 2010), something that will takes years or even decades to fully realize.

Table 1.1 Research Domain Criteria matrix

Domains/ Constructs	Units of analysis						
	Genes	Molecules	Cells	Circuits	Physiology	Behavior	Self-reports
Negative valence systems							
Fear/Extinction							
Stress/Distress							
Aggression							
Positive valence systems							
Reward seeking							
Reward/Habit learning							
Cognitive systems							
Attention							
Perception							
Working memory							
Declarative memory							
Language behavior							
Cognitive (effortful) control							
Systems for social processes							
Imitation, theory of mind							
Social dominance							
Facial expression identification							
Attachment/ Separation fear							
Self-representation areas							
Arousal/ Regulatory systems							
Arousal and regulation							
Resting state activity							

Comments References

Charney, D., Barlow, D., Botteron, K., Cohen, J., Goldman, D., Gur, R., *et al.* (2002). Neuroscience research agenda to guide development of a pathophysiologically based classification system. In D. Kupfer, M. First and D. Regier (eds.), *A research agenda for DSM-V*. Washington, DC: American Psychiatric Association, pp. 31–84.

Cuthbert, B. and Insel, T. (2010). The data of diagnosis: new approaches to psychiatric classification. *Psychiatry,* **73**(4), 311–14.

Feighner, J. P., Robins, E., Guze, S. B., Woodruff, R. A., Jr., Winokur, G. and Munoz, R. (1972). Diagnostic criteria for use in psychiatric research. *Archives of General Psychiatry,* **26**(1), 57–63.

First, M. (2006). Beyond clinical utility: broadening the DSM-V research appendix to include alternative diagnostic constructs. *American Journal of Psychiatry,* **163**(10), 1679–81.

First, M., Pincus, H., Levine, J., Williams, J., Ustun, B. and Peele, R. (2004). Clinical utility as a criterion for revising psychiatric diagnoses. *American Journal of Psychiatry,* **161**(6), 946–54.

Hyman, S. E. (2003). *Forward*. In K. Phillips, M. First and H. Pincus (eds.), *Advancing DSM: dilemmas in psychiatric diagnosis*. Washington, DC: American Psychiatric Association, pp. xi–xix.

Hyman, S. E. (2007). Can neuroscience be integrated into the DSM-V? *Nature Reviews Neuroscience,* **8**, 725–32.

Hyman, S. E. (2010). The diagnosis of mental disorders: the problem of reification. *Annual Review of Clinical Psychology,* **27**(6), 155–79.

Insel, T., Cuthbert, B., Garvey, M., Heinssen, R., Kozak, M., Pine, D., *et al.* (2010). Research Domain Criteria (RDoC): Toward a new classification framework for research on mental disorders. *American Journal of Psychiatry,* **167**(7), 748–51.

Insel, T. R. and Cuthbert, B. N. (2009). Endophenotypes: bridging genomic complexity and disorder heterogeneity. *Biological Psychiatry,* **66**, 988–9.

Kendler, K. S. and First, M. B. (2010). Alternative futures for the DSM revision process: iteration v. paradigm shift. *British Journal of Psychiatry,* **197**(4), 263–5.

Kraemer, H. C., Kupfer, D. J., Narrow, W. E., Clarke, D. E. and Regier, D. A. (2010). Moving toward DSM-5: the field trials. *American Journal of Psychiatry,* **167**(10), 1158–60.

National Institute of Mental Health (2008). *The National Institute of Mental Health Strategic Plan.(NIH Publication 08–6368)*. Bethesda, MD: National Institute of Mental Health.

Sanislow, C. A., Pine, D. S., Quinn, K. J., Kozak, M. J., Garvey, M. A., Heinssen, R. K., *et al.* (2010). Developing constructs for psychopathology research: Research Domain Criteria. *Journal of Abnormal Psychology,* **119**(4), 631–9.

Sartorius, N., Kaelber, C., Cooper, J., Roper, M., Rae, D., Gulbinat, W., *et al.* (1993). Progress toward achieving a common language in psychiatry. Results from the field trial of the clinical guidelines accompanying the WHO classification of mental and behavioral disorders in ICD-10. *Arch Gen Psychiatry,* **50**(2), 115–24.

Spitzer, R., Endicott, J. and Robins, E. (1978). Research diagnostic criteria: rationale and reliability. *Archives of General Psychiatry,* **35**, 773–82.

Spitzer, R., Forman, J. and Nee, J. (1979). DSM-III field trials: I. initial interrator diagnostic reliability. *American Journal of Psychiatry,* **136**, 815–17.

Zanarini, M. and Frankenburg, F. (2001). Attainment and maintenance of reliability of axis I and axis II disorders over the course of a longitudinal study. *Comprehensive Psychiatry,* **42**(5), 369–74.

Chapter 2

Introduction

Kenneth S. Kendler

Peter Zachar addresses the perennial problem of whether progress has been made in the classification of psychiatric disorders. Typical of his writing, he provides a balanced and thoughtful review from a range of perspectives. He frames the question as a search for a more valid psychiatric disorder. That is, he suggests reasonably that one way to monitor progress is to determine whether the current diagnostic criteria are more valid than their predecessors. This, of course, puts great weight on the central but oft debated concept of the diagnostic validity of psychiatric disorders.

Zachar quickly moves away from the position that there is one overarching concept of validity that should dominate this discussion—validity with a "capital" "V." Rather, and correctly in my mind, he suggests that we need "validity pluralism." Due to (1) the complex structure of psychiatric disorders, which can be viewed from some many perspectives, and (2) the existence of so many different things that people want from these diagnoses, the idea that one overarching validity concept could work is unrealistic. This is unsatisfying but probably cannot be helped. It is in the nature of psychiatric nosology to be dealing with highly multifactorial syndromes and trying to serve multiple masters.

One useful way that Zachar frames the problem reflects the dominant research traditions of the two great disciplines of psychology and psychiatry, which care most about these problems. Psychiatrists, as he notes, are most often concerned with external and predictive validity (i.e., does this diagnosis predict course, treatment, or family history?), while psychologists are often concerned with more internal and psychometric concepts of validity (does the disorder reflect a single dimension; do the individual criteria perform well?).

He only briefly alludes to a problem that has not perhaps received enough attention—that is the difference between "absolute" validity and "contrastive" validity. The former is what would be relevant if we are considering a new disorder. How well does it need to perform to be worth inclusion in the manual? The second arises when you are looking at changes to already established criteria. That is, does my new set of criteria for disorder X perform better than the criteria for disorder X listed in DSM-IV? The latter—"contrastive" validity—is a simpler problem. We just have to decide what "better" means, which is usually straightforward. The former—"absolute" validity—is just harder, as the threshold of "how much data is enough" can be quite hard to define.

Zachar briefly reviews the radical critiques of psychiatric nosology (that it represents "ad hoc pseudoscience"), which interestingly has been far more often targeted at the DSM than the ICD system. The rhetoric here can get pretty hot. For my money, neither pole (psychiatric nosology is pure science untainted by any social, economic or personal concerns versus all members of DSM and ICD committees are money hungry peons of the drug companies) is very close to the truth. Serious study of how social and personal concerns of the less malignant variety have impacted on psychiatric nosologic deliberations has, with very few exceptions, yet to be written.

Soundly, Zachar turns briefly to historical examples to try to see how science progresses toward better (equals more valid) models. He introduces two useful concepts of calibration (for an excellent example on the development of the thermometer see Chang (2004)) and multiple standards. It is, however, hard to see how some standards that have played a strong role in the history of science—such as predicting the existence of unobserved entities—would ever work for psychiatry. (While we might be able to predict treatment response, or course of illness, imagine that some advanced psychometric model predicts the existence of an unobserved psychiatric disorder, which is then subsequently discovered! Not in my lifetime, for sure.) Even for much harder sciences than psychiatry, major scientific decisions involved many factors that had to be carefully weighted in reaching a decision. Recall that the Copernican model was for many years unable to address the problem of the lack of parallax of stars seen from Earth at different seasons. Instrumentation was not then up to the needed accuracy to detect the parallax given the very great distances involved. Nonetheless, the Copernican model triumphed as more weight was given to other observations (moons of Jupiter, phases of Venus, etc.). So, inevitably, we have multiple standards, the importance of which has to be debated.

Zachar then turns briefly to the problem of realism versus non-realism in psychiatry. Few issues in the philosophy of psychiatric nosology are more weighty. Are psychiatric disorders things we construct, or things we discover? If it were clearly one or the other, this problem might have been solved some time ago. What makes this question so difficult, in my view, is the nuanced combination of factors from genes through culture that impact on our diagnoses.

In his concluding section, Zachar proposes four possible strategies for psychiatric nosology going forward: conservative, incremental, bold, and cautious progressivism. These nicely capture the range of views about the path forward for psychiatric nosology. As might be expected in our field, we have consensus neither on where we should be heading nor on how fast we should try to get there. However, Zachar crisply lays out these alternatives providing a balanced view of their strengths and limitations.

Introduction Reference

Chang, H. (2004). *Inventing Temperature: Measurement and Scientific Progress* New York: Oxford University Press.

Chapter 2

Progress and the calibration of scientific constructs: the role of comparative validity

Peter Zachar

2.1 Introduction

Has psychiatry made progress in the classification of psychiatric disorders? This is an important question, because if it has not done so then the scientific legitimacy of psychiatric taxonomy would be called into doubt.

In the early 20th century it was claimed that the greatest scientific achievements regarding our understanding of humanity were made by Copernicus, Darwin and Freud. In the latter part of that century, however, the DSM-III abandoned the Freudian metapsychology for what was argued to be a more scientifically legitimate approach based on operationalized diagnostic criteria. With each new edition of the manual come similar claims. The authors of the DSM-IV asserted that psychiatric diagnostic categories, developed on the basis of professional opinions rather than research results, could be improved upon if all changes were "evidence-based" (Widiger et al. 1991). Some architects of the DSM-5 contend that the categorical approach to classification is scientifically inadequate. Psychiatric phenomena, they claim, are really dimensional; therefore, many DSM categories should be replaced with a more scientifically valid dimensional approach. (Hyman 2010; Krueger et al. 2005; Smith and Combs 2010; Widiger and Trull 2007).

This raises two questions. First, can such large shifts in emphasis be considered cumulative scientific progress? Second, does every generation of psychiatrists have to denigrate the "illegitimate science" of the past in the name of progress?

Several thinkers (P. J. Caplan 1995; Kirk and Kutchins 1992; Kutchins and Kirk 1997) assert that the much vaunted scientific progress in psychiatry is an illusion. They state that the scientific support behind psychiatric constructs has been manipulated and marketed in the same way that political campaigns promote their candidates. In this view, the denigration of the past is a political strategy. Such critics also claim that many constructs for psychiatric disorders are not real entities, but ad hoc creations of psychiatrists who have been allocated positions of influence.

Such criticisms should not be ignored or dismissed, but taken seriously and carefully explored. The charge that psychiatric classification represents ad hoc pseudo-science is worthy of critical evaluation. Although these thinkers do not seem to be denigrating the validity of psychiatric classification in the manner of the Scientologists, the differences between the two can be subtle. In both cases, scientific validity is the issue.

In what follows, I will explore the questions raised by Kutchins, Kirk, Caplan and other critics by focusing on the relationship between progress and scientific validity. I begin with some general considerations from the history of science before turning to psychiatry proper.

2.2 **A historical perspective on scientific validity**

Turning to the history of science to look at both progress and validity, it is apparent that evaluations of progress and of scientific validity go hand-in-hand. *To say that progress has been made is to also say that current theories are more valid than their predecessors.* For example, the Copernican theory of the solar system is considered to be more valid that the Ptolemaic theory and also considered to represent scientific progress. The same is true with respect to particulate versus blending models of inheritance, prototype versus classical conceptions of folk categorization, and conceptualizing autism as a biologically-influenced developmental disorder rather than a child's psychological reaction to impersonal mothering. In all cases, theories that were once attributed scientific validity were improved upon by what came to be seen as more valid theories. Historically considered, criteria for validity are also criteria that allow us to say that one scientific theory is better than or an improvement on another theory.

People often write as if they know what validity really is. Occasionally, it is defined somewhat vacuously as "validity means that the disorder really exists." The notion that validity is a present versus absent property that constructs possess could be called validity with a *big* "V." An alternative perspective, called *validity pluralism*, construes validity as a matter of degree—based on a comparative assessment of multiple validity indicators. Often these indicators are formulated as precise questions, many of which are empirically testable. Examples of such questions are

♦ Is our construct appropriately correlated with an external criterion?

♦ Is the construct better modeled as a latent category or a latent dimension?

♦ Does our construct differentiate between samples in an expected way?

Many of these precise questions are articulated within one of two paradigms—the medical model of the psychiatrists and the psychometric model of the psychologists. Most thinkers view these two paradigms as overlapping. In some instances the perceived overlap is appropriate, but in others it is not.[1] Each paradigm has its own menu of validators (or criteria). Typical validators of the medical model include confirmed etiology, consistent time course, and family history. Typical validators of the psychometric model include internal consistency, predictive validity, and factorial validity.

The problem of validity is confusing because it is evaluated on multiple levels of abstraction and these changes of scope are not well tracked. I propose that it is better to accept a plurality of validity questions than seeking validity with a *big* "V." The notion of *comparative validity* that I will introduce in the next section is a *small* "v" notion.

2.3 **Validation and calibration**

In the physical sciences calibration refers to adjusting a measurement device so that the values it returns match a standard. In calibrating scales, technicians use a set of standard weights with known values (e.g., 10 grams, 1 gram etc.). Scales are routinely adjusted so that the scales' estimated value of a weight matches the known value of the weight. Scales can be calibrated to measure a variety of weights in a set. Scales are also calibrated with specific experimental uses in mind, and may be calibrated differently if the intended use shifts. For example, some experiments require that a scale be calibrated to measure very small amounts, whereas others do not.

A key fact about calibration of physical measures is that the values of many "weights" were selected by convention. At some point, the scientific community decided what should count as a standard meter, gram and second. Once these standards are fixed, whether or not the scale can meet them is *objectively specifiable*.

The validation of scientific constructs proceeds in an analogous fashion. They are expected to measure up to multiple standards, and what standards are relevant depend on how the construct will be used. An important regulative ideal is that the standards be defined in such a way that whether or not they are met is objectively specifiable. Because these standards are justified in what philosophers call the logical space of reasons, they are not arbitrary in the way that physical measurements of weight and length are arbitrary. Examples of standards that have been conventionalized in the history of science include the following include:

- ◆ The theory/construct predicts fact-events that have not been observed.
- ◆ The theory/construct explains diverse phenomena as manifestations of a single process (unification).
- ◆ Disorders must be understood in light of an accurate model of normal functioning.

It is worth noting that a proposed standard should only become conventionalized if it can be met. There is also no expectation that all intelligible standards can be met in all circumstances. Once conventionalized, however, such norms form part of the intellectual inheritance of subsequent generations.

The evolution of norms

Let me briefly provide more justification for the claim just made, namely, that validity/progress often involves the introduction of new standards of adequacy that can become conventionalized. One of the best known examples of this process is Shapin and Shaffer's (1985) study of the dispute between Robert Boyle and Thomas Hobbes over the role that experiment and demonstration of fact should play in natural philosophy.

Can a true vacuum (a space with no matter at all) exist? This was a widely-discussed question in the mid 17th century because it was seen to have important metaphysical implications, e.g., are there non-material events? Boyle is famous for using an air pump to create vacuums, with which he was able to study phenomena such as air pressure. In doing so, he avoided the question about the presence of matter and proposed that a vacuum refers to a space with air pumped out. According to Boyle, experiments that can be observed by others and replicated provide information about the kind of *facts* on which natural philosophy (the original term for "science") should be based. After achieving agreement among observers regarding the results of his experiments involving the addition and subtraction of quantities of air in a vessel, Boyle subsequently began talking about "air pressure" as a fact (not a construct).

Hobbes had many criticisms of this approach, and they cannot be easily summarized. Besides being a committed materialist (which he thought was incompatible with vacuums), Hobbes was concerned that grounding natural philosophy on observational agreement (experience) was too uncertain, and experiments too artificial. Hobbes claimed that demonstrative experiments are like magic tricks. As is true with magic tricks, he said that in experiments seeing should not be grounds for believing. Instead, Hobbes preferred the certainties of logic and reasoning. Many English scientists sided with Boyle and reports of experiments that allowed for replication and demonstration of fact became new scientific norms.

Another example of introducing new norms can be seen with the 1846 discovery of the planet Neptune. To understand this event, we have to return to the discovery of Uranus in 1781. Soon after its discovery, astronomers used Newton's equations to make predictions about Uranus's expected positions in the night sky as it orbited the sun (Kerrod 2000). Given that it takes about 84 years for Uranus to complete one orbit, it took some time to test these predictions. Over the next 65 years, it became evident Uranus's observed orbit did not match its expected orbit.

One of the earliest successes of the Newtonian model was Edmund Halley's 1705 prediction of the return of his famous comet, but the Newtonian model seemed to be unable to meet the Halley standard in the case of Uranus, i.e., to predict its future position in the night sky. In the middle part of the 19th century, some astronomers reasoned that if there was another planet orbiting the sun beyond Uranus, and if its gravitational pull on Uranus was taken into account, the failed predictions could be explained. Using the observed positions of Uranus throughout its orbit, Le Verrier in France and Adams in England independently made some calculations about where this planet would have to be in the night sky to make the predictions of Uranus's orbit agree with observation (Wilson 1997). The planet Neptune was quickly discovered to be about where the calculations said it should be.

Not only was the Newtonian model shown to match up to the Halley standard, it was also able to match up to a new, more impressive standard—*predicting the existence of as yet unobserved entities*. The prediction of Neptune's existence was not a simple demonstration of scientific validity, it was an argument for a new way of thinking about validity.

Just 30 years later, this new criterion of validity became important in another branch of science, namely, the atomic chemistry. When Mendeleev first put together his periodic table of elements, there were some obvious gaps in the table, for example, between and aluminum and indium. Mendeleev stated that such a gap pointed to an unobserved element (now called gallium). He also made some accurate predictions about this element's chemical properties (Scerri 2007). The periodic table's ability to measure up to the Newtonian standard of predicting the existence of new entities helped convince people of its validity.

The problem of multiple standards

It must be noted that predicting the existence of unobserved entities is only one relevant standard. Many such predictions have failed to be supported and are later ignored. Rather than meeting one magic bullet standard, the key issue is an overall judgment of how many standards a theory or construct is in coherence with.

For many constructs and theories, there is rarely a single standard. For example, claims about the progressive nature of the Copernican model were solidified once scholars, prodded by Galileo, came to accept that a valid model of the solar system must account for *both* retrograde motion and the phases of Venus (Sharratt 1996).

One of the great virtues of the Ptolemaic model was that it explained *retrograde motion* or the tendency of planets to move from east to west, then make a turn and move to the east for a time before switching directions again and continuing on as before. The Copernican sun-centered model offered an alternative explanation of this retrograde motion, and there was little reason to choose between the two theories. Galileo's discovery that Venus has phases (full, quarter, new) similar to the phases of the moon was readily explained along Copernican lines but a mystery for the Ptolemaic model. Galileo raised the bar and demanded that an adequate model of the solar system measure up to multiple standards.

Calibration is the molding of constructs to fit as many of the standards as possible, but it is not always possible to measure up to all rationally articulated standards. In some cases the various standards are weighted and the values of the weights can shift over time. Our goals for classification often influence how standards are weighted in terms of importance and even which standards are considered to be relevant at all. When this kind of selection process occurs, the resulting constructs are what I have called *practical kinds* (Zachar 2002, 2008).

A brief philosophical look at scientific progress: realism and non-realism

Ideally, the modification of constructs results in graduate improvement where constructs measure up to multiple standards. Kenneth Kendler (2009) construes progress as a process of cumulative *epistemic iteration*. For Kendler, epistemic iteration refers to the development of more stable, invariant truths from partial truths. Iteration is similar to Paul Meehl's notion of bootstrapping—which emphasizes developing valid indicators from an initial set of fallible indicators (Cronbach and Meehl 1955; Meehl 1995). In both cases, the assumption is that there is a fixed reality out there waiting to be known, and the job of the scientist is to detect the true signal and filter out the noise (Kraemer 2010).

In the history of science, judgments of successful approximation to reality are made by looking back and comparing past theories to currently accepted ones. Copernicus is compared to Ptolemy, Darwin to Lamarck, and the kinetic theory to the caloric theory. The idea of *comparative validity* is that the best scientific theories are "best" because they outperform competitors with respect to selected standards of validity.

According to the perspective of scientific realism, the comparative advantage of current theories over past theories, and the cumulative nature of this process, can be considered one of making successful approximations to reality. There is, however, a more minimalist and non-realist approach that says comparative validity (outperforming competitors with respect to rationally articulated standards of validity) is all that is needed to understand progress.[2] The key issue is getting theories/constructs calibrated with or in coherence with the relevant standards. Making metaphysical inferences to reality, says the non-realist, does not add anything substantial beyond being in coherence with the relevant standards.

It should be noted that getting into coherence is itself a high standard, especially if the criteria are themselves rigorous. To illustrate, calibrating a theory of evolution so that it is consistent with physics, geology, the fossil record, the rules of inheritance, comparative morphology and biogeography is no simple feat. Near the end of his life, Darwin actually de-emphasized natural selection because at that time it was not consistent with physical theories about the age of the earth or scientific theories of inheritance (Desmond and Moore 1991). In the 1940s it became evident that the physics and genetics of the 1880s were flawed. The realization that evolution by means of natural selection could be coherent with the findings of physics and especially genetics led the scientific community to, for the first time since its proposal, assert the validity of Darwin's initial theory.

Let me also emphasize that *basic realism* holds that there is a world external to human beings (independent of our beliefs about it), that the world is somehow the cause of our ideas about it, and that some ideas/beliefs are better than others. Both scientific realists and non-realists accept basic realism. The disagreement between them is in their views about the relationship between our scientific theories/constructs and "reality." The scientific realists say that good theories literally represent reality (at least potentially), and that is why we make progress. Non-realists adopt a more pragmatic approach and say that say that good theories allow us to successfully predict and/or make things happen with respect to our goals. For the non-realist, rather than being something that is represented literally in our theories, the world out there is something we bump up against when we meet resistance, trouble and doubt. We do not need special metaphysical inferences about "reality" in addition to "outperforms competitors" to understand progress.

To summarize our historical and philosophical exploration: making claims about progress requires adopting assumptions about validity. New standards of validity are often introduced as criteria of progress. Being able to cohere with as many rationally articulated standards of validity as possible is important, but not always possible. With this understanding in place, let us now return to the problem of psychiatric classification.

2.4 **Selling science: the role of claim-making**

In *The Selling of DSM*, Kirk and Kutchins (1992) make an analogy between the DSM-III revolution and a political campaign. Politicians often identify crises that need to be solved as a strategy for getting elected. Examples of common crises include inadequate national security and burgeoning budget deficits. During the election the problem is discussed in simplistic and dramatic terms, partly to appeal to voters' emotions. After the election, when the victors have to solve the crisis that they marketed, a couple of options are available. They can pass new laws and claim that the problem will now be solved or greatly improved. They can also abandon the simplistic story in favor of a more nuanced interpretation, at which point the problem becomes "too complicated" to easily resolve.

Kirk and Kutchins describe how the politician's strategy was used by the architects of the DSM-III to make the problem of reliability into a crisis. Robert Spitzer and colleagues, they say, used the newly developed kappa statistic to claim that the inter-rater reliability of the DSM-II ranged from "poor" to at best "only satisfactory"—which they identified as a state of crisis. Prior to the final adoption of the DSM-III, the architects claimed that the new operationalized criteria had resulted in great improvements, even a solution to the reliability problem. After the manual was published and inter-reliability proved to be disappointing, the problem of reliability was quietly set aside.

Without question, many of the unsavory aspects of the social process of science have manifested themselves in the various DSM revisions, up to and including DSM-5. From these observations, however, we cannot conclude that the politics of diagnosis represent nothing less than the corruption of science. What I suggest is that, to some extent, what Kirk and Kutchins call "claim-making" is a normal and even necessary part of scientific classification.

How could this be? It has to do with progress and the validity question. When scientists claim that progress has been made, they are also claiming that the new approach is more valid than previous approaches. This involves making a rationally persuasive argument about which standards should be used to evaluate scientific success, or to which measures a good theory must be calibrated. It is not possible to design an experiment to discover which set of standards should be given priority, therefore, advocating for new or altered standards requires claim-making.

Being able to shift the standards to which a scientifically adequate theory or construct must conform is part and parcel of scientific progress. Spitzer and his colleagues' claims about the importance of reliability for a scientifically adequate diagnostic system was an example of rational claim-making [3].

The importance of claim-making is also more than a historical observation; it is ongoing. No better example of claim-making can be given than the current push toward dimensional models in psychiatry. For example:

- There are too many NOS (not otherwise specified) diagnoses in the current system—a more scientifically adequate model will provide better diagnostic coverage.
- The current manual has artificially raised comorbidity rates—a more scientifically adequate manual will reduce these rates.

These are not the only standards that have been articulated, but they are prominent among the various standards against which the new manual is going to be expected to measure up. The more committed someone is to the progressive nature of the dimensional model revolution, the more likely it is that they will see these standards as raising the bar.

2.5 **Making-up disorders**

Next we turn to the assertion that psychiatrists make people "crazy" by labeling them as such (P. J. Caplan 1995; Kirk and Kutchins 1992; Kutchins and Kirk 1997). More specifically, the claim is that nosologists invent disorders by observing a pattern of behavior and giving it a name (what philosophers call a baptismal event). The name/label may also encode an explanatory conceptualization of the pattern. If successful, this name-and-explanation becomes an accepted convention. Mental health professionals then use it as a guide—and take an observed instance of the behavioral pattern as confirmatory evidence that the explanatory construct is descriptively correct.

The notion behind the "making them crazy" claim is that such naming is a type of wild diagnosis. A famous example of a wild diagnosis is drapetomania—described in the Antebellum south as an irrational compulsion to escape from slavery (A. L. Caplan et al. 2004). More recent candidates for wild diagnoses are masochistic personality disorder (P. J. Caplan 1995) and multiple personality disorder (McHugh 2008). In both cases a pattern of behavior was observed and named. These names in particular are theoretically loaded explanatory constructs—and arguably flawed explanations.

For instance, the term "masochistic" and its successor "self-defeating" serve as guides for interpreting behaviors such as *chooses to be with people who lead to disappointment* and *rejects attempts of others to help*. If such constructs were to become diagnostic conventions, then others would learn to interpret the behaviors in the same way. What makes such diagnoses wild is that better interpretations are available. For example, according to Caplan (1985) such behaviors are expectable reactions of powerless people to ongoing abuse and/or mistreatment. Placating the abuser, especially when it is not safe to leave, is often a rational survival strategy, not a pathological attempt to maintain access to a pathological form of gratification. "Making-up disorders" functions more as a slogan for referring to theories that are outperformed by one or more competitors.

Noticing patterns, classifying them and trying to explain them are legitimate scientific activities. How then, can psychiatrists distinguish more valid from less valid naming? They do so by turning to accepted validity criteria (selections from the general validity menu), and occasionally by introducing additional criteria. New constructs have to be calibrated with respect to these criteria—and outperform any competitors that exist.

One thing for certain is that the problem is not that psychiatry lacks criteria. In addition to all the standards of the psychometric model and the medical model, the following list of conceptual norms for validating disorders is also available (Stein et al. 2010).

- ◆ Occurs in the person
- ◆ Results in impairment
- ◆ Results in distress
- ◆ Manifestation of a dysfunction
- ◆ Involuntary.

These are all rationally articulated standards for what counts as a good disorder. Candidate disorder constructs should measure up to some of these standards, but it is unlikely that they will measure up to all of them. For these reasons, disorder constructs will be more or less good—the hard question is what counts as good enough? This represents a deep, important problem and forms part of what has been referred to as the incredible insecurity of psychiatric nosology (Kendler and Zachar 2008).

2.6 **Four approaches to validation**

How are we to proceed if no precise standard or pre-selected menu of standards is "the answer" to the validity problem? Four different strategies can be articulated. One is a conservative strategy, the second is an incremental strategy, the third is a bold strategy and the fourth is cautiously progressive.

The conservative strategy

The conservative strategy is favored by many critics of psychiatric classification. This strategy would limit psychiatry to the classification of high consensus, serious mental illnesses. According to these critics, a mistake was made in the early 20th century when the neuroses were taken out of neurology and combined with the severe disorders of the alienists to create the field of psychiatry. They argue that with the inclusion of neurotic conditions, the level of distress that is needed to be considered medically relevant was lowered and it is being lowered further with each addition of the manual. In various forms, these are the complaints of Szasz (1961), Horwitz and Wakefield (2007), Caplan (1995) and Kutchins and Kirk (1997).

According to such critics, the standards to which valid disorders have to be calibrated include the following.

◆ There is an empirically confirmable distinction between normal and abnormal.
◆ Every symptom is inherently pathological.
◆ The construct refers to a real entity that is causally related to the symptoms.
◆ The person with the condition can justifiably be allowed to adopt the sick role.

An important advantage of such a conservative approach to psychiatric nosology is that it would reduce the power of mental health professionals to casually describe patterns of maladaptive behavior as disordered, thereby curtailing both wild diagnosis and diagnostic fads.

The incremental strategy

The incremental strategy would not limit psychiatric classification to serious mental illnesses. Its purpose is to prevent wild diagnosis by constraining both the addition of new constructs and the revision of criteria for existing constructs (Pincus et al. 1992). The origin of this strategy can be detected in some of the excesses of the DSM-III and the DSM-III-R, the development of which represented a revolutionary period where new diagnostic categories were readily proposed and modified. At this time the nosological process skirted the line of being too wild, and the psychiatric authorities decided to constrain its future development.

According to the incremental strategy, any changes must be based on evidence that it would be an improvement. Also relevant to this strategy is Michael First's (Chapter 7, this volume) claim that a change that looks good on paper is less likely to be helpful unless it responds to a felt clinical need. Based on past experience, incrementalists are keen to avoid unforeseen harms (Frances 2009, 2010). This strategy emphasizes the virtue of being socially responsible, but like all virtues, both a deficiency and an excess is problematic. In excess, a socially responsible concern with avoiding unforeseen harms can lead to inaction and paralysis.

The bold strategy

The bold strategy claims that classification must be pushed forward by raising the bar.

> Concepts which have proved useful for ordering things easily assume so great an authority over us, that we forget their terrestrial origins and accept them as unalterable facts. They then become labeled as "conceptual necessities," "a priori situations," etc. The road of scientific progress is frequently blocked for long periods by such errors (Albert Einstein 1916, quoted in Fine, 1986, pp. 15–16).

Harkening back to the tradition of Descartes and Galileo, this bold strategy is more likely to be associated with the denigration of the past, often seen in claims that the current model is so flawed that progress is unlikely, and a re-boot is needed (Livesley 2003; Smith and Combs 2010; Widiger and Trull 2007). The boldest claims regarding the DSM-5 in this respect refer to the comparative superiority of dimensional models to categorical models.

The advocates of boldness are also more willing to emphasize a crisis of confidence in the existing taxonomy. Crisis talk is seen both in claims about the dire consequences for psychiatry if this problem is not solved and in hints that the current classification system is little better than pseudoscience.

One problem here is that the more revolutionary thinkers talk about the reification of diagnostic categories, but if their proposals are accepted, the resulting dimensions are also likely to be reified (Zachar and Kendler 2010). Throughout history, advocates of revolutionary change have also been vulnerable to fads, fashions and promulgation of unforeseen harms. All the same, both the history of science and the history of ideas in general teach that the achievers of progress are not uniformly prudent in their outlook: new and bold thinking is important. Reflecting on the strengths and weaknesses of the bold strategy leads to the fourth approach.

Cautious progressivism

Cautious progressivism takes into account 400 years of scientific history that was not available to Descartes and Galileo. With this history in mind, its advocates are less likely to simply denigrate the past, or to engage in exaggerated crisis talk, or to imply that one or two new standards will be magic bullets for solving the validity problem.

They do, however, understand the importance of raising the bar in the service of progress. The question is how to best do so. Rather placing all their hopes in Karl Popper-like bold conjectures, they contend that, practically speaking, variations that are somewhat continuous with the previous generation's standards have a better chance of being accepted. For example, they would not fail to emphasize that unidimensional constructs could (potentially) have greater reliability and also create new opportunities for identifying homogeneous groupings of cases. These ties to the concerns of the DSM-III generation give the claims of the dimensional model advocates additional weight. Progress can also be understood by emphasizing the continuity that exists rather than emphasizing revolution.

One assumption of cautious progressivism is that psychiatrists' compasses about disorders are more legitimate than both the conservative and the bold critics acknowledge (Kendler and Zachar 2008). Consider temperature, weight and length. We have some native abilities to detect these phenomena, however crude. Something similar, albeit more conceptually complex, may be true for detecting aberrant behavioral patterns (supplemented by some widely shared assumptions about normal functioning).

Over the last 150 years, many different disorder constructs have been proposed and systematized. Some of them represent fads and fashions, but some of them have remained fairly constant. The importance of authentic, empirically discovered stability is that it is something to hang our hats on over time—the achievement of which is an important goal of Ken Kendler's (Chapter 15, this volume) process of epistemic iteration. Although with progress comes change, if we were able to look into a crystal ball and get a glimpse of the diagnostic system used in 100 years, the cautious progressives would not be surprised to discover that many of the current constructs would still be recognizable in that system.

2.7 **Conclusion**

In this chapter I looked to the history and philosophy of science to explore the claim that psychiatric classification is invalid, and that the appearance of progress is an illusion. Rather than offering a single magic bullet solution to the validity problem, or defining validity as vacuously as meaning "a disorder really exists," I argued that a plurality of validities should be accepted. Among this plurality is the notion of comparative validity that emphasizes the rationally justified criteria we use to say that current theories/models are improvements on past theories/models. The calibration approach views validation as a process of developing constructs and theories that cohere with as many standards as possible—or cohere with standards that are given higher weights. Successfully molding diagnostic constructs so that they cohere with multiple standards should be considered an impressive achievement. Occasionally, progress involves taking a new look at validity by proposing a new rationally articulated standards of adequacy.

Almost no one would claim that the validity of psychiatric classification is satisfactory, or that the process of revising the classification is free from economic and political considerations This, however, is not unique to psychiatry and clinical psychology. The same is true of any socioculturally important scientific research program—from Galileo and Darwin right up to the present day. Without defending the current system, I argued that the process of making scientific progress often includes the kind of claim-making that some critics decry in psychiatry. Throughout history, scientific communities have identified crises as a way of justifying their new claims about adequacy, and have to work to get others to adopt those claims. Scientific progress often result in shifts in emphasis, but the past does not have to necessarily have be denigrated in order for one to improve upon it. In science, flaws and mistakes are important ingredients for making progress, not impediments to it.

What I referred to as the conservative and the bold approaches are expressions of dissatisfaction with the ambiguities of the current system. Their proponents would retreat from these ambiguities by adopting what they see as more certain (better justified) standards. The middle grounds of incrementalism and cautious progressivism, rightly or wrongly, are more tolerant of the current system. The main difference between the two is in how much risk they are willing to take in order to make progress.

Acknowledgments

Thanks to Andrea Solomon, Ken Kendler and Rachel Cooper for helpful comments.

Endnotes

1 For example, requiring that a group of psychiatric disorders constructs have a simple structure in the factor analytic sense may reduce the descriptive-phenomenological accuracy of the construct.

2 This notion of progress resulted from ideas discussed by Arthur Fine, *The Shaky Game: Einstein, Realism, and the Quantum Theory* (Chicago, IL: University of Chicago Press, 1986) and David L. Hull, *Science as a Process: An Evolutionary Account of the Social and Conceptual Development of Science* (Chicago, IL: University of Chicago Press, 1988).

3 Especially in measurement, reliability and validity are distinct concepts. Reliability is, however, a relevant factor in evaluating comparative validity. Kaplan, R. M. and Saccuzo, D. P. (2005) *Psychology Testing*. Belmont, CA: Wadsworth.

Chapter References

Caplan, A. L., McCartney, J. J. and Sisti, D. A. (2004). *Health, disease, and illness: Concepts in medicine*. Washington, DC: Georgetown University Press.

Caplan, P. J. (1985). *The myth of women's masochism* (1st ed.). New York: Dutton.

Caplan, P. J. (1995). *They say you're crazy: How the world's most powerful psychiatrists decide who's normal*. Reading, MA: Addison-Wesley.

Cronbach, L. J. and Meehl, P. E. (1955). Construct validity in psychological tests. *Psychological Bulletin*, **52**(4), 281–302.

Desmond, A. J. and Moore, J. R. (1991). *Darwin*. New York: Warner Books.

Fine, A. (1986). *The shaky game: Einstein, realism, and the quantum theory*. Chicago, IL: University of Chicago Press.

Frances, A. (2010). A warning sign on the road to DSM-V: Beware of its unintended consequences. *Psychiatric Times* (updated May 5, 2010) http://www.psychiatrictimes.com/dsm-5/content/article/10168/1425378 (accessed 5 May 5).

Frances, A. (2010). DSM in philosophyland: Curiouser and curiouser. *AAPP Bulletin*, **17**(2), 3–7.

Horwitz, A. V. and Wakefield, J. C. (2007). *The loss of sadness: How psychiatry transformed normal sorrow into depressive disorder.* New York: Oxford University Press.

Hull, D. L. (1988). *Science as a process: an evolutionary account of the social and conceptual development of science.* Chicago, IL: University of Chicago Press.

Hyman, S. E. (2010). The diagnosis of mental disorders: The problem of reification. *Annual Review of Clinical Psychology,* **6**, 155–79.

Kendler, K. S. (2009). An historical framework for psychiatric nosology. *Psychological Medicine,* **39**(12), 1935–41.

Kendler, K. S. and Zachar, P. (2008). The incredible insecurity of psychiatric nosology. In K. S. Kendler and Josef Parnas (eds.), *Philosophical issues in psychiatry: Explanation, phenomenology, and nosology.* Baltimore, MD: Johns Hopkins University Press, pp. 368–85.

Kerrod, R. (2000). *Uranus, Neptune, and Pluto.* Minneapolis, MN: Lerner Books.

Kirk, S. A. and Kutchins, H. (1992). *The Selling of DSM: The Rhetoric of Science in Psychiatry.* Hawthorne, NY: Aldine de Gruyter.

Kraemer, H. C. (2010). Concepts and methods for researching categories and dimensions in psychiatric diagnosis. In T. Millon, R. F. Krueger and E. Simonsen (eds.), *Contemporary Directions in Psychopathology.* New York: Guilford, 337–49.

Krueger, R. F., Watson, D. and Barlow, D. H. (2005). Introduction to the special section: Toward a dimensionally based taxonomy of psychopathology. *Journal of Abnormal Psychology,* **114**(4), 491–3.

Kutchins, H. and Kirk, S. A. (1997). *Making Us Crazy: DSM: The Psychiatric Bible and the Creation of Mental Disorders.* New York: Free Press.

Livesley, W. J. (2003). Diagnostic dilemmas in classifying personality disorder. In K. A. Phillips, M. B. First, and H. A. Pincus (eds.), *Advancing DSM: Dilemmas in psychiatric diagnosis.* Washington, DC: American Psychiatric Association, 153–89.

McHugh, P. R. (2008). *Try to remember: Psychiatry's clash over meaning, memory, and mind.* New York: Dana Press.

Meehl, P. E. (1995). Bootstraps taxometrics: Solving the classification problem in psychopathology. *American Psychologist,* **50**(4), 266–75.

Pincus, H. A., Frances, A. J., Davis, W. W, First, M. B. and Widiger, T. A. (1992). DSM-IV and new diagnostic categories: Holding the line on proliferation. *American Journal of Psychiatry,* **149**(1), 112–17.

Scerri, E. R. (2007). *The Periodic Table: Its Story and its Significance.* New York: Oxford University Press.

Shapin, S. and Schaffer, S. (1985). *Leviathan and the Air-pump: Hobbes, Boyle, and the Experimental life.* Princeton, NJ: Princeton University Press.

Sharratt, M. (1996). *Galileo: Decisive Innovator.* Cambridge: Cambridge University Press.

Smith, G. T. and Combs, J. (2010). Issues of construct validity in psychiatric diagnosis. In T. Millon, R. F. Krueger and E. Simonsen (eds.), *Contemporary directions in psychopathology.* New York: Guilford, 205–22.

Stein, D. J., Phillips, K. A., Bolton, D., Fulford, K. W., Sadler, J. D. and Kendler, K. S. (2010). What is a mental/psychiatric disorder? From DSM-IV to DSM-V. *Psychological Medicine,* **40**(11), 1759–65.

Szasz, T. S. (1961). *The myth of mental illness.* New York: Harper & Row.

Widiger, T. A. and Trull, T. J. (2007). Plate tectonics in the classification of personality disorder: Shifting to a dimensional model. *American Psychologist,* **62**(2), 71–83.

Widiger, T. A., Frances, A. J., Pincus, H. A., Davis, W. W. and First, M. B. (1991). Toward an empirical classification for the DSM-IV. *Journal of Abnormal Psychology,* **100**(3), 280–8.

Wilson, R. (1997). *Astronomy Through the Ages: The Story of the Human Attempt to Understand the Universe.* London: Taylor & Francis.

Zachar, P. (2002). The practical kinds model as a pragmatist theory of classification. *Philosophy, Psychiatry, & Psychology,* **9**(3), 219–27.

Zachar, P. (2008). Real kinds but no true taxonomy: An essay in psychiatric systematics. In K. S. Kendler and J. Parnas (eds.), *Philosophical issues in psychiatry: Explanation, phenomenology, and nosology.* Baltimore, MD: Johns Hopkins University Press, pp. 327–67.

Zachar, P. and Kendler, K. S. (2010). Philosophical issues in the classification of psychopathology. In T. Millon, R. F. Krueger, and E. Simonsen (eds.), *Contemporary directions in psychopathology.* New York: The Guilford Press, pp. 126–48.

Progress and the calibration of scientific constructs: a new look at validity

Rachel Cooper

In commenting on Peter Zachar's rich and interesting paper I am first going to set out what I hope is a fair reconstruction of Zachar's key claims before moving on to raise some queries and concerns.

2.8 A reconstruction of Zachar's claims

In his paper, Zachar asks a big question: has psychiatry made progress in the classification of psychiatric disorders? We can say that progress has been made if current theories are more valid than their predecessors. In assessing validity we have multiple standards that can be applied. For example, at a very general level, we might take the following to be indicators of the validity of a theory:

+ Novel predictions
+ Self-consistency
+ Coherence with other accepted theories.

Turning to psychiatry, and to the question of whether some particular diagnostic category is a valid disorder we again find that multiple standards are offered. For example, a valid disorder might be one that is characterized by the following:

+ Manifestation of a dysfunction
+ Results in distress
+ Low comorbidity with other conditions.
+ Predicts treatment response
+ Is clearly distinguished from normality
+ Runs in families.

Zachar reminds us that history and politics play a role in determining the standards for validity that a scientific community comes to accept. Each standard will be put forward by proponents at some particular point in time. For example, Zachar discusses the work of Kirk and Kutchins on the use of the kappa-statistic for inter-rater reliability that was used by the proponents of DSM-III. Political-style lobbying is required to get a standard accepted. This is because empirical evidence cannot be used to prove that introducing a new standard is a good idea.

Scientists will aim to get their constructs to meet as many of the generally accepted standards for validity as possible. Scientific progress can occur when a construct is adjusted over time so that more of the standards for assessing validity are satisfied. Zachar suggests that we can understand progress in psychiatry as consisting of such "calibration" and that we do not need to commit ourselves to scientific realism.

Very often, despite attempts at revision, a putative disorder that meets some of the possible criteria for validity will not meet all of them. In this case the various standards must be weighted. Different scientists might weight the criteria differently, and the accepted weightings can vary over time.

Within psychiatry it can clearly be seen why it is important to have standards for establishing validity. Mental health professionals are frequently accused of "making-up disorders"—that is of labeling people who are not disordered. It is reasonable to worry that invalid diagnostic categories might be included in schemes such as the DSM—and standards of validity are needed to root out such categories (or at least to prevent new invalid categories being added).

When a psychiatric classification can be seen to be only moderately successful, i.e., many putative disorders only meet some of the standards for validity, Zachar identifies four stances that a community might adopt. They might go conservative and only classify those conditions that do manage to meet all, or most, possible standards for validity. At the other end of the spectrum, they might act boldly, and seek to establish and apply brand new standards for validity. In between, they might adopt policies of "cautious progressivism" or "incrementalism," and only revise the existing classifications in such a way that revisions are more or less likely to increase validity. Though he does not explicitly say so, the discussion suggests that Zachar himself has most sympathy with cautious progressivism.

2.9 **Queries**

Zachar versus Kuhn

In many ways Zachar's account is reminiscent of claims made by Thomas Kuhn in *The Structure of Scientific Revolutions* (1962). Kuhn claims that normally science is conducted within a paradigm. Those who work within a paradigm share basic assumptions. Within a paradigm there will be broad consensus about basic theoretical claims, appropriate research questions, methodology and how to assess evidence.

During periods of "normal science" all of those working in some particular subdiscipline will work within one particular paradigm. While things go well, progress on various research questions will be made. However, over time various anomalies will build up; there will be phenomena that the paradigm can't explain, and research problems that stubbornly resist solution. Once the build-up of anomalies reaches a critical point, the community of scientists will perceive itself to be in crisis. Scientists will begin to doubt that the paradigm in which they have been trained is actually the right approach to addressing the questions in which they are interested. They will begin to cast around for alternatives. Alternative frameworks may develop, and if a new paradigm seems to do better than the old, then scientists will defect to it en masse. A new period of "normal science" will then begin, with new generations of scientist being trained into the new ways of thinking.

Importantly, on Kuhn's account, standards for assessing evidence vary with paradigm. To use examples from psychiatry, the adherents of some paradigms may think that theoretical claims must at least be consistent with first-person phenomenological reports, while other paradigms will dismiss such evidence as unimportant. As standards for assessing evidence vary with the paradigm, and all scientists work within one paradigm or other, there is no neutral stance from which paradigms can be compared. To use Kuhn's term, paradigms are "incommensurable."

The big problem for Kuhn's account is whether it is compatible with notions of scientific progress (in the final chapter of his book, Kuhn attempts to give an account of scientific progress but many are unconvinced that it works). The problem is that paradigms differ in what they count as a good theory, but can only be fairly judged on their own terms. It looks like there is no way of objectively determining whether one paradigm is better than another. How then can progress be judged?

In so far as Zachar's account is similar to Kuhn's I worry whether Zachar can genuinely give an account of scientific progress. Zachar notes that different scientific communities may adopt different standards of validity, and also weight those standards that they do share in different ways. With this in mind, Zachar's "calibration" looks like a very limited type of progress that will occur within a single paradigm and impress only the advocates of that paradigm. Consider again debates between paradigms in the mental health sciences that seek to take first person phenomenology seriously as evidence and those that do not. Those who rate phenomenological evidence highly can calibrate different varieties of phenomenological evidence all they like but they still will not impress the adherents of paradigms that do not see such data as evidence at all.

Problems with determining whether a condition is a valid disorder

Zachar asks how we can determine whether a condition is a valid disorder. In much of his discussion he avoids distinguishing two questions that I think are best kept separate. I think we can usefully distinguish two types of problem:

1. Is condition X genuinely a different kind of condition from condition Y? For example, is multiple personality disorder really the same condition as hysteria?

2. Is condition X genuinely a disorder—as opposed to some type of non-disorder condition? For example, is "complicated grief" a disorder as opposed to a normal human reaction? Is Asperger's syndrome a disorder as opposed to a valuable manifestation of neurodiversity?

My own view is that while questions of type 1 are scientific questions, those of type 2 are in large part ethical and political. This claim might be disputed, but the important point is that the questions are distinct.

In thinking through the implications of the difference, we might usefully borrow a suggestion from Derek Bolton's book *What is Mental Disorder?* (2008). Bolton suggests that systems such as the DSM might seek to include conditions that are valid in so far as they are distinct from other conditions. The tough questions of whether these "conditions of interest" are really disorders might be put to one side.

For comparison, suppose we set out to classify weeds (where weeds are defined as unwanted plants, or bad plants, or some such). We will face many difficult questions. Are daisies weeds? What about blackberries? A classification that sets out to list all and only weeds will become mired in controversy. However, many of the problems can be avoided if we instead compile a list of "plants that are sometimes taken to be weeds." Of course, we will still face some difficult questions—are blackberries really distinct from raspberries, for example? How should hybrid berries be classified? However, many tough choices can thus be avoided.

Scientific realism and psychiatry

In his paper Zachar cites some of the literature on scientific realism, and suggests that we might sensibly avoid committing ourselves to scientific realism when thinking about mental disorders. Instead, he thinks we can afford to be non-realists. I am worried about Zachar's suggestion that we might use non-realist accounts from the philosophy of science, which I think were originally developed mainly with the puzzles posed by theoretical physics in mind, to think about mental disorders. Physics and psychiatry are very different sciences, and debates about realism will play out very differently in the two areas.

Let's remind ourselves of the types of problem that led to the development of non-realist and anti-realist positions in the philosophy of science. First, some theoretical entities in physics have very odd properties—electrons are said to be both waves and particles, for example. Such odd properties mean that we cannot afford to be realists about electrons in a very robust sense; we can not think of electrons as being a bit like common sense physical objects like golf balls only much, much tinier.

Second, realist accounts in the philosophy of science have been challenged by the pessimistic induction (Laudan 1981). Consider the history of science. At least if we think of the history of well-developed and theoretically-oriented sciences, like physics and chemistry, what we see is a succession of theories that, while apparently successful in their day, have since been rejected. The pessimistic induction suggests that present scientists, like their predecessors, will turn out to be wrong. Given that so many past theories have been set aside, what reason do we have for thinking that our own current best theories will work any better? (Note that getting a version of the pessimistic induction to work for psychiatry is hard—there isn't much history, and there's even less past success).

The philosophical debates about scientific realism have developed with physics (and to a lesser extent chemistry) in mind. The most plausible examples have been taken from these sciences, and many of the accounts that have developed can only really be applied to these sciences. John Worrall's structural realism is an extreme example but illustrates the problem (Worrall 1989). Structural realism is offered as a type of partial realism that can deal with the pessimistic induction. Worrall looks at the history of theories about light. Over time there is much change—first light is thought to be a wave, then particles, then both. Still, Worrall points out the equations that describe the propagation of light remain the same. As a consequence, according to Worrall, we should believe in the "structure" of theories but not commit ourselves to their particular ontological claims. Worrall's "structure" is basically mathematical equations. His account might work for physics, but God only knows how it might be applied to a science like psychiatry.

Debates about scientific realism have talked in general terms about "science" but I suggest that participants in these debates have had physics in mind, and that the debates cannot be straightforwardly applied to a science like psychiatry. The concerns of someone who doubts the reality of electrons or superstrings are very different from the concerns of someone who doubts the reality of schizophrenia or multiple personality disorder. If I worry whether some particular mental disorder is "real" I'm not worrying about posited weird properties, or the pessimistic induction. Rather, and in line with my earlier suggested distinction between worrying about whether a condition is a valid disorder (as opposed to a non-disorder state) and worrying whether it is a condition distinct from others, I may have one or more of the following types of concern (amongst others): is this condition a disorder as opposed to a moral failing? Is it a disorder as opposed to the mislabeling of some range of normality? Is it is distinct condition or merely a variant of something else?

To reinforce my point about the different forms that concerns about realism take when one is concerned with psychiatry as opposed to physics we can make use of J. L. Austin's classic comments about the term "real." Austin reminds us that when we ask whether something is "real" we implicitly have some contrast in mind.

> . . . a definite sense attaches to the assertion that something is real, a real such-and-such, only in the light of a specific way in which it might be, or might have been, not real (Austin 1962, p. 70).

Thus, real cream is made from milk rather than vegetable oil, and a real Van Gogh was painted by Van Gogh rather than being a fake. Turning to debates about scientific realism, when people worry whether electrons are real, spelling out exactly what the contrasting possibilities are is tricky, but it is something like that electrons might be merely useful theoretical fictions. When people worry whether a mental disorder is real the contrasting possibilities are quite different. This means that forms of non-realism, developed by philosophers of science with physics in mind, can not sensibly be imported into the philosophy of psychiatry.

Approaching the problem from a different angle, suppose we accept that some disorder is real. Let's take Down syndrome as example that almost everyone will accept. When I say that Down syndrome is a real condition I mean the following: there are people with Down syndrome who form a kind. In important respects people with Down syndrome are similar to each other. They tend to have a characteristic physical appearance, and to have intellectual disabilities. In addition there are characteristic genetic abnormalities that cause Down syndrome. What's more, Down syndrome is plausibly a real disorder—the symptoms of Down syndrome are involuntary, they are not the result of a moral failing or of faking. The symptoms are also undesirable and so Down syndrome cannot simply be regarded as a normal variation. This is what I mean when I say that Down syndrome is real.

Zachar thinks that being a realist is risky and unnecessary, and that one can instead be a non-realist. I think that he has illegitimately imported both his concerns and his solution from the philosophy of physics. Psychiatry is different, and if Zachar wants us to be non-realists in this area he needs to spell out exactly what non-realism in the philosophy of psychiatry entails. This involves making it explicit what he thinks it would mean to be a realist about mental disorders, and also to flesh out the contrast that his non-realist urges us to accept instead.

Comments References

Austin, J. (1962). *Sense and Sensibilia*. Oxford: Clarendon Press.

Bolton, D. (2008). *What is Mental Disorder?* Oxford: Oxford University Press.

Kuhn, T. (1962). *Structure of Scientific Revolutions*. Chicago, IL: University of Chicago Press.

Laudan, L. (1981). A confutation of convergent realism. *Philosophy of Science*, **48**, 19–49.

Worrall, J. (1989). Structural realism: The best of both worlds? *Dialectica*, **43**, 99–124.
    Reprinted in D. Papineau (ed.) (1996). *The Philosophy of Science*. Oxford: Oxford University Press, pp. 139–65.

Chapter 3

Introduction

Josef Parnas

There are at least two ways to read Dr Ghaemi's chapter: as a reflection on philosophy of psychiatry and psychiatric nosology (more specifically the DSM) or as a reflection on the psychiatry's condition as a branch of medicine (or as a combination of both). The commentary by Derek Bolton takes up the task of disentangling philosophical and scientific issues.

Ghaemi sees his own position in continuation with the humanistic, rational tradition of Enlightenment, anchored in scientific realism. As a contrast, he invokes "postmodernism," beginning with Nietsche and Kirkegaard and more recently embodied by figures like Heidegger, Lacan, and Foucault. Post-modernism, which is an umbrella term, is credited with a sort of nihilism or extreme value relativism, antirealism and a deprecating attitude towards science.

Ghaemi thinks that a rational psychiatric nosology should classify psychiatric "diseases," rather than "disorders," and the borders of such diseases should be defined by biological etiological research. Schizophrenia and bipolar illness are obvious prime candidates for achieving a disease status. Adhering to the Hippocratic principle, psychiatry should only concern itself with treatable diseases: "all diseases are not treated: only those that are treatable, based on scientific knowledge, are treated; untreatable diseases, which have no cure or little basis for improvement, and self-limiting diseases, which improve naturally, are untreated." That does not mean that psychiatry should not alleviate suffering for the untreatable, but rather that psychiatry should consider itself from start as a medical profession. The post-modernist/non-Hippocratic DSM-IV is, says Ghaemi, guided by short-term concerns that bypass scientific considerations. It focuses on symptoms rather than on disease entities and many of its categories are pragmatic responses to extra-scientific needs and pressures. Reliability is the ultimate goal rather than a means.

As noted earlier, Ghaemi's text may also be read as a call for psychiatry to regain its identity as a medical discipline through a refusal and opposition to dispersing itself with countless varieties of psychological malaise, of which we have no etiological clue and for which we have no effective treatments. This is an important issue, because our profession is, in fact, increasingly burdened by disguised social problems, controversial behaviors or varieties of psychological reactions, previously unnamed, and simply belonging to a "permissible repertoire" of human existence.

Chapter 3

Taking disease seriously: beyond "pragmatic" nosology

S. Nassir Ghaemi

I think I differ from some of my colleagues on some basic assumptions about the nature of the medical profession, psychiatry as a discipline and the concepts of health and illness. I will not fully justify my positions, but simply state them to highlight differences in basic conceptual assumptions between me and other contributors, and then I'll relate them to my specific recommendations about the DSM.

3.1 The Hippocratic tradition

This school of thought is often misquoted as being just about "first do no harm" and being cautious in treatment. The Hippocratic school viewed medicine as an art, a skill one learns, based on a science. Medicine is not just art; it is not just science; it is both. The science of medicine has to do with the bodily basis of disease states, which manifest as symptoms. The art of medicine has to do with tracing symptoms back to disease, and individualizing the science to the patient (Jouanna 1999).

The basic Hippocratic approach, therefore, rejects from the beginning what is the common basis of psychiatric practice today: treatment of symptoms. In the Hippocratic tradition, symptoms are not treated; they must first be converted to syndromes, which represent diseases. Even then, all diseases are not treated: only those that are treatable, based on scientific knowledge, are treated; untreatable diseases, which have no cure or little basis for improvement, and self-limiting diseases, which improve naturally, are untreated. The concept of *Primum non nocere,* thus, meant *knowing when to treat and when not to treat, based on what kind of disease one diagnosed* (Jouanna 1999).

This tradition demonstrates the intimate connection between nosology, science and treatment. They all go together; they can't be separated. Our science determines what our nosology is based on clinical research about syndromes and biological research about diseases. Our science also determines how large the realm of treatable disease is. Science is the glue that holds the Hippocratic nosology together, and both clinical and treatment research are central to it.

Contrast this approach with many contemporary assumptions: At the conference, my colleague Derek Bolton states that science will go on, irrespective of our nosology. This is not true: if we get our clinical nosology wrong, our biological research will fail. Genetics will not produce results if our phenotypes are false; biological markers will fail to distinguish artificially chosen syndromes; drug studies will fail to show robust benefits in heterogeneous populations.

We cannot separate clinical and biological research. We hear, over and over again, that eventually biological markers will be found, or we will suddenly "discover" some diseases, and then our clinical descriptions will miraculously change. This has never happened in the history of medicine. Miracles are not to be awaited.

This is why the DSM-revision process is so central to all of psychiatry.

3.2 **Non-Hippocratic traditions in psychiatry**

Despite superficial fealty, the profession of medicine rejected the Hippocratic tradition described earlier for most of the past two millennia. Non-Hippocratic assumptions run deep among us. The basic non-Hippocratic view can be summarized as follows: (1) We should treat symptoms. (2) We should use our theory to justify our treatments.

The most common theory in the past that justified symptom treatment in medicine was Galen's humoral theory. In modern psychiatry, one can see Freud's libido theory as a similar approach. Currently, the "chemical imbalance" neurotransmitter models, increasing or decreasing monoamines with drugs, is similar. The non-Hippocratic tradition is also reflected in today's popular trend of social constructionist theory (Berrios and Porter 1999; Healy 2008), whereby the past is seen as little relevant to the present, and where the biological reality of most current diagnoses, and the utility of most current drugs, are rejected (Whitaker 2010).

In the conference, Paul McHugh made an excellent point that I would link to this discussion. The key problem with DSM-III, which was initially a strength, is its rejection of etiology. By being "atheoretical," DSM-III unwittingly implemented a theory of eclecticism: anyone is free to choose any theory he or she wants, or to use no theory at all. This approach dovetailed nicely with the post-modernism behind the social constructionist critique, and it flowered in the avowedly post-modernist philosophy of the DSM-IV leadership, which I will describe later in this chapter.

By not specifically committing to a Hippocratic disease model, while admitting the limitations of our current state of knowledge about many diseases, DSM-III onwards has put us on a path that, I fear, is a dead end. We don't know what represents disease, and, just as importantly, what mental symptoms do *not* represent disease. And what's worse, many of our colleagues conclude from this confusion that it doesn't matter.

3.3 **Defining mental illness**

A common critique of psychiatric nosology is that we don't have a general definition of mental illness.

I wonder if it may not be the case that *this* doesn't matter. The wish for general definitions is old-fashioned Platonic philosophy, a search for metaphysical essences and definitions that sounds important but in fact is meaningless. Many analytic philosophers have joined in this mantra, forgetting that the basis of Anglo-American philosophy—in the original work of Russell and Wittgenstein and Ayer—was all about rejecting such false general metaphysical questions.

We don't need a general definition of mental illness to identify specific psychiatric diseases, just as we don't need a general definition of physical illness to identify specific medical diseases. In the last chapter of *General Psychopathology* (Jaspers 1998),

Karl Jaspers, who many nosologists cite in support of skepticism about disease models, discussed this matter at great length, and came to the same conclusion as Russell and Wittgenstein would have: we don't have or need a general definition of mental illness (in general), but we can still construct a nosology of mental illnesses (plural). (I have reviewed Jaspers's discussion in this chapter at length elsewhere) (Ghaemi 2009a).

So I respond thus to the part of the commentary by Derek Bolton in which he views a definition of mental disease as central to my viewpoint. Specific diseases will be identifiable as they always have been, as *an abnormality of the body, often in an organ, which leads to a stereotypic syndrome presentation and a typical clinical course.* This suffices. We need not make false abstract claims, such as the common claim that *all* mental illness is mulifactorial (it isn't) and therefore nosology can't be disease-based, or that therefore we need complex models of illness, like the biopsychosocial model. This is all part of the atheoretical eclecticism which is the underlying ideology of current psychiatry (Ghaemi 2009a). We can reject all these views and go back to the tradition of Hippocrates and the *medical humanism* of William Osler and think of diseases as abnormality of the body interpreted through human experience, or alternatively, non-diseases as problems of human experience that get expressed as bodily symptoms.

3.4 Excursus on post-modernism

These are some of the philosophical assumptions on which I think I differ from some of my colleagues. By becoming atheoretically eclectic, DSM-III opened the door to post-modernist nihilism. It was my experience at this conference that I should probably try to explain what I mean by the concept of post-modernism. Our most insidious assumptions are those which we don't understand. So I hope readers will tolerate a brief excursus here; after we see how we've gone wrong, it will be clearer how we might right these wrongs.

Post-modernism is a general phrase which does not mean one thing, but yet has some meaning (Ashley 1997). A good analogy might be socialism, which was a broad cultural movement, with impact in politics and economics and throughout the humanities and intellectual life; it ranged from mild versions, like British Labour, to extreme fanatics, like Lenin and Stalin's totalitarianism. It could be the source of true and useful insights into economics, for instance, or it could be a completely false and distorting ideology of intellectual repression.

These analogies hold for post-modernism, but perhaps more so, in that socialism at least was an explicit political movement, while post-modernism is more of an unconscious, and hence unrecognized, cultural climate of opinion. To the extent that it is explicit, we can date its roots to the 19th century Romantic reaction to the rise of science, led in philosophy by Kierkegaard and Nietzsche. Post-modernism then gained steam after World War I burst the bubble of Victorian optimism about progress (Ashley 1997). Jaspers and Heidegger arose in the 1920s, explicitly describing post-modernist themes in a new philosophy of existentialism. After the horrors of World War II, with both atom bombs and Nazi genocide, post-modernism took off in defeated France, and, since then, it has spawned a slew of key French theorists, foremost among them Michel Foucault. In the student revolts of 1968, the spirit of post-modernism exploded in the Western world, and in many ways, the countercul-ture movement of that era represents the social flowering of post-modernism (Bloom 1988). Since then, the Western world has been living a tense mixture of post-modernist ideas along with older traditional religious or Enlightenment attitudes.

Psychiatry has followed this cultural tide. Kraepelin was a classic 19th-century, posi-tivist Enlightenment believer in science and progress. Freud grew out of that tradition but took the first steps toward post-modernist disillusion. Foucault launched a direct attack on psychiatry's rationalist and Enlightenment heritage, ingeniously describing the social construction of insanity (and many other medical conditions) (Foucault 1973), and when DSM-III declared that no theory was right, the post-modernist destruction of all theories succeeded. Since then social constructionist thinking, which is de rigeur ideology in most university humanities departments (Gross and Levitt 1997), has seeped over into the sciences, with psychiatry being one of the first to succumb.

3.5 The false "pragmatism" of DSM-IV

The relevance of post-modernism has become apparent to me in the course of some recent Internet-based debates with the leader of DSM-IV, (http://www.psychiatric-times.com/mood-disorders/content/article/10168/1642824). In what follows, I am directing my critique towards what I understand to be his views, but this should not be misinterpreted in a personal way as one person disagreeing with another. My interlocutor is only the most explicit representative, I think, for a general way of thinking that reflects the conceptual assumptions involved with DSM-III and DSM-IV.

In these debates, the term "pragmatism" is not the philosophical concept (devel-oped by Charles Sanders Peirce and William James in the 19th century), but the sim-ple English usage that practical consequences are what matter. (This is the same concept as pure utilitarianism.) Truth becomes reduced to expedience. This view dovetails with post-modernism because it is non-problematical only if we don't believe there is such a thing as truth, separate from expediency. This is a basic tenet of post-modernist philosophy. When applied to psychiatry, as it has most clearly by Foucault and his acolytes, it means either that there is no mental illness at all, or that we can't know what mental illnesses are. In either case, we make things up. This false pragma-tism (false because it betrays the actual ideas of Peirce and James), when applied to psychiatric nosology, becomes nothing different from psychiatric gerrymandering: DSM committees nip and tuck definitions as they wish; if interpreted benignly, they do so in the best interests of all involved (doctors, patients, the profession, the public, the government); if interpreted less benignly, they do so following their own personal opinions and biases (my counterpart, for instance, is explicit in wishing to avoid the diagnosis of bipolar disorder wherever possible, effectively broadening the diagnosis of "major depressive disorder" (MDD)).

There are some rationalizations for this gerrymandering, each of which is refutable: the pharmaceutical companies are constantly trying to take advantage of our diagnoses, it is claimed, so we should construct our nosologies so as to make it harder for those companies to market their deadly drugs to us. In practice, this "pragmatic" belief justifies opposition to any broadening of diagnoses to mild symptoms. My response: if only we could outsmart the pharmaceutical companies so easily.

The claim is made that science is always provisional, and thus rarely are we able to "close the discussion" by reference to definitive scientific evidence, especially in psychiatric nosology. Hence pragmatism trumps science. My response: the problem is not about closing the discussion with science; we aren't even opening our discussions with scientific content. This obsession with pragmatism typically involves ignoring, in effect, what scientific evidence we have, since it is always presumed to be so inadequate.

If a consensus of the scientific community of investigators (which is what Peirce meant by pragmatic truth) is presented in favor of a certain nosological view, this consensus is rejected since the "experts" are always trying to expand their diagnoses. Science receives only lip service, the least important criterion for psychiatric diagnosis: in practice, it is ignored.

3.6 **Misconceptions of nosologists**

Besides pragmatism, there are other specific assumptions, some of which were presented at the conference by Dr Jablensky, which seem to have driven past DSM nosologies. They may appear self-evident, but I think they are questionable and further muddy any attempt to create a scientifically valid nosology:

1. *Treatment response is nonspecific.* This is not the case. In fact, some treatments are specific, such as lithium for prevention of manic and depressive episodes (Goodwin and Jamison 2007). No other agent has been shown do so in monotherapy in scientifically valid research designs (Goodwin and Jamison 2007). Sometimes it is not treatment response, but rather treatment *non-response*, or (more generically) treatment *effects*, which are specific. Thus, antidepressant induced mania is quite specific to bipolar disorder as opposed to MDD, occurring in only 0.04% of persons with MDD versus 10% of those with bipolar disorder, according to recent huge randomized studies of over 3000 patients (Perlis et al. 2011; Sachs et al. 2007). A meta-analysis of over 3000 patients, including many non-randomized studies, was more variable, but still found that antidepressants were over 10 times as likely to cause mania in bipolar disorder than in MDD (Vazquez et al. 2011).

2. *Clinical syndromes tend to overlap so that there is no "point of rarity."* Overlap does not mean that conditions cannot be distinguished. In the Roscommon family study of schizoaffective disorder (Kendler et al. 1993), for instance, the lifetime risk of schizoaffective disorder in family members of probands with schizoaffective disorder was only about 3%, the same as with probands of schizophrenia or mood disorder, whereas the risks of both schizophrenia (6%) and mood disorder (54%) was much higher. Schizoaffective illness did not breed true. When the frequency of schizoaffective disorder was assessed in the community in the National Comorbidity Survey, the prevalence of all non-affective psychosis, including schizophrenia, was

0.7%. Schizoaffective disorder was a fraction of this overall number (Kessler et al. 1994). Mood disorder was diagnosed in about 10% of the sample. Thus, the community prevalence of schizoaffective disorder is consistent with the chance co-occurrence of schizophrenia and mood disorder, just as the genetic data show. There is overlap, there is no clear point of rarity, but this does not mean that the two conditions cannot be distinguished. This overlap is considered by some, like Crow (1998), as definitive contradiction of the schizophrenia/affective illness dichotomy. But some overlap exists between many biologically different groupings. An exception is not disproof; knowledge is probabilistic, not absolute.

3. *We have no agreed upon definition of mental disorder* "which implies that we have failed to establish prior agreement on the essential characteristics of that which we are trying to identify" (Kendell and Jablensky 2003). But there are no *essential* characteristics of mental disorder, and there is no need for a general metaphysics of it, as described previously.

4. *Symptoms lead to other symptoms producing either multiple diagnoses or "arbitrary hierarchies."* But hierarchies are not inherently arbitrary; they can be quite empirically sound. For instance, a half century of research has proven that psychotic symptoms per se do not imply the diagnosis of schizophrenia; they empirically occur in about 25–50% of patients with mania and 15–25% with depression (Goodwin and Jamison 2007; Pope and Lipinski 1978). These patients do not have any of the other features of schizophrenia, either by course or genetics or treatment effects. Thus, we can state, with empirical near-certainty, that a hierarchy for psychotic symptoms is justified in which mania and depression are above schizophrenia.

By making these assumptions, nosologists make matters more complex than they are, and then they conclude that we need complex nosologies. In fact, specific clear mental diseases can be identified—at least sometimes—with clear clinical syndrome distinctions, differential treatment effects and empirical hierarchies. Other times, this is not the case, but this need not mean that in all cases we are ignorant and confused. Let's know what we know, and know what we don't know, and stop using the latter to deny the former.

3.7 **What do we want our nosology to do for us?**

I think we can all agree that, in the end, all the activities of our profession are aimed at improving the lot of our patients. And all would also agree that the best way to improve patients' outcomes is to be able to treat them effectively. And I think most would agree that if we could know what diseases caused patients' symptoms, we could treat them most effectively. If these premises are accepted, it seems to me to follow clearly that the main goal of our nosology should be to help us find out what diseases are causing the symptoms experienced by our patients.

This would be my main goal: some might see it as a "research" perspective; I don't. Research improves clinical care; clinical care informs research; the two go together. One cannot get good clinical outcomes unless one produces and uses good research.

So this goal for nosology—to find out which diseases exist—is also a goal which has the best practical outcomes: patients will get the best treatments when we know which diseases exist.

3.8 **A pragmatic test for DSM-IV pragmatism**

I will next try to explain that the "pragmatism" underlying our nosology prevents us from understanding which conditions are diseases with primarily biological sources, and which conditions are social constructions, with primarily social or psychological sources.

I noticed that many of my colleagues, including some at the conference, seem to assume that this is not the case. Derek Bolton said that science will proceed however it wants to proceed, irrespective of how we define mental disorders. I hear, over and over again, especially by those tired of these debates, that science will eventually give us biological markers or genes, and then we will finally know how to classify mental disorders.

I note that most nosologists are not themselves researchers, and thus perhaps they don't realize the extent to which DSM definitions permeate the whole research process in psychiatry. If you want to do a study of genetics of schizophrenia, for instance, you might pick all kinds of candidate genes, but what will be your phenotype? DSM-defined schizophrenia. If you want to do a study of biological markers in depression, you can have all kinds of interesting neuroscientific possibilities, but what definitions will you use to define a clinical case to see if those markers are present versus controls? DSM-defined "major" depression. Our biological research is only as good as our clinical definitions. If our clinical definitions are wrong, if they distort the reality of disease, then our biological studies will be wrong.

Neither God nor Nature, whichever you would like to credit as defining reality, is likely to follow the gerrymandered definitions of a DSM committee.

I don't mean to criticize individuals here, although it is natural for those human beings who have been members and leaders of those committees to take umbrage with this criticism. But ideas deserve criticism, whether they are right or wrong. If wrong, to be discarded, if right to be defended. These "pragmatic" assumptions of DSM nosology have gone unexamined too long. If I am mistaken, I hope to be corrected. But a critical examination of these ideas needs to happen sometime.

In effect, this is a pragmatic test of DSM pragmatism: Has it produced good practical results in our understanding and treatment of mental illnesses?

I fear the answer is negative. In fact, my own arrival at this conclusion came in the other direction. First, as with many, I noticed how we have failed in our genetic and biological research in the past three decades (Kendler 2006). More recently, I've noticed how we've failed with our treatment research for depression in particular, with much less benefit with our drugs than many believed (Ghaemi 2008).

The common conclusion was to blame the drugs (they just don't work well) or to blame the brain (it's just very complicated to study). After appreciating the purely post-modernist belief-system of some of the leaders of DSM-IV, the suspicion dawned on me that perhaps the blame is misplaced: it is not our drugs nor our brain that is at fault—it is our DSM nosology.

3.9 **Reliability and validity**

The claim was always made, and I accepted it too, that DSM-III in particular at least enhanced the reliability of psychiatric diagnoses. We could all speak the same language, at least, even if we weren't certain if our definitions reflect reality; then by using the same definitions, research studies could be better compared with each other, and, over time, we could evolve, based on data, towards closer and closer approximations of reality. Reliability was a precursor to validity. This was how some DSM-III leaders, like Gerald Klerman, defended their views in the early 1980s (Klerman et al. 1984).

Something changed by the time DSM-IV came along in the mid 1990s. The pragmatic post-modernist criterion put aside any claim or interest in diagnostic reality. Scientific data were rejected or ignored, and no gradual evolution towards more scientifically true criteria occurred. Once science became the least important criterion, rather than the most, this link between reliability and validity was severed. Reliability became an end in itself, rather than a way-station to validity. Now all we have is a common language, a discourse in the sense that Foucault meant it, a pure fiction that represents the hegemony of our society. We may view this hegemony as benign; we may try to rig it so that the pragmatic results are "good," in our opinions. But it still is a fiction, one that has no correspondence with any reality or truth independent of our social structures and personal preferences.

3.10 **The DSM of internal medicine**

Psychiatry would do well to follow the example of internal medicine, which had its own DSM, leading to great scientific progress. Without stethoscopes or tuning forks or reflex hammers, much less blood tests or genetic causes, psychiatry today is quite similar to internal medicine or neurology in the 19th century. Let's apply the pragmatic test and see how they produced practical consequences that are so much better than psychiatry has managed in the last half century.

The internal medicine approach might be summarized thus: it began in a state as chaotic as current psychiatry—in the late 19th century, there were many treatments and little knowledge of disease. William Osler, observing the scene, despaired (Osler 1932). One needed to teach the practitioners not to treat syphilis or pneumonia or angina, while at the same time teaching the researchers how to go about identifying the causes of syphilis or pneumonia or angina. Osler's *Principles and Practice of Medicine* (Osler 1912), which outlived its author and dominated medical teaching from 1900 to about 1950, taught generations of clinicians to be therapeutically conservative and diagnostically precise. It was the DSM of internal medicine, before that profession knew the causes of most of its diseases; Osler's DSM was based purely on the most scientifically sound clinical observation of syndromes. About a decade after Osler's death, Ronald Fisher invented the concept of randomization (in agriculture) as a means of testing whether something causes something else in biological research. Two decades later, Alexander Fleming, working in basic science, discovered that penicillin killed bacteria. Three decades later, A. Bradford Hill put it all together and conducted the first randomized clinical trial, proving that streptomycin specifically cures tuberculous pneumonia (Ghaemi et al. 2009b).

The circle—from diagnosis to research to treatment—was closed.

In sum, careful clinical observation, without any other consideration, produced the best practical results in the long-term, because only in that way can clinical work link up with biological science.

We have historical evidence that this process applies to mental illnesses too. Syphilis proves that psychiatric diseases can be real biological entities in the natural world. In its early and middle stages, for decades at times, one cannot distinguish the mania, depression, and psychosis of neurosyphilis from what Kraepelin then called dementia praecox (DP) and manic-depression (MDI). Yet by careful clinical description, psychiatrists were able to identify those with general paralysis of the insane (GPI), and later when syphilis tests were developed and the spirochetes identified, studies of blood and brain in these patients showed that they had syphilis, in contrast to MDI and DP patients (Shorter 1997). If psychiatry had applied the DSM-pragmatic test in 1900, those GPI patients would have been mixed with the MDI and DP patients, and the later syphilis tests would have been all over the place; those biological studies would have been negative, and neurosyphilis would not have been identified. Some say there will never be another spirochete; others at the conference, in response to my critiques about ignoring the disease concept, said that if we had a spirochete, we would use a disease concept. But this is self-fulfilling prophecy: if we continue to take this false pragmatic, post-modernist approach to DSM nosology, we will never know whether or not there is any other spirochete to be found. (We might be surprised, just as happened with *Helicobacter pylori* for peptic ulcer disease.)

The larger lesson from internal medicine is that science should matter—first, middle and last—in nosology. It can be done; it has been done, even with classic mental illness syndromes.

3.11 **What do we mean by science?**

I have observed that a final, deep-seated resistance to some of these ideas reflects a profound cynicism about science. I reject false pragmatism and pure social constructionism. But this does not make me, as an audience member at the conference commented, a "Platonist." Just because one rejects post-modernism, it does not mean that one is stuck in 1860s-era positivistic science-worship. I also agree with Karl Marx (Foucault is not needed) that economic and political forces shape all our beliefs, including scientific ideas. I agree with Peirce and James and Jaspers and Nietzsche and Quine that facts do not exist in isolation but are influenced by our hypotheses and theories (Fulford et al. 2006). I agree with all of them that our knowledge of reality and truth is not a simple process, and that science does not produce Absolute knowledge, with a capital A, nor complete certainty, but rather probabilistic knowledge.

I accept all this, and I say so clearly, so readers will not misconstrue my critique of post-modern nihilism as meaning that I belong to the other absolutist extreme.

Some critics, both within the DSM process and without, reject science as a basis for defining our nosology because they see science as corrupted—by the pharmaceutical companies and by desire for status and power: pure post-modernist social construction. I think we need to appreciate that this is an extreme ideological view.

With all the caveats just given, I do believe that science can obtain true knowledge, with truth defined as above as probabilistic. This truth reflects reality, not in a "naïve" sense that I think any old fact is absolute reality, but in the sense which Peirce meant, and which James in his later writings described: that reality exists independent of specific human beings, and that our knowledge of that reality is conditioned by it. Reality draws the scientific inquirer closer and closer towards it. Modern philosophers call this "scientific realism," the notion that scientific work, properly conducted, with all its limitations, engages with realities of the world (Fulford et al. 2006).

3.12 **Recommendations for DSM-5 and beyond**

My recommendations for the DSM process, based on the considerations discussed, are as follows:

1. Remove false "pragmatism" as the primary consideration in constructing diagnostic definitions.

2. Scientific research in clinical nosology, using classic epidemiological validators (symptoms, course, family history, treatment response, biological markers) should be the foremost consideration at all times in defining diagnostic definitions. Where there is consensus among scientific experts in a diagnosis, diagnostic considerations should be changed. The definition of consensus does not mean complete certainty, since this is impossible in science. Rather, the definition of how much scientific evidence is needed to change criteria should reflect the scientific evidence on which our current criteria are based. If new evidence exceeds the data on which current criteria are based, then those new data should be utilized to change diagnostic criteria.

3. Where more or better evidence does not exist, or where significant controversy holds among experts, then practical considerations can be taken into account as a lower-level priority upon which to decide to change or not change diagnostic definitions.

4. Remove the word "disorder" from DSM and replace it with "disease" for those conditions for which a biological basis in etiology and pathogenesis is either known, or well supported, by research. This would represent about a dozen or so diseases, I think, beginning with schizophrenia and bipolar disease.

5. Replace "disorder" with "condition" or "syndrome" for all the other clinical constructs that do not have a well-supported etiological and pathogenetic basis in biology. These socially constructed clinical syndromes are no less "real" than biological diseases, but they are non-biological in their etiologies: their social and psychological sources are important and deserve separate attention, as opposed to being lumped with biological "disorders" as they are now.

If these recommendations were adopted, I think the manual could also be greatly shortened by removing altogether many clinical constructs that have no disease basis and which have little nosological evidence based on scientific data (such as some of the personality disorders).

My view here is method-based (in the tradition of Karl Jaspers), not eclectic nor dogmatic (Ghaemi 2007). The post-modern eclectic mix of arbitrary preferences has proven its barrenness. But dogmatic responses are not helpful. Unfortunately many biological researchers dogmatically try to fit all clinical conditions into the biological disease model, even when their scientific research does not objectively support that view. Just as unfortunately, most social constructionists dogmatically try to deconstruct biologically validated diseases like manic-depressive illness, based on the social and cultural contexts of those diseases. We need to be clear when we are faced with diseases, and when not. Mixing and matching pragmatically will not do; taking only one approach is hardly better. Real scientific work, conducted honestly in awareness of this distinction, will allow us to classify what is what.

3.13 **Conclusions**

Psychiatry sits in the same place scientifically as medicine did at the end of the 19th century. If we are to experience the advances that medicine achieved, we would do well to study and follow the example of historical success. The first step would be to reclaim the Hippocratic tradition based on taking the concept of disease seriously. We could then hold that mental diseases are those conditions about which we now know (as with neurosyphilis), or will know (as with schizophrenia and manic-depressive illness), the specific biological abnormalities of the body and its organs which cause the illness, and control its course and response to treatment.

The next step would be to explicitly reject and move beyond those post-modernist beliefs that have caused stagnation in psychiatric nosology. Instead, we should work vigorously to describe our psychiatric syndromes to the best of our current scientific ability, much as Osler did for medicine in his textbook. If that work is done objectively and honestly, then such definitions will promote and link to future advances in neuroscience and biology, unlike our past "pragmatic" diagnoses. Then, research will clarify which of our clinical conditions are diseases of the body, and which are primarily social constructions of culture and the human condition.

Chapter References

Ashley, D. (1997). *History without a subject: The postmodern condition*. Boulder, CO: Westview Press.

Berrios, G. and Porter, R. (eds.) (1999). *A history of clinical psychiatry*. London: Athlone Press.

Bloom, A. (1988). *Closing of the American mind*. New York: Simon and Schuster.

Crow, T. J. (1998). From Kraepelin to Kretschmer leavened by Schneider. *Archives of General Psychiatry*, **55**, 502–4.

Foucault, M. (1973). *Madness and civilization*. New York: Vintage Books.

Fulford, K. W. M., Thornton, T. and Graham, G. (eds.) (2006). *Oxford Textbook of Philosophy and Psychiatry*. Oxford: Oxford University Press.

Ghaemi, S. N. (2007). *The Concepts of Psychiatry*. Baltimore, MD: Johns Hopkins University Press.

Ghaemi, S. N. (2008). Why antidepressants are not antidepressants: STEP-BD, STAR*D, and the return of neurotic depression. *Bipolar Disorders*, **10**(8), 957–68.

Ghaemi, S. N. (2009a). *The rise and fall of the biopsychosocial model: Reconciling art and science in psychiatry*. Baltimore, MD: Johns Hopkins University Press.

Ghaemi, S. N. (2009b). *A Clinician's Guide to Statistics and Epidemiology in Mental Health: Measuring Truth and Uncertainty*. Cambridge: Cambridge University Press.

Goodwin, F. and Jamison, K. (2007). *Manic Depressive Illness* (2nd ed.). New York: Oxford University Press.

Gross, P. R. and Levitt, N. (1997). *Higher superstition: The academic left and its quarrels with science*. Baltimore, MD: Johns Hopkins University Press.

Healy, D. (2008). *Mania: A short history of bipolar disorder*. Baltimore, MD: Johns Hopkins University Press.

Jaspers, K. (1998). *General Psychopathology*. Baltimore, MD: Johns Hopkins University Press.

Jouanna, J. (1999). *Hippocrates*. Baltimore, MD: Johns Hopkins University Press.

Kendell, R. and Jablensky, A. (2003). Distinguishing Between the validity and utility of psychiatric diagnoses. *American Journal of Psychiatry*, **160**(1), 4–12.

Kendler, K. S. (2006). Reflections on the relationship between psychiatric genetics and psychiatric nosology. *American Journal of Psychiatry*, **163**(7), 1138–46.

Kendler, K. S., McGuire, M., Gruenberg, A. M., O'Hare, A., Spellman, M. and Walsh, D. (1993). The Roscommon family study I. *Archives of General Psychiatry*, **50**, 527–40.

Kessler, R. C., McGonagle, K. A. Zhao, S., Nelson, C. B., Hughes, M., Eshleman, S., *et al.* (1994). Lifetime and 12-month prevalence of DSM-III-R psychiatric disorders in the United States. Results from the National Comorbidity Survey. *Archives of General Psychiatry*, **51**(1), 8–19.

Klerman, G. L., Vaillant, G. E., Spitzer, R. L. and Michels, R. (1984). A debate on DSM-III. *American Journal of Psychiatry*, **141**(4), 539–53.

Osler, W. (1912). *The principles and practice of medicine*. New York: D. Appleton and Company.

Osler, W. (1932). *Aequanimitas (Third Edition)*. Philadelphia, PA: The Blakiston Company.

Perlis, R. H., Uher, R., Ostacher, M., Goldberg, J. F., Trivedi, M. H., Rush, A.J., *et al.* (2011). Association between bipolar spectrum features and treatment outcomes in outpatients with major depressive disorder. *Archives of General Psychiatry*, **68**(4), 351–60.

Pope, H. G., Jr. and Lipinski, J. F. (1978). Diagnosis in schizophrenia and manic-depressive illness. *Archives of General Psychiatry*, **35**, 811–28.

Sachs, G. S., Nierenberg, A. A. Calabrese, J. R., Marangell, L. B., Wisniewski, S. R., Gyulai, L., *et al.* (2007). Effectiveness of adjunctive antidepressant treatment for bipolar depression. *New England Journal of Medicine*, **356**(17), 1711–22.

Shorter, E. (1997). *A History of Psychiatry*. New York: John Wiley and Sons.

Vazquez, G., Tondo, L. and Baldessarini R. J. (2011). Comparison of antidepressant responses in patients with bipolar vs. unipolar depression: A meta-analytic review. *Pharmacopsychiatry*, **44**(1), 21–6.

Whitaker, R. (2010). *Anatomy of an epidemic: Magic bullets, psychiatric drugs, and the astonishing rise of mental illness in America*. New York: Crown.

What is psychiatric disease? A commentary on Dr Ghaemi's paper

Derek Bolton

There are many points of interest and worthy of discussion in Dr Ghaemi's paper. It discusses contrasts on a grand scale between Hippocratic and Gallean traditions in medicine; between post-modernism, pragmatism and realism in philosophy; and between the eventual clarity and therapeutic success of the 19th- and 20th-century disease models—and the apparent relative messiness of current psychiatry.

In this commentary I will focus on four points relevant to Dr Ghaemi's argument:

1. On the definition of disease, which is more problematic than Dr Ghaemi seems to suppose.

2. On the shift from the relatively clear 19th/20th-century disease models to the relatively complex, messy, models of contemporary models of psychiatric conditions, which Professor Ghaemi's presents in the context of, or even as, changes in philosophy—I will suggest, rather, that this shift has been in the science.

3. On why the current diagnostic classification manuals have operationalized criteria: this is a matter of scientific method, not (or not only) an expression of post-modernism.

4. Having discussed these points of disagreement, however, I will suggest that Professor Ghaemi is right when his points are interpreted as recommendations for a distinctive role of medical psychiatry within the broader domain of mental healthcare.

First then, consider the definition of disease. Professor Ghaemi is right that medical definitions of disease are straightforward, but that is because they typically help themselves to a concept like "abnormal"—as in "an abnormality of the body." So we are owed an account of "abnormal," which, to put a long story short, can run in three ways. Two of these are versions of naturalism: Boorse's biostatistical theory and Wakefield's evolutionary theoretic definition, both of which are highly problematic, as reviewed recently in Bolton (2008). But if we do not rely on these naturalist accounts of "abnormality," and hence "disease," we are left with various other approaches, such as what Professor Ghaemi calls the biological reductionist, the biopsychosocial approach, or medical humanism, which all keep the word "abnormal" or "disease" or some cognate term in them. We can break out of this circle of terms—disease, illness, abnormality, dysfunction, pathology, etc.—by invoking states of the body or mind that lead to poor outcomes, such as excessive distress, impairment of day-to-day functioning, or premature death. This constitutes the third main approach to the "definition" of disease, of the sort in fact employed in the DSM and ICD. Consistent with this approach, the more plainly a condition is associated with poor outcomes, and the more poor the outcomes, the more likely it is that its disease status will be uncontentious; conversely, if the association is weak, or the value of the outcome is ambiguous, or temporary, self-limiting, the more the disease status of the condition is questionable.

A general point here and one relevant to Professor Ghaemi's paper is that while "abnormality of the body" looks like an objective, independent fact, and the naturalist definitions in terms of statistical abnormality or evolutionary "design," seek exactly to preserve and validate this appearance, conceptualization of pathology in terms of poor outcomes no longer has the appearance of scientific fact. Our judgments as to what outcomes are harmful or not, and to what extent, and their weights one against another, are sensitive to social and personal contexts and interpretations.

My second main point concerns the shift from the relatively clear 19th/20th-century disease models to the relatively complex, messy, models of contemporary models of psychiatric conditions. While Professor Ghaemi gives a general and straightforward definition of disease (with the aid of the notion of abnormality), he gives the concept much more specific content by focusing on particular examples taken from 19th- and 20th-century biomedicine: tuberculosis and syphilis, caused by bacteria, and treatable, it turned out, by penicillin. In these conditions we have not only bodily processes leading to dismal outcomes, but also, and critically, both of the following features: a specific causal pathway leading to the poor outcomes, involving infection by specific toxins, and, a specific cure, one which targets and disrupts the causal pathway. In brief, there are one-to-one relations between etiology and disease, and between disease and cure. Professor Ghaemi calls us to search/research for such diseases in psychiatry, under the banner of philosophical realism, as opposed to post-modernism. However, and this is my main point, the issue here is not a philosophical one, it is a matter of what the phenomena are, a matter for the science, and we should judge it in these terms. Professor Ghaemi is right of course to say that the 19th/20th-century disease model has worked for some physical conditions, and did work for one psychiatric condition, syphilis, and there is no a priori reason why it should not apply to all or some more psychiatric conditions. There is certainly no a priori reason why it cannot apply, but equally there is no a priori reason why it should. It is simply not an a priori, philosophical issue, and not a matter whether we favor, in particular, philosophical realism rather than post-modernism. It may have turned out that major depressive disorder, plus or minus a bit, is like, in respect of the form of its causal modeling, tuberculosis and syphilis. So far is has not; but it is not just that we have not yet had a look, but rather we have had a decent look, and what we have seen so far is not like a univariate causal pathway amenable to a single kind of preventative strategy or treatment. This is the position I highlighted in my paper to conference, and in this volume—but it is not a philosophical position: it is not anti-realism, or post-modernism, or pragmatism, or any other philosophical or cultural-ism; it is just that these are the findings in the science so far.

My third point concerns the rationale for operationalizing the description of symptoms and syndromes in clinical observational terms, as in the current diagnostic classification manuals. The current position here, as for the other topics discussed earlier, is, I suggest again, not a matter of being in the throes of a post-modern disease, but rather a matter of applying scientific method. The rationale for using operationalized, clinical observational terms, as I referred to briefly in my paper to conference and in this volume, is to achieve good enough reliability. The approach may be criticized for letting in conditions that are not, in some sense, genuine pathology. The background to such a criticism is of course some independent notion of disease, independent of the approach in the current manuals. Dr Ghaemi proposes that we have let in conditions that are not real diseases. But how do we know this? And how are we to find out which of the conditions in the manuals are real diseases and which are not? Further, and this is the main question for the present purpose, what kind of classification system do we need while we are doing the necessary research to find out? One of the first issues to be addressed would be: how can we be confident enough that different groups are researching the same thing, replicating or failing to replicate each other's findings? In other words, the problem of reliability would have to be resolved enough, presumably by producing something looking very much like the current manuals; finding a solution to this problem of reliability cannot be avoided. Again, this is not a matter of a post-modern disease—it is rather that we have to have a reliable enough basis for the science of causes and treatments to proceed. The general point I am making here applies to any complaint that the current diagnostic manuals are overinclusive, that they have included not only genuine pathology, defined by some unapparent feature, but also other conditions, especially when the alleged overinclusiveness is laid at the door of the current use of observational criteria for diagnosis. Wakefield makes a similar complaint, and the point made earlier applies to it: while we do the science to sort out which of the conditions are and which are not genuine dysfunctions (understood in Wakefield's evolutionary theoretic sense), we would need a system of description of symptoms and syndromes at the observational level, much as in the current manuals (Bolton, 2007). Again, the rationale for this clinical observational approach to diagnosis is not philosophical or cultural, but is primarily rather a matter of what scientific method is to be used while the research on the nature of the conditions of interest and their etiology proceeds.

Philosophy and the diagnostic manuals aside, however, there are no doubt distinctions to be made among the psychiatric conditions, those conditions of body and mind associated with poor outcomes, and some of these distinctions may be marked by calling some diseases and others something else—and this brings me to my fourth and last point of commentary on Professor Ghaemi's paper (an addition in this volume to my commentary at conference).

Professor Ghaemi comments that he believes that research to date provides enough evidence for including only a few current psychiatric diagnoses as diseases, these few including schizophrenia, manic-depressive illness, melancholic depression and obsessive–compulsive disorder. It would no doubt be a complicated matter to work through the very large research literatures on each of these conditions, comprising large amounts on the many aspects of these conditions, including etiology and treatment, also bearing in mind areas of conflicting or otherwise contentious findings, to tease out what made these conditions diseases and others not. However, speaking of belief, I would believe that that if a family member or friend of mine had one of these conditions—and if, in the case of obsessive–compulsive disorder, a proper dose of the indicated psychological therapy had been tried and had failed—then the right health-care would include assessment by a psychiatrist for use of medication, and not only for first-line treatment, but for tailored algorithmic step-up through medications and combinations as indicated. I would suppose, on the basis of research evidence and experience, that psychological therapy may well be helpful in addressing many issues of the patient's attitude and adjustment to the illness, and recovery of a viable life, but, medical care, the strategies of medical care and medical-psychiatric interventions would be essential to have, or to at least consider. In brief, I would agree with characterizing some conditions, such as bipolar disorder, as genuine psychiatric diseases, if only to signal these crucial pragmatic, treatment considerations. One reading I have of the key message of Professor Ghaemi's paper is that psychiatry should not lose sight of its crucial role and responsibilities in the medical management of such conditions, should not lose itself in problems and approaches which can be otherwise managed. I find this reading of the paper interesting—not as a psychiatrist but as one concerned with mental health services—because it would echo recent concerns within the psychiatry profession in the UK and to some extent internationally that its role is becoming unclear (especially Craddock et al. (2008); also Katschnig (2010), and commentaries.)

Comments References

Bolton, D. (2007). The usefulness of Wakefield's definition of mental disorder for the diagnostic manuals. *World Psychiatry*, **6**(3), 165–6.

Bolton D. (2008). *What is mental disorder? An essay in philosophy, science and values*. Oxford: Oxford University Press.

Craddock, N., Antebi, D., Attenburrow, M.J., Bailey, A., Carson, A., Cowen, P., *et al.* (2008). Wake-up call for British Psychiatry. *British Journal of Psychiatry*, **193**, 6–9.

Katsching, H. (2010). *Are psychiatrists an endangered species? Observations on internal and external challenges to the profession. World Psychiatry*, **9**, 21–28. [With commentaries in the same issue.]

Chapter 4

Introduction

Kenneth S. Kendler

Rachel Cooper takes on a central issue for psychiatric nosology that is not often asked by nosologists themselves—that is: when is psychiatric diagnosis a source for good versus bad in the world? Furthermore, when this question comes to serious nosologists, it is often couched in such shrill terms by our strident critics that whatever substance is contained in the critique is often disregarded. It is therefore of particular value that she address the question of the possible benefit versus harm of a psychiatric diagnosis in a thoughtful, dispassionate and reasoned manner.

She quickly makes the useful distinction between a global condemnation of psychiatric diagnosis (best to get rid of the whole damn thing!) versus a more targeted critique (the application of conduct disorder to inner city minority youth often results in a pathologizing of subculturally normative behavior).

Dr Cooper's summary of the benefits of classification will be familiar to many. In a very practical way, classification is a bedrock part of the practice of medicine because so much of our approach to treatment is based on diagnosis. One good thing about classification is that it can tell you a lot of useful things about an individual so classified—treatment, prognosis, etc. As an aside, Dr Cooper has obviously received some pushback from her claim that some psychiatric disorders are natural kinds that she has retreated from her use of that "metaphysically encrusted" term to a simpler term: "repeatables." (For readers who want a quick tour of the long history and controversy about this term—look at the article on Natural Kinds in the Stanford Encyclopedia of Philosophy at http://plato.stanford.edu/entries/natural-kinds/).

She sensibly relates the value of classification of psychiatric disorders to "whether cases of a mental disorder are importantly similar to each other." The more similar they are, the more benefit to be gained from classification. She also briefly notes the problem, pondered by several other contributors to this volume, of too many classifications. If, as we know, there are many possible ways to classify psychiatric patients, how do we pick the best? Here she refers to the quite interesting work of the philosopher, John Dupré, who subscribes to a promiscuous sort of realism that emphasizes the inherent disorder of the world (Dupré 1993). Dupré and Cooper would, I think, agree with Zachar, who in this volume (Chapter 2) argues for "validity" pluralism for psychiatric disorders.

Then, Dr Cooper turns to the dangers of classification. My guess is that readers' reactions to this section will have a lot to do with their professional backgrounds. Physician-psychiatrists will probably be the least tolerant of these concerns. They are strongly socialized in a medical environment where having a diagnosis (hypertension, asthma, breast cancer) is widely accepted and generally not problematic. Why should psychiatry be different? Psychologists, however, often take a quite different perspective. If any readers have ever heard a psychiatrist and psychologist argue vigorously about the relative merits of the terms "patient" and "client," they will understand my point here. If I were to succinctly summarize my view on this question, it is that psychiatric disorders just strike "closer to home" than do medical disorders. If I do or do not have hypertension, that leaves me as the same basic person. I might take a pill every day and worry about my salt intake, but I am still me. However, if I have schizophrenia or antisocial personality, that illness comes to define me in a much more central way. That is, while I *have* hypertension, you might argue I *am* schizophrenic (or at least that is how others might view me).

Dr Cooper does approach this issue, particularly for antisocial personality, in a relatively novel way, with a focus on self-narratives. Her three possible responses ("challenge," "embrace," or "uncertainty") are useful concepts. Here, her discussion, especially if generalized to other psychiatric disorders, could profit from a link with the large literature in psychiatry on "insight" (Markova 2005). We know, for example, that patients with psychotic illness or mania, who challenge their diagnosis and do not regard themselves as ill, have (of course) lower medication compliance and poorer outcomes than those who recognize that their mind/brains are not always functioning optimally. That is, sometimes, challenging a psychiatric diagnosis can be an expression of personal strength but other times it can be a symptom of illness. Our response to such challenges should probably be quite different in these two scenarios.

So, given that classification can have benefits but may also cause harm, Dr Cooper's last section tries to balance these perspectives. She rejects the extreme solution of trashing the DSMs (and ICDs) altogether. She has some practical suggestions to minimize harm (e.g. the development of positive illness narratives). Furthermore, she appropriately raises a very hard question—one actively debated in the field—of whether some diagnostic categories ought not to be proposed because of the possibility of harm. She reviews the concerns about the "psychosis risk syndrome" in this light. She ends with a cautious optimism. Psychiatric classification can, in total, contribute to the relief of human suffering, but it would be naïve of us to think that this enterprise cannot cause harm. (I am pleased to note that current criteria in DSM-5 for the adoption of a new disorder specifically must address the question of possible harm). Seeking to maximize benefit and minimize harm is surely the correct way forward.

Introduction References

Dupré, J. (1993). *The Disorder of Things: metaphysical foundations of the disunity of science.* Cambridge, MA: Harvard University Press.

Markova, I. (2005). *Insight in Psychiatry* (1st ed.). Cambridge: Cambridge University Press.

Chapter 4

Is psychiatric classification a good thing?

Rachel Cooper

In this chapter I seek both to ask whether psychiatric classification is a good thing, and also to make it clear how this is an issue on which reasonable people can disagree. When I'm talking of "classification" I have in mind the type of classification facilitated by diagnostic systems such as the DSM.

We can question the wisdom of classifying mentally ill people either in general or in particular cases. At the general level, we might ask whether research programs such as that associated with the DSM are a force for good or evil. At the particular level, we may query the role of classification in some particular subdomain, currently, for example, personality disorders stand out as a particularly contested area. Questions at the two levels are, of course, linked. Those who are generally skeptical about psychiatric classification will worry about classification in many particular cases. Writers such as Thomas Szsaz (1974), for example, would accept only classifications of organic brain disorders as legitimate. At the other end of the scale, even those who are generally pro-classification will agree that some areas of human behavior should not be included in the DSM, for example, they might worry about the potential medicalization of normal grief (Horwitz and Wakefield 2007).

As tends to be the case with philosophical discussion, much of my argument will be at a fairly abstract level and will be couched in general terms—I shall consider why, in general, classification can be helpful, and what, in general, are the risks attached to classification. However, applying the discussion to particular cases is straightforward, and I shall also mention particular cases as the chapter proceeds. My overall claim will be that classification in psychiatry is frequently, but not always, a good thing. The chapter is split into three main sections. The first considers the benefits of classification, the second considers the harms that classification can produce, the third, and most tentative, section starts to consider how classificatory projects might best proceed in order to maximize the benefits and minimize the harms.

4.1 The benefits of classification

Classification can enable us to gain power over a domain. Where entities fall into groups that are genuinely similar to each other in theoretically important ways then classifying them into groups of like entities is a valuable part of scientific practice. As entities that fall into such natural groups are similar they can be expected to behave similarly. What is all this talk of "genuinely similar," "natural," "theoretically important" doing? Basically I just want to emphasize that in order for classification to yield power over a domain the similarities have to be significant and out there in the world. The classification that I am interested in is of the sort that has been used to such great advantage in chemistry and the biological sciences. All samples of an element have the same atomic number, and this ensures that their properties are alike. All members of a species are genetically similar and have similar developmental histories; as such they can be expected to thrive in the same sort of habitat, to eat the same food, to have similar life spans, and so on.

Those who favor classification frequently talk of "natural kinds." Members of a natural kind are alike, and natural laws mean that members of a kind will behave similarly. Depending on the author, other conditions have also been added. Natural kinds have been claimed to be universal (in the sense of occurring everywhere), discrete, to have essential properties, and so on and so forth (see, for example, the conditions imposed by Haslam (2003) and Zachar (2001)). In earlier work I talked in terms of natural kinds, and claimed that at least some mental disorders can be considered natural kinds (Cooper 2005). One of the problems I encountered is that the term "natural kind" has become encrusted with metaphysical baggage. When I talked about "natural kinds," intending to use the term with minimal commitments, I was heard as being committed to all sorts of things.

Now instead of talking of natural kinds I will talk of "repeatables." This makes clear the basic important idea; some entities in the world are alike, and will behave in similar ways. As applied to mental disorders, the idea that there may be repeatables is this: if we consider individual cases of mental disorder some can be seen to be similar to each other. Furthermore some of these similarities will be theoretically important, and in some cases patients who are grouped together will be alike in fundamental ways (maybe they all have the same genetic abnormality, or all have similar levels of some neurotransmitter, or all have similar relationships with their childhood caregivers). If we take cases of mental disorder as our domain and plot them onto a multidimensional quality space (as in cluster analysis) then we will find clusters of similar cases.

If we focus on the right properties, then the clusters that such a process generates will be inductively powerful. External validation on the basis of treatment response, family history, demographic correlates and so on can give additional reason to believe that patients who are being classified together are similar in genuinely important respects. If all goes well, a case that falls in a particular cluster can be expected to behave in ways that are similar to others of its class. The importance of such similarities is obvious if one thinks of treatments. The hope would be that a treatment that is found to work for one member of a class will work for others in that class too.

Note that the key question in looking for repeatables is whether cases of a mental disorder are importantly similar to each other. The question of whether varieties of mental disorder will turn out to be discrete or continuous turns out to be a side issue. It is the fact that there are similarities between entities that does all the work when it comes to making inductive inferences and grounding explanations. It is because "repeatables" all have similar properties that one will behave like the others of its type. Thus, classifications that vary along dimensions can be as powerful as those that rely on discrete categories. Think of alloys as an example. Knowing that a sample is a particular alloy is as useful, and useful in the same kinds of ways, as knowing that it is a 100% pure metal (if a sample is known to be 55% zinc and 45% copper, one can predict how the sample will behave just as well as if one knew it to be pure copper). There is reason to think that at least some mental disorders will be better mapped by a continuous rather than a categorical classification system. Draft versions of the DSM-5 suggest that classifications of personality disorders will go this way.

The idea that mental disorders are repeatables is a very weak claim. It says simply that cases of disorder can be grouped together on the basis of important similarities, and that cases that are grouped together can then be expected to behave in similar ways. One potential worry is that we might be able to pick out many, but inconsistent, potentially useful classifications. In his 1990 paper "Toward a scientific psychiatric nosology" Ken Kendler suggests that this might turn out to be the case with some mental disorders. Kendler takes the case of schizophrenia, and discusses evidence that the criteria that pick out subtypes that best predict treatment response may be different from those that best fit with familial aggregation.

Similar situations occur elsewhere in science, and occur because the world is messy and complex. Within biology, species can be delimited on multiple different criteria. Evolutionary theorists are chiefly interested in groups of organisms based on common descent. Ecologists are more interested in classifying on the basis of current behavior. Thinking about such cases, the philosopher John Dupré urges us to be realists, but "promiscuous realists" (Dupré 1981, 1990, 2001). His thought is that multiple different classification systems can be picked out, with different classification systems being most suitable for different purposes. Thinking in terms of a multidimensional quality space, on Dupré's picture we can discern different groupings if we focus in at different levels of resolution or restrict our attention to particular dimensions of the space. Dupré's suggestion is that we should let a thousand flowers bloom, and that each scientific subdiscipline should be permitted to classify as it finds most useful.

Returning to psychiatry, a promiscuous realist would suggest that if, for example, it is the case that one set of criteria best predicts treatment outcome while another set best predicts how disorders run in families, then researchers interested in different questions should use different criteria. Though Dupré tends to emphasize the advantages of embracing multiplicity, it should be noted that there is also a downside. If different researchers use different sets of criteria for different sorts of research, then seeking to combine their findings to make an overall judgment becomes problematic. Suppose that those working on schizophrenia did start to use multiple different sets of criteria. In effect, those interested in treatment would be talking about slightly different entities when they talked of "subtypes of schizophrenia" than would those looking at patterns of inheritance. As a consequence, "translation" would be required in those cases where data from both sorts of studies was required together. Recognizing multiple sets of repeatables will thus not be cost free and may not always be worthwhile. Still the key point can be upheld—the existence of competing classifications is compatible with a domain consisting of repeatables.

To summarize this section: classification will be useful in so far as mental disorders turn out to be repeatables, in the sense that all cases of a type of disorder are fundamentally similar. We should hope that mental disorders do turn out to be repeatables, as only with repeatability will it be possible to develop therapies that can be hoped to work for all cases of a kind of mental disorder.

4.2 **The dangers of classification**

And yet, a major tradition sees something problematic about classifying human beings. A sign outside the counselor's office at my university depicts tins of food and reads "Labels are for tins. Not people" in the same sort of tone that other posters warn of the evils of racism or domestic violence. One infers that labeling people is not a nice thing to do. The idea that classifying people is at least a little bit evil can also be found in the work of many of those who are opposed to "the medical model" (as found in antipsychiatry, critical psychiatry, postpsychiatry).

Diagnostic labels may cause harm in various ways. For example, in some cases, labels harm individuals by facilitating prejudice against them. Thus racial labels played a role in enabling the system of apartheid practiced in South Africa. Clearly labels can also harm through inaccurately reflecting the structure of reality. For example, when a classification system mistakenly lumps together disorders that are really distinct this may result in patients receiving suboptimal treatments. Though important, there is little of philosophical interest to say about such harms. In this section I focus on a different and philosophically underinvestigated variety of harm. These harms arise because diagnostic labels can enter the narratives by which people make sense of their lives and thereby limit the meaningful futures that a person can imagine. In discussing these harms I will draw on Alastair MacIntyre's (1981) ideas about the importance of narrative for human flourishing, Ian Hacking's (1995) work on the looping effects that affect human kinds, and Carl Elliott's (1999, chapter 7) work on diagnosis and identity.

Narratives are important for human flourishing. In recent years this claim has become a commonplace in both philosophy and medicine (MacIntyre 1981, Elliott 1999). Some go so far as to link the narratives that a person tells about themselves with a person's identity (MacIntyre 1981). I don't want to align myself with such radical views here, but I do think that the narratives that structure people's lives are important. At the very least such narratives help to shape what an individual thinks they might do and how they come to understand how they have acted in the past.

Both illness itself and the act of diagnosis can threaten our ability to narrate our lives. The fact that illness can compromise our narrative abilities, for example, through distracting us with pain, or by destroying our memory, should be underlined. I don't want to give the impression that I think it is only the talk of doctors rather than also the problems of bodies and minds that cause difficulties for narrative agency. Here though I shall focus on the problems that the act of diagnosis can itself produce.

The nub of the problem is this: we structure our lives with the help of narratives, but we are not the sole authors of our life stories. Others, too, play a role in shaping what we can sensibly say about ourselves. Some coauthoring occurs by negotiation, but some situations place us in a position similar to that of someone playing the "continue-the-story" game played by children. In the children's game someone writes the first few sentences of a story, they pass it on to the next player who adds a passage, who passes it on to a third, and so on. The challenge is to continue the story in a way that makes sense given what one's coauthors have said.

The interactions between a patient and a mental health professional as a diagnosis is made can be thought of in a similar vein. When a patient goes to a professional they tell them part of the story, the professional, in making a diagnosis, adds to it, and the patient is left to continue. Sometimes the effect of being diagnosed may be minimal, and arguably diagnosis may enable someone to practice reasonable planning and thus gain control over their life. Suppose I come to think of myself as having depressive tendencies. This may structure my actions in certain ways. Maybe I avoid drugs that have been found to trigger depression in those who are susceptible. Such actions may be reasonable and helpful for me.

However certain diagnoses are more problematic. Certain diagnoses will imply that one's assessment of reality is not reliable (schizophrenia), or that one is essentially manipulative (borderline personality disorder), or that one can never be trusted around children (pedophilia). Once one accepts such a diagnosis as accurate, telling a good story about one's life will become difficult. By telling a "good story" I mean both telling a story with narrative coherence, plot, etc. and also telling a story whereby one appears as a decent human being. Plausibly, people need to be able to tell stories about themselves that are good in both senses if they are to think well of themselves. To illustrate the problems that diagnoses can pose let's consider antisocial personality disorder (ASPD). This is an extreme example, in so far as a diagnosis of ASPD will be one of the toughest to incorporate into a good story about one's life; however, it will clearly illustrate the problems that diagnostic labels can pose.

According to the DSM, ASPD is characterized by a number of undesirable character traits—aggressiveness, irresponsibility, deceptiveness, and so on. In short, someone with ASPD is a bad person. In addition, a powerful tradition has it that that personality disorders are lifelong states that can be highly resistant to treatment. That is someone with ASPD is an irrecoverably bad person. Suppose one receives a diagnosis of ASPD. What does one do then? As I found it hard to imagine how one might respond to receiving such a diagnosis I looked at posts on an online support group for people with ASPD (http://www.psychforums.com/antisocial-personality). There seemed to be three basic ways to respond to diagnosis.

1. *Challenge the diagnosis.* Some refuse to believe the diagnosis. Either they give reasons for distrusting the individual clinician who diagnosed them, or they give reasons for thinking that all psychiatric diagnoses are unreliable. Given the esteem with which medicine is held in our culture, challenging a diagnosis will not always be a viable possibility.

2. *"Embrace the dark-side."* Some embrace the idea that they are evil. They have online names like "Lannibal Hector" and "Rage" and swap stories about torturing small animals and homeless people. Amongst such discussions the more sophisticated present themselves as being moral relativists, or think of themselves as Nietzschean supermen. The problem with this option is that it is morally unacceptable. Someone with ASPD who takes this option becomes worse than they were before.

3. *Uncertainty.* Some people don't know how to respond to their diagnosis. They have found themselves diagnosed and then, in some cases, abandoned by mental health professionals, and don't have any idea what they should do now they have come to think of themselves as people with ASPD.

Admittedly, the example of ASPD is an extreme one, and one might feel little sympathy for people who manifest the types of behaviors that tend to lead to them receiving such a diagnosis. Still the example of ASPD illustrates how the act of diagnosis can itself harm someone. Coming to believe that one is an untreatably bad person is difficult to live with.

Of course physical diagnoses also limit the narratives that patients can sensibly tell about their lives. Most clearly this is the case with diagnoses of terminal illness. However, diagnoses of mental disorder are perhaps particularly hard to incorporate into a good narrative about oneself, both because many mental disorders are chronic conditions, and also because in so far as mental disorders affect personalities, emotions and beliefs they affect a person considered as an agent more directly than do many physical disorders.

4.3 **What to do?**

Classifying mental disorders can be hoped to bring great benefits. If mental disorders are repeatables, then once a correct classification scheme is achieved, diagnosis can be expected to predict how a case will behave. In particular, a treatment that works for some members of a class can be hoped to work for others. However, classifying people can also harm them. Harms may come about in various ways, but here I have focused on the ways in which diagnostic labels enter into the narratives by which people make sense of their lives and can limit the range of imaginable future courses of action. In this final section I begin to consider how classification systems might be developed so as to maximize their potential benefits and limit the associated risks.

When considering the benefits and harms associated with classification, we can start by noting an unfortunate asymmetry. A classification system can only be expected to be useful if it is at least approximately correct, but it can harm people even if it is wrong. It is my *belief* that there is a disorder such as ASPD, and that I have it, which harms me.

How should we act in such a situation? When hypotheses will harm whether they are right or wrong, but only do good if they are roughly correct, it would be wise to proceed with modesty and caution. As we have seen by considering the case of ASPD, a classification system that makes the general claim "There are people of type X," and a diagnostician who makes the particular claim "You are a person of type X" can do harm. Such labels can enter the narratives that people tell about themselves and limit the possible futures that they can imagine. In such situations it is better that the doubts that surround the validity of classes in a classification system, or an individual's diagnosis, are made explicit. Where there are doubts, a classification system that makes it explicit that there are competing classifications, and that the validity of a category is disputed, will do less damage. How modest is the current DSM? Not very. The foreword to the DSM presents it as being a work in progress, but the language used in the main text suggests that the claims made in the DSM are definite truths rather than contested hypotheses. The harms produced by psychiatric classification could be reduced by making classifications such as the DSM more explicitly tentative.

The harms that result from diagnosis can also be minimized by making hopeful illness narratives—where such exist—more accessible. In general, individuals model the stories that they tell about themselves on those that are readily available in their culture. Publicizing examples of people who manage to tell good stories about themselves while living with condition X will thus make it more likely that those who are newly diagnosed with condition X will also come to be able to tell good stories about themselves. For example, in the past, telling a good life story that incorporated a diagnosis of schizophrenia was very difficult. In recent years it has become easier because hopeful narrative templates have become available via the Hearing Voices Network (http://www.hearing-voices.org/) and similar groups.

In so far as it is knowledge of psychiatric labels that causes harm, one might wonder if things would be better if classification systems were developed and diagnoses made in secret. Maybe the harms caused by psychiatric diagnosis occur because lay people and patients currently know too much, and a more secretive psychiatry would do less damage? Such a suggestion should be rejected however. Within the human sciences, rigid distinctions between those who classify and those who are classified have been linked with a sorry history whereby classification has come to be biased against the less powerful (for studies of gender and psychiatry see Lunbeck (1994), on race see Fernando (2002) and Cooper (2007 chapter 8)). The DSM itself has a history whereby categories have come to be included on dubious grounds—in the past, lobbying by special interest groups, and pressures from the insurance and pharmaceutical industries have played a role (Cooper 2005; Kutchins and Kirk 2003). It is plausible that more openness, rather than less, is needed to combat such tendencies (Longino 1990).

A secret psychiatry is undesirable; however, this doesn't mean that patients necessarily have to be told of their diagnosis. Consider the "don't ask, don't tell" policy adopted by many of those who deal with Huntington's disease. Huntington's disease is a horrible, untreatable, genetically-caused disorder that develops during middle-age. Genetic tests mean that those who will develop it can be identified. However, many of those who know they are at risk decline the tests. If they are going to die horribly they would rather not know. I think that it would be rational for those who suspect that they might be diagnosed with certain psychiatric disorders to similarly avoid finding out. Most notably, there is often going to be little value in being diagnosed with a personality disorder—as we have seen with the case of ASPD such diagnoses can leave patients in a position where they are unable to tell a coherent good story about themselves. Knowledge isn't always good thing.

Modesty, publicizing hopeful disorder narratives, and don't ask, don't tell policies will help limit the harms of diagnosis, but some damage will still be done. At the end of the day I suggest that whether one thinks that classifying some subdomain of mentally ill people is on balance a good or bad idea must depend on a weighing up of the costs and benefits. This approach is consistent with that which will be adopted by those drafting revisions to the DSM-5 where in the case of revisions "potential benefits. . .should outweigh potential harms" (Kendler et al. 2009). It should be noted that as diagnoses affect not only patients, but also their relatives and friends, and broader society, the costs and benefits to be considered need not be limited to those affecting the patient.

The idea that only revisions that are likely to do good should be included in the DSM has come in for criticism. In a recent piece in the Bulletin of the AAPP, Dr Ghaemi argues that the gerrymandering of categories will set back research (2010). He thinks that a classification should seek to mirror the natural structure of the domain of mental disorders, and that this will best enable research that will one day lead to pragmatic benefits. My suggestion is not that the DSM should lie about the nature of mental disorders, but rather that there may be conditions about which it should keep silent. The fundamental basis for my suggestion is that I think there may be truths that we are better off not knowing. This point is most easily made when one thinks of military research—there are facts about poisons that we do not need to find out. In so far as research in psychiatry can harm people there may similarly be areas where it is best not to conduct research.

Unfortunately, in practice determining whether a new category will be helpful can be extremely difficult. Consider current debates over the possible addition of psychosis risk syndrome (Moran 2009). Advocates argue that inclusion of the new diagnostic category will facilitate early treatment. Critics argue that the stigma that will be associated with the diagnosis, and the side effects that will result from drug treatment, outweigh any benefits. This case nicely brings out how very hard it is to determine whether a new category will overall do good or be harmful. Some of the consequences of introducing the new category are fairly predictable. Pharmaceutical companies would seek to market drugs for the treatment of such patients. Some employers, particularly those seeking recruits for high-stress jobs, would seek to avoid employing people with psychosis risk syndrome. Other consequences of introducing a new category are hard to predict. What would it be like to be diagnosed with psychosis risk syndrome? Would one spend one's time worrying about becoming psychotic? Or would one be pleased that one's condition was being monitored?

Trying to predict the effects of a new diagnostic category will always be difficult. We can, however, make some generalizations. Where a condition is mild and currently untreatable, patients will have little to gain from it being classified. If that condition affects traits close to an individual's core identity the potential for the classification to do harm may also be great. Prodromal personality disorders thus stand out as candidate disorders where classification could be expected to bring no net benefits for patients.

Although we can get some way thinking about whether classification is a good idea on a case-by-case basis, often the relevant issues will be very difficult, and so we will find ourselves falling back on considerations about the benefits and harms of classification in general. For example, whether one will think that adding some particular new, but currently untreatable, condition is worthwhile will depend in large part on whether one thinks that research is likely to result in a successful treatment being developed. And, one's judgment of the prospects of research will depend on whether one thinks that psychiatric research has generally managed to lead to useful treatments.

Although I am not as optimistic as some, I tend to optimism. I think that mental disorders may well turn out to be repeatables, and that as a consequence the development of successful class-based treatments (that is, treatments that will be effective for all those with a particular type of disorder) can be hoped for. On balance, and despite the harms it causes, I think that much, though not all, psychiatric classification is justifiable. However, I have shown how this is an issue on which reasonable people can disagree. Determining when classification can be hoped to bring more benefits than harms is far from clear-cut.

Acknowledgments

This paper has been presented at the conference 'Brain and Self. Psychiatric Nosology: Definition, History and Validity' at the Center for Subjectivity Research, Copenhagen November 2010, at the Philosophy of Psychiatry Work in Progress Day at Birmingham University in May 2010, and also at a philosophy seminar at Lancaster University. I am very grateful for the comments of those present.

Chapter References

Cooper, R. (2005). *Classifying Madness*. Dordrecht: Springer.

Cooper, R. (2007). *Psychiatry and Philosophy of Science*. Stocksfield: Acumen.

Dupré, J. (1981). Natural kinds and biological taxa. *The Philosophical Review*, **XC**, 66–90.

Dupré, J. (1993). *The Disorder of Things*. Cambridge, MA: Harvard University Press.

Dupré, J. (2001). In defence of classification. *Studies in History and Philosophy of Biological and Biomedical Sciences*, **32**, 203–19.

Elliott, R. (1999). *A Philosophical Disease: Bioethics, Culture and Identity*. New York: Routledge.

Fernando, S. (2002). *Mental Health, Race and Culture* (2nd ed.). Basingstoke: Palgrave.

Ghaemi. N. (2010). DSM-IV, Hippocrates, and pragmatism: What might have been. *AAPP Bulletin*, **17**, 32–5.

Hacking, I. (1995). The looping effect of human kinds. In D. Sperber, D. Premack and A. James Premack (eds.) (1995) *Causal Cognition: A Multidisciplinary Debate*. Oxford: Clarendon Press. pp. 351–83.

Haslam, N. (2003). Kinds of kinds: A conceptual taxonomy of psychiatric categories. *Philosophy, Psychiatry and Psychology*, **10**, 203–17.

Horwitz, A. and Wakefield, J. (2007). *The Loss of Sadness: How Psychiatry Transformed Normal Sorrow into Depressive Disorder*. Oxford: Oxford University Press.

Kendler, K. (1990). Toward a scientific psychiatric nosology. Strengths and limitations. *Archives of General Psychiatry*, **47**, 969–73.

Kendler, K., Kupfer, D., Narrow W., Phillips, K., and Fawcett, J. (revised 21.10.09). Guidelines for making changes to DSM-V. Available online at http://www.dsm5.org/ProgressReports/Documents/Guidelines-for-Making-Changes-to-DSM_1.pdf

Kutchins, H. and Kirk, S. (2003). *Making Us Crazy*. New York: Free Press

Longino, H. (1990). *Science as Social Knowledge: Values and Objectivity in Scientific Inquiry*. Princeton, NJ: Princeton University Press.

Lunbeck, E. (1994). *The Psychiatric Persuasion*. Princeton, NJ: Princeton University Press.

MacIntyre, A. (1981). *After Virtue*. London: Duckworth.

Moran, M. (2009). DSM-V developer weigh adding psychosis risk. *Psychiatric News,* **44**(16), 5.

Szasz, T. (1974). *The Myth of Mental Illness: Foundations of a Theory of Personal Conduct* (Revised ed.). New York: Harper & Row.

Zachar, P. (2001). Psychiatric disorders are not natural kinds. *Philosophy, Psychiatry and Psychology,* **7**, 167–81.

Diagnoses as labels

S. Nassir Ghaemi

Dr Cooper raises the question of whether psychiatric classification is a good thing. It is an ethical question: is nosology good? The author concludes it is a utilitarian judgment call. She allows for a previous epistemological discussion about how we can know that mental illnesses exist, and with the concept of repeatables, allows for such a possibility. But she avoids the metaphysical question: do mental illnesses in fact exist? This is the source, I believe, of the debate. People who think it all comes down to a utilitarian judgment call often do so because, deep down, they doubt the reality of mental diseases.

The best counterexample to such doubts about whether classification is "good" is the history of medicine: those who believe classification is "bad" will need to explain why Benjamin Rush, who agreed with them, was correct. Rush held that there is only one illness (variations on the four humors) and one treatment (variations on bloodletting). So are we to go back to this? What other alternatives do critics suggest? And how are those alternatives "better" than our current, albeit flawed, commitment to science (with all its complexities)? Post-modernists will proclaim their ideologies about the history of medicine, but this is like Marxists criticizing discussions of economics. It does not convince anyone who thinks for himself.

Some raise the issue of "labeling" as a harm of nosology. But, labels do not have to be dehumanizing; the author seems to presume this is the case. Sometimes labels are quite humanizing. When psychoanalysts refused to label patients with manic-depression, who actually had that disease, and gave them daily psychoanalysis for years on end, without any effect except prolongation of patients' torture and decimation of their bank accounts, psychoanalysts were dehumanizing their patients. When those patients received the correct "label" of their disease, and then were markedly improved with lithium, they were handled humanistically. One can be biologically reductionistic and humanistic at the same time. Many assume the opposite, without acknowledging any of these real examples from medical history.

Often critics presume the dehumanizing use of labels in the phrase "You are" as opposed to the phrase, "You have." My teacher Leston Havens, a great humanist psychotherapist, taught the difference. Our patients may or may not have diseases, but it is certainly false to say they are their diseases.

Discussions of ethics often are confined to utilitarian views. The main problem with the utilitarian approach, of course, is knowing the outcomes. Sometimes this is clear; I am not opposing utilitarian grounds always. But, people sometimes do not acknowledge sufficiently that frequently, if not usually, the outcomes are not clear, and false utilitarian judgments are made.

Our colleagues often mentioned, in the conference, the "unforeseen" or "unexpected" consequences of DSM-IV. That is exactly the problem: why are we engaging in these "pragmatic" and utilitarian judgments when we really cannot foresee the future?

One could take duty-based or virtue-based approaches that would lead to different judgments. For instance, I may see it as my duty to know and find and tell the truth. Or one may see it as the virtue of being a doctor or the virtue of science to know and find and tell the truth. I would hold that these approaches produce the best results, in the long run, even on "pragmatic" or utilitarian grounds.

Part II

The historical development of modern psychiatric diagnoses

Chapter 5

Introduction

Josef Parnas

This chapter takes its reader on a journey through the past and current complexities of psychiatric classification in the domain of major psychoses. The chapter is not easy to introduce briefly because it's a very dense, content-rich review of the topic. It is written by one of the founding figures behind the World Health Organization's (WHO's) International Pilot Studies on Schizophrenia. Nearly every relevant aspect of psychiatric classification is touched upon here. We move through the concepts such as "disease" and "disorder," the issue of category versus dimension, the shakiness of commonly accepted criteria of validity of psychiatric entities, the permutations of the classification of psychoses since the original institution of Kraepelinian dichotomy to the future versions of DSM and ICD, and we end with general reflections on the likely future of psychiatry. The important message of the chapter, elegantly summarized through a quotation from Jaspers, is that classifications are provisional and pragmatic tools, which carry with them a danger of unwarranted reifications.

There are two issues brought up by Jablensky that I wish to draw the reader's attention to. One is related to the very origins of the dichotomy between schizophrenia and affective illness. Jablensky points to the description of the course of illness as playing a pivotal role in this dichotomy, specifically through the notion of incurability (for schizophrenia). Here, as Jablensky points out, we are confronted with all kinds of transitional states between curability and incurability, a muddled picture, additionally complicated by (a non-random) therapeutic option and therapeutic response. An important result from the International Pilot Study of Schizophrenia follow-up studies, quoted by Jablensky, demonstrates that a substantial percentage of the patients diagnosed with schizophrenia recover with time, and the likelihood of that recovery is, to a no-trivial degree, independent of the initial definition of the schizophrenia diagnosis (broad versus narrow).

The second issue that merits special attention is the relation between the concepts of *validity* versus *utility* (see also Schaffner, Chapter 9, this volume). Jablensky laments unclarity of the concept of validity, which he believes is imported to psychiatry from psychometrics. He refrains from defining it himself but refers instead to Robins and Guze's familiar list of criteria of validity: familial aggregation, syndromic distinctiveness, outcome, para-clinical measures (biological correlates), etc. Jablensky believes that validity is a dichotomous or binary feature: a diagnosis is either valid or invalid, like, says Jablensky, you are either pregnant or not pregnant. I believe that this binary view of validity mainly applies to the validity concept in logic: a syllogism (an argument) is either valid or not, depending on whether it follows (or not) from a premise

Here, "valid" is not identical with "true." An argument can be logically valid but false if the premise is false. It seems to me that in the medical model, validity is similar to a relation of reference between a concept and its referent, an object in nature, e.g., between the word "cat" and this particular cat or cat as a species. It is a function of reference to pick up its object correctly. Since our knowledge is always finite and perspectival (e.g., dictated by our pragmatic concerns), we do not access an absolute reality with its objects as it is "in itself" (in Kantian terms, a "noumenal" reality). Moreover, our expectations to find reality neatly divided into natural kinds have diminished considerably over the recent decades. Therefore, I think, we can only expect validity to behave in a graded way. It comes to resemble what Jablensky calls as "utility."

Chapter 5

The nosological entity in psychiatry: a historical illusion or a moving target?

Assen Jablensky

By *nosology* we do not only mean the set of classification categories, but also—and above all—we have in mind the underlying theory about the nature of the conditions that are being classified and the principles and rules of the classifying process. Are we dealing with discrete, discontinuous entities, or with graded continuous phenomena to which we can apply a sliding rule of thresholds in order to separate "pathology" from "normal variation" and determine the need for treatment? What is the relationship between the clinical manifestations of a presumed "disorder" and the pathological processes or genetic aberrations, partial aspects and fragments of which are being progressively uncovered by research?

Questions like these have been asked and answered—variously—since the earliest stages of clinical research in psychiatry in the second half of the 19th century. Yet, notwithstanding the impressive recent achievements in the neuroscience and genetics of psychiatric disorders, many of the present day's answers to these basic questions are, in fact, variations on themes that have been played and replayed in the earlier periods of scientific psychiatry. This suggests that there may be inherent shortcomings in the mainstream nosological paradigm adopted in clinical psychiatry since the beginning of the 20th century that need to be critically examined and, possibly, transcended with the help of concepts and methodological tools that are available today. In my discussion of these issues I will focus primarily on the taxonomy of the major psychoses since their history epitomizes many of the controversies, conjectures and refutations that continue to cast a long shadow on the present juncture of classification revision involving both DSM and ICD.

5.1 Classification in science

The term classification denotes "the activity of ordering or arrangement of objects into groups or sets on the basis of their relationships" (Sokal 1974); in other words, it is the process of *synthesizing* categories out of the raw material of sensory data. Classification in science, including medicine, can be defined as the "procedure for constructing groups or categories and for assigning entities (disorders or persons) to these categories on the basis of their shared attributes or relations" (Millon 1991). The act of assigning a particular object to one of the categories is *identification* (in medical practice this is diagnostic identification). Diagnosis and classification are interrelated: choosing a diagnostic label usually presupposes some ordered system of possible labels, and a classification is the arrangement of such labels in accordance with certain specified principles and rules. The term *taxonomy*, often used as a synonym for classification, should refer properly to the meta-theory of classification; in medicine the corresponding term *nosology* denotes the concepts and theories that support the classification of symptoms, signs, syndromes and diseases, whereas the term *nosography* refers to the act of describing and naming such entities. The names jointly constitute the *nomenclature* within a particular field of medicine.

The classical taxonomic strategy, exemplified by grand systems of classification in the natural sciences, such as the Lynnaean systematic of plants or the Darwinian evolutionary classification of species, assumes that *substances* (i.e., robust entities that remain the same in spite of change in their attributes) exist "out there" in nature. When properly identified by sifting out all accidental characteristics, some substances reveal themselves as the *phyla* or *species* of living organisms and thus provide a "natural" classification. In medicine, an essentialist view of diseases as independently existing agents causing illnesses in individuals was proposed by Sydenham in the 18th century (Scadding 1996); its vestiges survive into the present in some interpretations of the notion of "disease entity."

5.2 **What is the unit of classification in psychiatry?**

Medical classifications are created with the primary purpose of meeting pragmatic needs related to diagnosing and treating people experiencing illnesses. Their secondary purpose is to assist in the generation of new knowledge relevant to those needs, though progress in medical research usually precedes, rather than follows, improvements in classification. Simply stating that medical classifications classify *diseases* (or that psychiatric classifications classify *disorders*) begs the question since the status of concepts like "disease" and "disorder" remains obscure. As pointed out by Scadding (1996), the concept of "disease" has evolved with the advance of medical knowledge, and at present, is no more than "a convenient device by which we can refer succinctly to the conclusion of a diagnostic process which starts from recognition of a pattern of symptoms and signs, and proceeds, by investigation of varied extent and complexity, to an attempt to unravel the chain of causation." The diagnostic process in psychiatry has been summarized succinctly by Shepherd et al. (1968): "the psychiatrist interviews the patient, and chooses from a system of psychiatric terms a few words or phrases which he uses as a label for the patient, as to convey to himself and others as much as possible about the aetiology, the immediate manifestations, and the prognosis of the patient's condition."

"Disease," therefore, is an explanatory construct integrating information about: (1) statistical deviance from the population "norm"; (2) characteristic clinical manifestations; (3) characteristic pathology; (4) underlying causes; and (5) the extent of reduced biological fitness. For a constellation of observations to be referred to as "a disease," these parameters must be shown to form a "real-world correlational structure" (Rosch 1975) which is stable and also distinct from other similar structures. Two issues are of

relevance here. First, the typical progression of knowledge starts with the identification of the clinical manifestations (the *syndrome*) and the deviance from the "norm";
understanding of the pathology and etiology usually come much later. Secondly, there
is no fixed point or agreed threshold beyond which a syndrome can be said to be "a
disease." Today, Alzheimer's disease (AD), with dementia as its clinical manifestation,
specific brain morphology, tentative pathophysiology and at least partially understood
causes, is one of the few conditions in psychiatric classifications that are already
defined by their pathology rather than their syndrome. There is a clear tendency for
the pathologically defined disorder, such as AD, to be subdivided into a series of
genetically defined variants, as in other branches of medicine. Schizophrenia, however, is still better described as a syndrome (Kendell and Jablensky 2003).

5.3 **The hypothesis of the nosological entity**

The basic unit of discourse underlying the present classifications of the psychoses is
the notion of the *nosological entity*, remaining more or less in the form in which it was
first formulated by Kahlbaum (1863). This notion postulates a close correspondence
between etiology, brain pathology, symptom patterns and outcome as a criterion for
assuming that seemingly disparate clinical states and syndromes belong together as
manifestations of a single "disease." As it is well known, this hypothesis later enabled
Kraepelin (1899) to group together several clinical syndromes into the nosological
entities of manic-depressive insanity and *dementia praecox* respectively, and to lay
down the foundation for the dichotomy of the major psychoses which, *grosso modo*,
has been adopted by the majority of psychiatrists in the world until the present.

However, two aspects of the original nosological hypothesis need to be emphasized:
first, that among the several criteria defining the nosological entity, the criterion of
outcome reigned supreme; and, secondly, that outcome was defined, by and large, in
terms of "curability" and "Incurability." To quote Kraepelin (1899), "the course of
dementia praecox is generally a steadily progressive one. . .The common outcome of
all severe forms of dementia praecox is dementia. . .The prognosis of manic-depressive
insanity is favourable for the individual attack. . .even after very long duration of
excitement or depression, one may still hope with great probability for complete res-
toration." Looking back to Kraepelin's early writings, it becomes clear that the criterion of outcome as the cornerstone of his system was largely a matter of convenience—he
realized that knowledge of etiology and brain pathology at the time could offer little
guidance, while outcome was a variable easily accessible to the clinician and could be
described with considerable refinement.

Kraepelin was aware of the provisional nature of his system, and critics, such as
Berze (1912) and Hoche (1912), who violently opposed his "nosological dogmatism,"
actually induced him to re-think radically some of his basic premises. Kraepelin's last
papers contain entirely new points of view on the problem, to which I shall refer later.
Notwithstanding Kraepelin's late revisionism (1920), the nosological system based
on the "disease entity" concept established itself firmly in the mainstream of clinical
psychiatry, where it remains to the present day. Notably, Bleuler's (1911) revision of
the concept of dementia praecox and re-naming it as *schizophrenia* (the term was
also adopted by Kraepelin) did not change substantially the underlying nosological

principle, although it extended somewhat the diagnostic boundaries of the entity by suggesting that "the group of schizophrenias" could include non-psychotic, or pre-psychotic variants, such as "latent schizophrenia."

5.4 **Shortcomings and contradictions of the "classical" nosological model**

In the last century, clinical psychiatry has been witness to a number of major attempts at developing alternative approaches to the systematics of psychotic disorders, but none of them has been as successful as the classical (Kraepelinian) nosological theory, broadly defined. The building blocks of the latter can be grouped into two categories: (1) phenomena accessible to clinical observation—symptoms, syndromes, patterns of course, and a range of outcomes; (2) non-clinical correlates, which in turn can be subdivided into such describing primarily individuals (e.g., biological variables or behavioral characteristics), and such describing populations (e.g., epidemiological or culture-related). The essential task in the construction of a nosology of discrete disease entities is to identify internally cohesive clinical groupings based on established high-level inter-correlations between symptoms and syndromes (the cross-section) and patterns of course and outcome (the longitudinal aspect). The ultimate test of the nosological validity of such groupings is the degree to which they correlate with variables of potential etiological significance, pathogenetic mechanisms, treatment response, and the degree of stability they possess vis-à-vis demographic and cultural variation.

The nosological entities, defined in this way, and the "entity" of schizophrenia in particular, soon met with multiple contradictions and difficulties. The requirement that there should be a close correspondence between the features of the cross-section, i.e., the symptoms and syndromes of the disorder, and the characteristics of its course and outcome, was never fully met. The criterion of "curability" versus "incurability" proved to be too crude, and attempts to identify in the initial stages of a schizophrenic illness syndromes that would reliably predict its ultimate outcome, have on the whole failed. It was, furthermore, demonstrated that, on one hand, a proportion of the "typical" schizophrenias recover completely, and, on the other hand, a proportion of "typical" manic-depressive illnesses run a chronic and disabling course. These observations were incompatible with the assumptions of the "dichotomy" model, not because of the rare exceptional cases but due to the sheer magnitude of the proportions of cases whose longitudinal patterns of course ran contrary to the original hypothesis. The inadequacy of the "curability" criterion became even more obvious after the introduction of psychopharmacological treatment which had the effect of creating a huge "gray zone" of outcomes that could not be clearly classified as either "recovery" or post-psychotic "defect." This led to a situation, pithily described by Leonhard and von Trostorff (1964, p. 7):

> If two psychiatrists have different diagnostic opinions about an endogenous psychosis, the decision can be reached only through a catamnesis, or not at all. If one of them diagnoses a manic-depressive illness, then only the demonstration of a defect can prove him wrong; according to the prevailing opinion, this outcome is not found in such cases. The other,

who diagnoses schizophrenia, cannot be refuted at all. He may stick to his diagnosis, even if the catamnesis shows no evidence of defect.

Those who argue that recovering schizophrenias are not "true" specimens of the disorder, and ought to be retrospectively re-diagnosed if full and lasting recovery occurs, might be interested in the data from the two major WHO studies: the International Pilot Study of Schizophrenia, IPSS (1979) and the subsequent Ten-country Study on Determinants of Outcome of Severe Mental Disorders (Jablensky et al. 1992). In the IPSS, cases were diagnosed in the strictest possible way, by applying three sets of criteria: (1) clinician's diagnosis according to ICD-8; (2) computer diagnosis using the CATEGO algorithm (Wing et al. 1974); and (3) empirical grouping of cases by cluster analysis, according to maximum shared characteristics. Patients who met simultaneously the three sets of criteria were designated as the "concordant" group of schizophrenia. This group was expected to be more homogeneous than the rest of the cases, including course and outcome. However, the data did not reveal any significant differences in course and outcome between the group of "concordant" cases and the group of "non-concordant" cases. This finding casts considerable doubt on the prognostic value of a "restrictive" diagnosis of schizophrenia. Moreover, the less explicitly structured clinicians' diagnoses of the schizophrenia subtypes indicated some consistent prognostic trends.

These findings do not stand alone in the recent literature. A number of well-designed follow-up studies in the last 20 years confirm the notion that severe deterioration is not the "typical" outcome of schizophrenia, even if a very long (10–65 years) follow-up period is considered. Moreover, some of these studies have shown that many of the symptoms and syndromes that are often regarded, in the early phase of a schizophrenic illness, as indicators of a poor prognosis, or as irreversible impairments, actually undergo a reversal in a significant proportion of cases. This was strikingly demonstrated by the long-term follow-up of the patients of the WHO International Pilot Study of Schizophrenia (prevalence cohort, follow-up at 26 years after the episode of inclusion) and the WHO Ten-Country Study of Schizophrenia (incidence cohort, follow-up at 15 years after the first psychotic episode). To quote from the WHO report (2007):

> The most striking overall finding. . . is that the current global status of over half of these subjects—56% of the incidence group and 60% of the prevalence group—is rated as 'recovered'. Nearly half have experienced no psychotic episodes in the last 2 years of follow-up. . .These percentages accord fairly well with ratings of both current symptoms and functioning.

The "classical" nosological hypothesis could be salvaged if it could be demonstrated that within the broad range of possible outcomes, particular patterns could be predicted by specific constellations of symptoms and signs. Of course, this would amount to a fragmentation of the "disease" schizophrenia into a number of nosological minientities. Such efforts have been undertaken, e.g., by Leonhard (1999) among others, but with uncertain success. In the WHO studies, a major attempt was undertaken to identify predictors of different patterns of outcome by using multivariate statistical techniques, such as stepwise multiple regression analysis (WHO 1979; Jablensky et al.

1992). Two conclusions were drawn from these analyses. First, the low percentage of the variance explained by predictors (56 variables) suggests that either the set of potential predictors was incomplete, and potentially important variables were left out, or unidentified factors intervened after the initial assessment and had an impact on the outcome that was at least equal to that of the tentative potential predictors. Secondly, among the variables of prognostic significance, only a few were mental state variables—most of the predictors were indicators of long-standing personality characteristics and of the social situation of the patient. Both conclusions point to a view of the prognosis of schizophrenia is an open-ended process whose direction can, within limits, be modified at any point, rather than as a preformed development determined by the initial manifestations of the illness. I should point out that presumed "characteristic" or quasi-pathognomonic psychopathological phenomena, such as the Schneiderian first-rank symptoms (Schneider 1959), which were associated with initial diagnostic decisions favoring schizophrenia, did not appear to have prognostic significance (Jablensky et al. 1992). If anything, the Schneiderian symptoms tended to reappear in subsequent episodes of psychosis but they were definitely not associated with a poor prognosis.

Another shortcoming of the "classical" nosological system is its failure to separate consistently the two major entities of schizophrenia and affective disorders. This has been known for a long time but the difficulty was thought to reside in the imprecise definition of the diagnostic criteria, rather than in the existence of a large group of conditions which simply defied the dichotomy and exhibited the features of a clinical "hybrid" in every possible respect. This group has attracted a variety of diagnostic labels, including "schizoaffective disorder" (Kasanin 1933), or "unsystematic schizophrenias" (Leonhard 1999), and has been classified alternately with the schizophrenias and with the affective disorders, but never found a comfortable place in either category. A number of investigators then espoused the idea of a "third major psychosis" (Leonhard 1999), re-adopting the categorical principle of classification but abandoning the original dichotomy. The existence of a sizeable group of psychoses which are intermediate between the schizophrenic and affective psychoses—at least in terms of course and outcome—poses the problem of defining the borderline between the two nosological entities. This remains today as an open question of how much one could stretch the boundaries of one or the other condition in order to accommodate the "intermediate" or "atypical" cases without damaging beyond repair the internal cohesiveness of the diagnostic groups. Alternative solutions to the boundary shifting are: (1) the designation of a third group of psychoses, and (2) treating the "poor prognosis" schizophrenia and the "good prognosis" affective disorders as the two extremes on a clinical (and presumably genetic) continuum which could accommodate all of the intermediate forms.

A third problem for which the "classical" nosological theory has failed to find a generally acceptable solution is the classification of the sub-threshold, practically non-pathological forms of cognitive and affective deviations and the unusual personalities which are encountered among biological relatives of schizophrenia patients. Their importance and frequency were recognized by Bleuler (1920) who coined the term "latent schizophrenia." There is a bewildering variety of diagnostic labels proposed for these conditions: "abortive schizophrenia"—Bleuler (1920); "ambulatory schizophrenia"—Zilboorg (1941); "pseudoneurotic schizophrenia"—Hoch and Polatin (1949); "borderline schizophrenia"—Kety (1988), but none among them has been universally accepted, nor the diagnostic criteria have been unequivocally defined. Subsequent evidence has provided a good deal of support for a genetic link to schizophrenia, which has strengthened the concept of a schizophrenic "spectrum" (Kendler et al. 1994). However, both the place of these conditions in the psychiatric classification and their definition are still a matter of contention. The DSM-III solution, which removed the non-psychotic syndromes from the category of schizophrenia and assigned them, as "schizotypal personality disorder," to the personality disorders, runs counter to the principle that conditions of a presumably common origin should be classified together. The scarcity of diagnostic and follow-up studies in this field is indeed a hindrance, although the few focused studies on this condition suggest that they rarely develop into an overt psychosis.

The "borderline" or "spectrum" forms related to the affective psychoses have so far received less attention than the non-psychotic satellites of schizophrenia, but the recognition of a syndrome of "masked depression" (Kielholz 1979), and the well established notion of an affective or cyclothymic personality disorder suggest that similar problems also exist on the affective side of the "classical" diagnostic dichotomy of the major disorders. At present, the "borderline" forms are of limited therapeutic interest, since most cases do not require pharmacological treatment, and there is little evidence that, if provided, treatment is effective. Their theoretical and research importance, however, is considerable, especially from the point of view of the genetics of the major psychoses. If, along with the manifest major psychoses, the existence of clinically subliminal disorders produced by a shared genotype could be demonstrated, the search for endophenotypic traits and mechanisms would be facilitated. In this sense, the study of the "borderline" disorders may hold the key to a better understanding of the pathogenetic aspects of the major psychiatric syndromes.

To recapitulate the main issues and contradictions within the argument about the difficulties encountered by the "classical" nosological model of psychiatric illness, the following points may be relevant:

1. The criterion of "curability" (recovery) versus "incurability" (irreversible decline) which in the past served as a prognostic and nosological watershed between the affective and schizophrenic disorders is totally inadequate from a contemporary practical and theoretical point of view. A large proportion of the schizophrenic illnesses, diagnosed by present criteria, do not develop the chronic deteriorating course predicted by the "classical" nosological model; on the other hand, chronicity and significant impairment are present in a non-negligible proportion of the affective disorders.

2. The correlation between the initial cross-section of the illness, in terms of symptoms and syndromes, and the longitudinal aspects of the disorder, in terms of frequency and duration of psychotic episodes, remissions and levels of social functioning, is not sufficiently strong to support the notion of a "prognostic diagnosis" and of a classification based on the assumption that the early symptoms of the disorder can reliably predict its course and outcome.

3. The categorical dichotomy of schizophrenic and affective disorders is difficult to maintain in view of the undisputed existence of symptomatological transitions between the two, and the growing evidence that transitions are also present in the course and outcomes of the disorders.

4. In addition to the problem of the "borderline" between the two major groups of disorders, a further complication is presented by their "borderline" to non-psychotic "spectrum" conditions essentially manifesting as personality traits, genetically linked to schizophrenia or bipolar affective disorder.

5.5 **Post-Kraepelinian remedial approaches**

The difficulties referred to in previous sections have been suspected and occasionally brought to light in clinical psychiatry over the last several decades, leading to attempts at appropriate adjustments to the classification of the psychiatric disorders while still retaining the basic notion of the nosological entity as the mainstay of the whole system. Such revisions have taken three different approaches.

The first approach has involved the shifting of the boundary of the dichotomy in such a way as to absorb the majority of "atypical" cases within a modified version of the one or the other group of disorders. This approach has produced a variety of "narrow" and "broad" re-definitions of the scope of schizophrenic and affective disorders. Examples are Langfeldt's (1937) notion of "nuclear" schizophrenia and "schizophreniform" disorders; and the antithetic suggestion that most "atypical" schizophrenic illnesses are, in fact, phenotypic variants of the affective psychoses (Pope and Lipinski 1978). More recently, the Feighner criteria (1972), and subsequently DSM-III, formulated a restrictive definition of the category of schizophrenia, retaining implicitly the old idea that "true" schizophrenia is a condition whose hallmark is a tendency to a deteriorating course, and shifting a large proportion of cases into an ever expanding intermediate category of schizoaffective disorders. This strategy would be justified if it were possible to demonstrate that re-defining the categories on symptomatological grounds would yield more homogeneous patient populations in terms of course and outcome. Several studies, including the WHO IPSS (1979), have compared the prognostic implications of alternative diagnostic definitions of schizophrenia based on varying scope of the category. The results have, by and large, demonstrated only marginal advantages for some of the examined sets of diagnostic criteria which were insufficient for the practical purposes of prognostic diagnosis.

The second approach has consisted in attempts at a wholesale rejection of the dichotomy and, instead, in fragmenting the large group of psychoses into multiple "micro-nosological" entities for which symptomatological, prognostic, genetic and treatment response validating criteria were to be sought. This strategy is best represented by the Wernicke–Kleist–Leonhard tradition (Leonhard 1999) which defined a large "third" group of "cycloid" psychotic disorders. Within the affective disorders, this approach introduced the split between "bipolar" and "unipolar" disorders (Leonhard 1999) which later became generally adopted. A similar development in Scandinavian psychiatry has been the evolution of the concept of "psychogenic" or "reactive" psychoses (Strömgren 1987). The common feature of these undertakings is that they retain both the categorical approach to the subdivision of the field and the "classical" criteria of the nosological entity, while rejecting or ignoring the original dichotomy. However, the degree to which this approach captures real biological discontinuities among the multiple entities remains uncertain.

The third approach, represented in French psychiatry by Ey et al. (1923), was a more radical departure from the Kraepelinian nosology, as it has never been bound by the notion of "curability" versus "incurability," nor has it ever fully accepted the dichotomy of psychotic disorders. Instead, the classification of psychoses involves two major axes: (1) the depth and locus of psychotic disorganization ("disorders of consciousness" and "disorders of personality"); and (2) the distinction between acute and chronic courses of the conditions.

5.6 **Was the nosological entity, after all, an illusion?**

None of the approaches described in previous sections to re-shaping the nosology of the major psychiatric disorders has been entirely successful. Yet there can be no doubt that the "classical" nosological hypothesis proved to be a major step forward by introducing order and parsimony in a field that had previously been chaotic or arbitrarily subdivided. As Jaspers (1963) pointed out, "the idea of the disease entity is in truth an idea in Kant's sense of the word: the concept of an objective which one cannot reach since it is unending; but all the same it indicates the path for fruitful research and supplies a *valid* point of orientation for particular empirical investigations." The least that could be said is that the nosological hypothesis helped to formulate clearly and to bring into focus issues which subsequent critics could oppose or endorse, in an antinomial fashion, thus contributing to a diversity of viewpoints that was healthy and necessary for a developing discipline such as psychiatry.

A more fundamental re-thinking and re-shaping of the nosological theory underlying the classification of psychotic disorders would require, on one hand, overcoming and resolving the kind of contradictions outlined earlier and, on the other hand, developing concepts that would allow a better interdigitation of clinical, neurobiological, genetic and behavioral data. Some basic premises of such an approach to the nosology of the major psychiatric disorders were outlined by no other than Kraepelin in one of his last articles, entitled "Die Erscheinungsformen des Irreseins" (1920). Addressing the future of psychiatric research, Kraepelin's position can be summarized in the following four points:

1. It is necessary "to turn away from arranging illnesses in orderly well-defined groups, and to set ourselves the undoubtedly higher and more satisfying goal of understanding their essential structure."

2. "The affective and schizophrenic forms of mental illness do not represent the expression of particular pathological processes, but rather indicate the areas of our personality in which these processes unfold. . .We must, then, accustom ourselves to the idea that the phenomena of illness which we have hitherto used are not sufficient to enable us to distinguish reliably between manic-depressive illness and schizophrenia in all cases. It must remain an open question whether this is due to general human psychological mechanisms operating in combination with

pathological changes, or whether hereditary factors make certain areas more susceptible and accessible to pathological stimuli."

3. "The various syndromes of illness may be compared with the different registers of an organ, any of which may be brought into play according to the severity or extent of the pathological changes involved. They impart a characteristic tone to the illness quite irrespective of the mechanism which has brought them into play." Schizophrenic and affective symptoms were to be regarded, according to this view, as two among the possible "registers" of psychopathology.

5.7 **The present state of the nosological issues in psychiatry: DSM-IV and ICD-10**

Classifying involves forming categories or *taxa* for ordering natural objects or entities and assigning names to these. Ideally, the categories of a classification should be jointly exhaustive to account for all possible entities, and mutually exclusive. In biology, despite continuing arguments between proponents of evolutionary systematics, numerical taxonomy and cladistics, there is agreement that classifications reflect fundamental properties of biological systems and constitute "natural" classifications. This is not so with psychiatric classifications. First, the objects being classified in psychiatry are not "natural" entities but explanatory constructs. Secondly, the taxonomic units of "disorders" in DSM-IV and ICD-10 do not form hierarchies and the current classifications contain no supraordinate, higher-level organizing concepts. Therefore, DSM-IV and ICD-10 are certainly not systematic classifications in the usual sense in which that term is applied in biology. A closer analogue to current psychiatric classifications can be found in the so-called indigenous or "folk" classifications of living things (e.g., animals or plants) or other material objects. "Folk" classifications (Blashfield 1986) do not consist of mutually exclusive categories and have no single rule of hierarchy (but contain many rules that can be applied ad hoc). Such naturalistic systems retain their usefulness because they are pragmatic and well adapted to the needs of everyday life. Essentially, they are augmented nomenclatures, i.e., lists of names for conditions and behaviors, supplied with explicit rules about how these names should be assigned and used. As such, they are useful tools of communication and should play an important role in psychiatric research, clinical management and teaching.

5.8 **The "reification" problem**

Today, many clinicians are aware that diagnostic categories are simply concepts, justified only by whether or not they provide a useful framework for organizing the complexity of clinical experience in order to make predictions about outcome and to guide treatment decisions. However, once a diagnostic concept like schizophrenia has come into general use, it tends to become "reified" (Hyman 2010) as an entity of some kind which can be invoked to explain the patient's symptoms and whose validity need not be questioned. Even though the authors of DSM-IV may be careful to point out that "there is no assumption that each category of mental disorder is a complete discrete entity," the mere fact that a diagnostic concept is listed in an official classification and provided with a precise operational definition tends to encourage this insidious reification (Kendell and Jablensky 2003).

5.9 **The ambiguous status of the classificatory unit of "disorder"**

The term "disorder," first introduced as a generic name for the unit of classification in DSM-I (1952), has no clear correspondence with either the concept of disease or the concept of syndrome in medical classifications. It conveniently circumvents the problem that the material from which most of the diagnostic rubrics in psychiatry are constructed consists primarily of reported subjective experiences and patterns of behavior. Some of those rubrics correspond to syndromes in the medical sense, but many appear to be sub-syndromal and reflect isolated symptoms, habitual behaviors, or personality traits. The ambiguous status of the "disorder" creates conceptual confusion and hinders the advancement of knowledge. Apart from the "reification fallacy," the fragmentation of psychopathology into a large number of "disorders," of which many are merely symptoms, leads to a proliferation of comorbid diagnoses which clinicians are forced to use in order to describe their patients. This blurs the important distinction between true comorbidity (co-occurrence of etiologically independent disorders) and spurious comorbidity masking complex but essentially unitary *syndromes*. It is, therefore, not surprising that disorders, as defined in the current versions of DSM and ICD, have a strong tendency to co-occur, which suggests that "fundamental assumptions of the dominant diagnostic schemata may be incorrect" (Sullivan and Kendler 1998).

5.10 **Reinstating the concept of syndrome**

Although the range and number of possible etiological factors—genetic, toxic, metabolic or experiential—that may give rise to psychiatric disorders is practically unlimited, the range of psychopathological syndromes, reflecting the brain's responses to a variety of *noxae*, is limited. Since a variety of etiological factors may produce the same syndrome (and conversely, an etiological factor may give rise to a spectrum of different syndromes), the relationship between etiology and clinical syndrome is an indirect one. In contrast, the relationship between the syndrome and the underlying pathophysiology, or specific brain dysfunction, is likely to be much closer. This was recognized long ago in the case of psychiatric illness associated with somatic and brain disorders where clinical variation is restricted to a limited number of "organic" brain syndromes, or "exogenous reaction types" (Bonhoeffer 1912). In the complex psychiatric disorders, where etiology is multifactorial, future research into specific pathophysiological mechanisms could be considerably facilitated by a sharper delineation of the syndromal status of many current diagnostic categories. This provides a strong rationale for reinstating the syndrome as the basic unit of future versions of psychiatric classifications. Indeed, this was proposed by Essen-Möller (1961), the original advocate of multiaxial classification:

> At the present state of knowledge, there appears to be a much closer connection between aetiology and syndrome in somatic medicine than in psychiatry. . .while in somatic

medicine it is an advantage that aetiologic diagnoses take the place of syndromes, in psychiatric classification aetiology can never be allowed to replace syndrome. . .a system of double diagnosis, one of aetiology and one of syndrome, has to be used.

5.11 **Validity and "validators"**

While the reliability of psychiatrists' diagnoses may be substantially improved, due to the acceptance and use of explicit diagnostic criteria, their *validity* remains contentious. What is meant by validity of a diagnostic concept in psychiatry is rarely discussed and few studies have addressed this question explicitly and directly. There is no simple measure of validity of a diagnostic concept that is comparable to the well-established procedures for the assessment of reliability. The types of validity often mentioned in the context of psychiatric diagnosis—construct, content, concurrent and predictive—are all borrowed off the shelf of psychometric theory in psychology. However, few diagnostic concepts in psychiatry meet these criteria at the level of stringency normally required of psychological tests. Despite such ambiguities, a number of *procedures* have been proposed to enhance the validity of psychiatric diagnoses in the absence of a simple measure. Thus, Robins and Guze (1970) outlined a program with five components: (1) clinical description; (2) laboratory studies; (3) delimitation from other disorders; (4) follow-up studies; and (5) family studies. This schema was later elaborated by Kendler (1980) who distinguished between antecedent validators (familial aggregation, premorbid personality, precipitating factors); concurrent validators (e.g., psychological tests); and predictive validators (diagnostic consistency over time, rates of relapse/recovery, response to treatment). Andreasen (1995) has proposed "additional" validators, such as molecular genetics, neurochemistry, neuroanatomy, neurophysiology and cognitive neuroscience, and suggested that "the validation of psychiatric diagnoses establishes them as 'real entities'."

These procedural criteria implicitly assume that psychiatric disorders are distinct entities; the possibility that disorders might merge into one another with no clear boundary in between is rarely considered. There is increasing evidence of overlapping genetic predisposition to schizophrenia and bipolar disorder, as well as to seemingly unrelated disorders, such as autistic spectrum, intellectual disability, and, possibly, epilepsy. It is equally likely that the same environmental factors contribute to several different syndromes (Kendell and Jablensky 2003). Should such findings be systematically replicated, their repercussion on future psychiatric classifications will be considerable. Variations in psychiatric symptomatology might indeed better represented by "an ordered matrix of symptom-cluster dimensions" (Widiger and Clark 2000) than by a set of discrete categories. However, it would be premature at this time to discard the current categorical entities. Although there is a mounting assumption that many (or most) of the currently recognized psychiatric disorders are not disease entities, strictly speaking this has never been demonstrated, mainly because few studies of the appropriate kind have ever been designed and conducted.

5.12 **Validity and utility**

It is crucial to maintain a clear distinction between *validity* and *utility* (Kendell and Jablensky 2003); at present these two terms are often used as if they were synonyms. A diagnostic rubric may be said to possess utility if it provided nontrivial information about prognosis and likely treatment outcomes, and/or testable propositions about biological and social correlates. The term "utility" was first used in this sense by Meehl (1959) who wrote that:

> The fundamental argument for the utility of formal diagnosis. . . amounts to the same kind of thing one would say in defending formal diagnosis in organic medicine. One holds that there is a sufficient amount of aetiological and prognostic homogeneity among patients belonging to a given diagnostic group, so that the assignment of a patient to this group has probability implications which it is clinically unsound to ignore (p. 92).

Many though not all, of the diagnostic concepts listed in contemporary nomenclatures such as DSM-IV and ICD-10 are extremely useful to clinicians, whether or not the category in question is valid, as they provide information about the likelihood of future recovery, relapse, deterioration, and social handicap; they guide treatment decisions; they describe symptom profiles and their evolution over time; and they guide research on the etiology of the syndrome. However, there is a critical difference between validity and utility. Validity is an invariate characteristic of a diagnostic category—there may be uncertainty about its validity because of lack of relevant empirical information—but in principle, a category cannot be "partly" valid (Kendell and Jablensky 2003). Either it is or it is not valid, and its validity does not depend on the context. *Utility*, on the other hand, is a graded characteristic that is partly context specific. Schizophrenia may be an invaluable concept to practicing psychiatrists, but of little use to scientists exploring the genetic basis of psychosis. The existence of several rival definitions of a syndrome, overlapping the same patient populations, raises the suspicion that it is not a valid category since these rival definitions suggest that symptom variation is continuous and no identified boundary of the syndrome can be drawn. Alternatively, if all the rival definitions identify almost identical patient populations, then there is no important difference between them and the category may well be valid. Only one definition can be valid, unless the alternatives identify virtually the same population of individuals. On the other hand, several alternative definitions can all be *useful* and can have different utilities in different contexts. For example, the DSM-IV definition of schizophrenia is particularly useful for predicting outcome, because some degree of chronicity is in-built. But a much broader definition, covering a heterogeneous "schizophrenia spectrum," is more useful for defining a syndrome with high heritability (Jablensky and Kendell 2002; Kendell and Jablensky 2003).

5.13 **Structural issues: categories versus dimensions**

There are many different ways in which classifications can be constructed. The fundamental choice is between a categorical and a dimensional structure, and it is worth recalling the observation by the philosopher Carl Hempel (1961) 50 years ago that, although most sciences start with a categorical classification of their subject matter, they often replace this with dimensions as more accurate measurements become possible. The requirement that the categories of a typology should be mutually exclusive and jointly exhaustive has never been fully met by any psychiatric classification, or, for that matter, by any medical classification. Psychiatric classifications are eclectic in the sense that they are organized according to several different classes of criteria, e.g., presenting symptoms or traits, age at onset, course, pathology and causes, without a clear hierarchical arrangement. One or the other criterion may gain prominence as knowledge progresses or contextual (e.g., social, legal, service-related) conditions change. However, despite their apparent logical inconsistency, medical and psychiatric classifications survive and evolve because of their essentially pragmatic nature. Their utility is tested almost daily in clinical decision making and this ensures a natural selection of useful concepts by weeding out obsolete ideas (Jablensky and Kendell 2002).

Categorical models or typologies are the traditional, firmly entrenched form of representation for medical diagnoses. They are thoroughly familiar, and most of the present knowledge of the causes, presentation, treatment and prognosis of mental disorders was obtained, and is stored, in the categorical format. Furthermore, they are easy to use under conditions of incomplete clinical information and have the capacity to "restore the unity of the patient's pathology. . . into a single, coordinated configuration" (Millon 1991). The main disadvantage of the categorical model is its propensity to encourage a "discrete entity" view of the nature of psychiatric disorders. If it is firmly understood, though, that diagnostic categories do not necessarily represent discrete entities, but are simply a convenient way of organizing and presenting information, there should be no fundamental objection to their continued use.

Dimensional models, on the other hand, have the major conceptual advantage of introducing explicitly quantitative variation and graded transitions between forms of disorder, as well as between "normality" and pathology. This is important not only in areas of classification where the units of observation are traits (e.g., in the description of personality disorders) but also for classifying patients who meet the criteria for two or more categories simultaneously, or who straddle the boundary between two adjacent syndromes. They allow the diagnosis of "sub-threshold" conditions which constitute the bulk of mental ill-health seen in primary care settings.

Whether psychotic disorders can be better described dimensionally or categorically remains an open question for research. The difficulties with dimensional models of psychopathology stem from several sources. First and foremost is the absence of an established, empirically grounded metrics. Most existing scales of symptom severity are of a psychometrically low level of measurement: they are either nominal or ordinal, where one is simply able to state that $a>b>c. . .>n$ on some property, assigning numbers which indicate rank order and nothing more. It seems unlikely that *equal-interval* scaling, or *ratio* scales (which possess an absolute or natural zero) will ever be developed for reported subjective *symptoms*. Although intelligence, aptitude and personality test scores are also, strictly speaking, ordinal, some of them approximate interval equality fairly well (Kerlinger 1973). Secondly, there is no sight of an agreement on the number and nature of dimensions required to account adequately for clinical variation. Lastly, dimensional models are too complex and cumbersome for everyday clinical practice. These considerations seem to preclude, for the time being, a radical restructuring of psychiatric classification from a predominantly categorical to a predominantly dimensional model. However, categorical and dimensional models need not be mutually exclusive, as demonstrated by so-called mixed or class-quantitative models which combine qualitative categories with quantitative trait measurements. For example, there is increasing empirical evidence that a retained (and refined) categorical clinical description of the syndrome of schizophrenia can be supplemented with selected quantitative traits, such as measurements of sustained attention, memory dysfunction, amplitudes and latencies of event-related brain potentials, and volumetric deviance of cerebral structures as intermediate or "endophenotypes" (Jablensky 2009). There is a growing body of clinical and neuroscience data suggesting a possibility to develop nosological models which might combine the advantages of the categorical clinical approach (cognitive ease of use) with the refinement provided by research on endophenotype-based dimensions. Modern statistical techniques offer a variety of ways to handle multifactorial and multidimensional data and, therefore, any number of "axes" in such nosological model is conceivable.

5.14 **DSM-5, ICD-11 and beyond**

In the present process of revision of the DSM and ICD, both the APA and WHO are confronted with a dilemma. The revision process has generated requests to alter the criteria defining many individual disorders, to eliminate some and to add new "disorders," and so on. In many cases the reasons for such changes, viewed in isolation, seem cogent. However, all definitional changes have serious disadvantages: they are confusing to clinicians; they create a situation in which the relevance of all previous clinical and epidemiological research into disorders as currently defined is uncertain; and they involve tedious and sometimes costly changes in the content and wording of diagnostic interviews, as well as in the algorithms to generate diagnoses from clinical ratings. A series of such changes—from DSM-III to DSM-IIIR to DSM-IV to DSM-5, for example, risks discrediting the whole process of psychiatric classification.

It is important to maintain awareness of the fact that most of psychiatry's disease concepts are merely working hypotheses and their diagnostic criteria are provisional. The present evolutionary classification in biology would never have been developed if the concept of *species* had been defined in rigid operational terms, with strict inclusion/exclusion criteria.

The same may be true of complex psychobiological entities like psychiatric disorders. Both extremes—a totally unstructured approach to diagnosis and a rigid operationalization—should be avoided. Defining a middle range of operational specificity, which would be optimal for stimulating critical thinking in clinical research, but also rigorous enough to enable comparisons between the results of different studies in different countries, is probably a better solution. None of the attempts at reshuffling and re-defining the ICD or DSM classification rubrics without sufficient and compelling evidence has so far been successful, and further attempts may be arbitrary and premature. This should not mean that we must wait until better, robust biological markers and indicators become available to the clinician or the epidemiologist. On the contrary, experimenting with research-oriented classifications and diagnostic tools linked to emerging "research domain" neurobiological and genetic criteria (Cuthbert and Insel 2010) is necessary and urgent. A more fundamental re-thinking and re-shaping of the nosological theory underlying the classification of psychotic disorders would require, on one hand, overcoming and resolving the kind of contradictions outlined above and, on the other hand, developing concepts that would allow a better interdigitation of clinical, neurobiological, genetic and behavioral data. Although the majority of psychiatric disorders appear to be far too complex from a genetic point of view than it was assumed until recently, molecular genetics and neuroscience will play an increasing role in understanding their etiology and pathogenesis. However, the extent of their impact on the diagnostic process and on the classification of psychiatric disorders is difficult to predict. The eventual outcome is less likely to depend on the knowledge base of psychiatry per se, than on the social, cultural and economic forces that shape the public perception of mental illness and determine the clinical practice of psychiatry. A possible, but unlikely, scenario is the advent of an eliminativist "mind-less" psychiatry (Eisenberg 2000), driven solely by biological models. It is much more likely that clinical psychiatry will retain psychopathology—the systematic analysis and description of subjective experience and behavior—as its core. It is also likely that classification will evolve towards a system with at least two major axes: one etiological, using neurobiological and genetic organizing concepts, and another syndromal or behavioral-dimensional. The mapping of two such axes onto one another will provide a stimulating research agenda for psychiatry for many years to come.

It may be appropriate to conclude this excursion into the history of psychiatric nosology and the speculation about alternatives that might do better in the near future, with a quotation from Jaspers (1963) which pointedly summarizes the main message of this paper:

> When we design a diagnostic scheme. . . we abandon the idea of disease entity and once more have to bear in mind continually the various points of view (as to causes, psychological structure, anatomical findings, course of illness and outcome), and in the face of the facts we have to draw a line where none exists. . .a classification therefore has only a provisional value. It is a fiction which will discharge its function if it proves to be the most apt for the time (p. 605)

Chapter References

Andreasen, N. C. (1995). The validation of psychiatric diagnosis: new models and approaches (editorial). *American Journal of Psychiatry*, **152**, 161–2.

Berze, J., (1912). *Die primäre Insuffizienz der psychischen Aktivität*. Leipzig: Deuticke.

Blashfield, R. K. (1986). Structural approaches to classification. In T. Millon and G. L. Klerman (eds.) *Contemporary Directions in Psychopathology: Towards the DSM-IV*. New York, The Guilford Press, pp. 363–80.

Bleuler, E. (1911). *Dementia praecox oder die Gruppe der Schizophrenien*. In G. Aschaffenburg (ed.), *Handbuch der Psychiatrie*. Leipzig: Deuticke, pp. 124–243. (English translation: Dementia Praecox, or the Group of Schizophrenias. New York: International Universities Press (1950).

Bleuler, E. (1920). Lehrbuch der Psychiatrie. *Dritte Auflage*. Berlin: Julius Springer.

Bonhoeffer, K. (1912). Die Psychosen im Gefolge von akuten Infektionen, Allgemeinerkrankungen und inneren Erkrankungen. In G. Aschaffenburg (ed.), *Handbuch der Psychiatrie*. Leipzig, Deuticke, pp. 1–110.

Cuthbert, B. N. and Insel, T. R. (2010). Toward new approaches to psychotic disorders: the NIMH Research Domain Criteria Project. *Schizophrenia Bulletin*, **36**, 1061–62.

Eisenberg, L. (2000). Is psychiatry more mindful or brainier than it was a decade ago? *British Journal of Psychiatry*, **176**, 1–5.

Essen-Möller, E. (1961). On the classification of mental disorders. *Acta Psychiatrica Scandinavica*, **37**, 119–26.

Ey, H., Bernard, P. and Brisset, C. (1923). *Manuel de psychiatrie* (6th ed.). Paris: Masson.

Feighner, J. P., Robins, E., Guze, S. B., Woodruff, R. A., Winokur, G. and Munoz, R. (1972). Diagnostic criteria for use in psychiatric research. *Archives of General Psychiatry*, **26**, 57–63.

Hempel, C. (1961). Introduction to problems of taxonomy. In J. Zubin (ed.), *Field Studies in the Mental Disorders*. New York, Grune & Stratton, pp. 3–32.

Hoche, A., (1912). Die Bedeutung der Symptomkomplexe in der Psychiatrie. *Zeitschrift für die gesamte Neurologie und Psychiatrie*, **12**, 540–51.

Hoch, P. H. and Polatin P. (1949). Pseudoneurotic forms of schizophrenia. *Psychiatric Quarterly*, **23**, 248–76.

Hopper, K., Harrison, G., Janca, A. and Sartorius, N. (2007). *WHO Recovery from Schizophrenia. An International Perspective*. New York: Oxford University Press.

Hyman, S. E. (2010). The diagnosis of mental disorders: the problem of reification. *Annual Review of Clinical Psychology*, **6**, 155–79.

Jablensky, A. (2009). Endophenotypes in psychiatric research: focus on schizophrenia. In K. Salzinger and M. R. Serper (eds.), *Behavioral Mechanisms and Psychopathology*. Washington DC: American Psychological Association, pp. 13–40.

Jablensky, A. and Kendell, R. E. (2002). Criteria for assessing a classification in psychiatry. In M. Maj, W. Gaebel, J. Lopez-Ibor and N.Sartorius (eds.), *Psychiatric Diagnosis and Classification*. Chichester: John Wiley & Sons, pp. 1–24.

Jablensky, A., Sartorius, N., Ernberg, G., Anker, M,. Korten, A., Cooper J. E., *et al.* (1992). Schizophrenia: manifestations, incidence and course in different cultures. A World Health Organization ten-country study. *Psychological Medicine*, Monograph Supplement, **20**, 1–97.

Jaspers, K. (1963). *General Psychopathology* (J. Hoenig and M. W. Hamilton trans.). Chicago, IL: The University of Chicago Press, pp. 569–605.

Kahlbaum, K. L. (1863). *Die Gruppirung der psychischen Krankheiten und die Einteilung der Seelenstörungen*. Danzig: Kafemann.

Kasanin, K. (1933). The acute schizoaffective psychoses. *American Journal of Psychiatry*, **90**, 97–126.

Kendell, R. and Jablensky, A. (2003) Distinguishing between the validity and utility of psychiatric diagnosis. *American Journal of Psychiatry*, **160**, 4–12.

Kendler, K. S. (1980). The nosologic validity of paranoia (simple delusional disorder): a review. *Archives of General Psychiatry*, **37**, 699–706.

Kendler, K. S., Gruenberg, A. M. and Kinney D. K. (1994). Independent diagnoses of adoptees and relatives as defined by DSM-III in the provincial and national samples of the Danish Adoption Study of Schizophrenia. *Archives of General Psychiatry*, **51**, 456–68.

Kerlinger, F. N. (1973). *Foundations of Behavioral Research* (2nd ed.). London: Holt, Rinehard & Winston, pp. 426–41.

Kety, S. (1988). Schizophrenic illness in the families of schizophrenic adoptees: findings from the Danish national sample. *Schizophrenia Bulletin*, **14**, 217–22.

Kielholz, P. (1979). The concept of masked depression. *Encephale*, 5 (5 Suppl), 459–62.

Kraepelin, E. (1899). *Psychiatrie. Ein Lehrbuch für Studirende und Aerzte.* 6. Auflage. Leipzig: Barth.

Kraepelin, E. (1920). Die Erscheinungsformen des Irreseins. (English translation: *Patterns of Mental Disorder.* In S. R. Hirsch and M. Shepherd (eds.) *Themes and Variations in European Psychiatry.* Bristol: John Wright & Sons, pp. 7–30.)

Langfeld, G. (1937). The prognosis in schizophrenia and the factors influencing the course of the disease. *Acta Psychiatrica et Neurologica Scandinavica Supplementum,* **13**, 1–228.

Leonhard, K. (1999). *Classification of Endogenous Psychoses and their Differentiated Etiology* (H. Beckmann ed.) (2nd ed.) Vienna: Springer.

Leonhard, K. and von Trostorff, S. (1964). *Prognostische Diagnose der endogenen Psychosen.* Jena: Gustav Fischer, 7.

Meehl, P. E. (1959). Psychodiagnosis. In *Selected Papers*, Minneapolis, MO: University of Minnesota Press.

Millon, T. (1991). Classification in psychopathology: rationale, alternatives, and standards. *Journal of Abnormal Psychology*, **100**, 245–26.

Pope, H. G. and Lipinski, J. F. (1978). Diagnosis in schizophrenia and manic-depressive illness: a reassessment of the specificity of "schizophrenic" symptoms in the light of current research. *Archives of General Psychiatry*, **35**, 811–28.

Robins, E. and Guze, S. B. (1970). Establishment of diagnostic validity in psychiatric illness: its application to schizophrenia. *American Journal of Psychiatry*, **126**, 983–7.

Rosch, E. (1975). Cognitive reference points. *Cognitive Psychology*, **7**, 532–47.

Scadding, J. G. (1996). Essentialism and nominalism in medicine: logic of diagnosis in disease terminology. *Lancet*, **348**, 594–6.

Schneider, K. (1959). *Clinical Psychopathology.* New York: Grune & Stratton.

Shepherd, M., Brooke, E. M. and Cooper, J. E. (1968). An experimental approach to psychiatric diagnosis. An international study. *Acta Psychiatrica Scandinavica Supplementum*, **201**, 7–89.

Sokal, R. R. (1974). Classification: purposes, principles, progress, prospects. *Science*, **185**, 1115–23.

Strömgren, E. (1987). The development of the concept of reactive psychoses. *Psychopathology*, **20**, 62–7.

Sullivan, P. F. and Kendler K. S. (1998). Typology of common psychiatric syndromes. An empirical study. *British Journal of Psychiatry*, **173**, 312–19.

Widiger, T. A. and Clark L. A. (2000). Towards DSM-V and the classification of psychopathology. *Psychological Bulletin*, **126**, 946–63.

Wing, J. K., Cooper, J. E. and Sartorius, N. (1974). *Measurement and Classification of Psychiatric Symptoms.* London: Cambridge University Press.

World Health Organization. (1979). *Schizophrenia. An International Follow-up Study.* Chichester: Wiley.

Zilboorg, G. (1941). Ambulatory schizophrenia. *Psychiatry*, **4**, 149–55.

The Kraepelinian pipe organ model (for a more dimensional) DSM-5 classification

Darrel A. Regier

The Jablensky chapter addresses the fundamental underlying theory about the nature of mental disorders. In fact, the choice of the name as *disease*, *syndrome* or *disorder* indicates a certain selection bias for a particular theory. *Disease* implies an underlying cause, clinical manifestations, deviations from norms and a prognosis of reduced biological fitness. In contrast, *syndromes* are simply clinical manifestations of something and deviations from norms without any specific causal attributions. *Disorders* aren't actually defined but appear to be some hybrid—less precise than a disease and more indicative of discrete pathology than a syndrome.

The more important consideration is the conceptual approach to these entities as discrete, discontinuous phenomena versus graded, continuous phenomena to which we can apply a sliding threshold to separate pathology from normal variation. Jablensky suggests at the onset that there are "inherent shortcomings in the mainstream nosological paradigm adopted in psychiatry since the beginning of the 20th century. An essentialist view of diseases as independent agents causing illnesses."

Kraepelin (1920) espoused this essentialist disease entity concept and chose "outcome" as the primary validity criterion—using it to separate dementia praecox from manic-depressive insanity. Even Bleuler's 1911 revision of schizophrenia, which included schizotypal disorder as Kety (1985) did in his schizophrenia spectrum concept, still relies on a categorical "disease concept."

Jablensky notes that the major problem of conceptualizing manic depressive or bipolar disorder as a separate "categorical disease" from schizophrenia has been the failure of these to separate consistently. The result is a frequent hybrid referred to as schizoaffective disorder, and there are also a good number of relatives with subthreshold schizotypal disorder. Hence, the population genetics and the variable outcomes associated with the specific constellations of symptoms, signs, and their respective durations (the syndrome) fail to correlate as one would expect with independent disease entities.

One of the more fascinating observations noted in the Jablensky paper is the report that Kraepelin actually turned toward a more dimensional model in one of his last papers in 1920 (Kraepelin 1920, p. 26). The three concepts discussed in this paper included: (1) a decision to turn away from orderly, well-defined groups in order to understand the essential function that was disturbed; (2) a conclusion that hereditary factors make certain areas of personality more susceptible and accessible to pathological stimuli; and (3) the illustrative comparison between various syndromes to the different registers of an organ—any of which may be brought into play according to the extent of the pathological changes involved. In this parallel, one can visualize the multiple components of schizophrenia and bipolar syndromes as independent pipes (symptoms/traits) or even different registers (domains).

As the spouse of a professional organist with whom I have spent countless hours in church organ lofts, pulling stops or watching her kick on presets for multiple combinations of diapasons, flutes, strings, or reeds like the krumhorn or fagotto pipes, Kraepelin's late-breaking pipe-organ analogy rings true to my clinical experience with patients who don't fit neatly into categorical diagnoses. Although some syndromes have a very distinct categorical presentation (like the krumhorn or the trumpet stop on the organ), many are characterized by a recognizable blend of symptom presentations much like the mixtures that blur the distinct sounds of the organ. Indeed, there is a common complaint among medical students and psychiatry residents that patients don't seem to read or exhibit the DSM or ICD diagnostic criteria when they present for treatment. Kraepelin's pipe-organ analogy also represents a prescient anticipation of our more recent understandings that there may be hundreds of independent molecular genetic contributions to many common mental disorders.

Within the DSM-5 developmental process, the group most attuned to this approach has been our Personality and Personality Disorders Work Group. They have recognized that the 10 personality disorders in DSM-IV don't exist as neatly differentiated diagnostic entities, as indicated by the finding that not otherwise specified (NOS) is the most common personality diagnosis and that even those with a specific personality diagnosis often qualify for several others as well. Hence, there is great interest in identifying fewer distinct syndromes (disorder types) and greater interest in identifying the combinations of traits/symptoms that seem to cluster most frequently in what are referred to as domains, such as emotional dysregulation (including mood, anger, anxiety traits), detachment, antagonism, disinhibition, and schizotypy. Each of these domains consists of 5–10 specific symptoms that tend to present together in individuals when large groups of people are tested. Where clinically significant impairment in personality function qualifies an individual for a personality disorder, it would be possible to characterize the disorder as "trait specified" by displaying a severity profile of applicable trait domains. The more frequently recognized combinations of these domains are seen as the criteria for the syndromes which are currently recognized as disorders.

Not only can the individual symptom traits be conceptualized as the independent organ pipes in the Kraepelin analogy, but the trait domains may also be seen as expressions of the underlying heredity factors that make certain areas of personality more susceptible and accessible to pathologic stimuli—the second observation in Kraepelin's late conceptual approach. This is in fact the approach that Robert Krueger, PhD, has taken in identifying internalizing and externalizing disorders through latent trait analyses of co-morbidity rates of mental disorders in epidemiological and clinical population groups (Krueger 1999; Krueger et al. 1998).

Jablensky notes that the mental disorders in ICD-10 and DSM-IV are not jointly exhaustive to account for all entities; nor are they mutually exclusive. Subsequently, we have an excess of comorbidity and NOS diagnoses. There are also no superordinate or higher-level organizing concepts at present; the adoption of a disorder grouping that linked internalizing and externalizing disorders together would begin to provide such a concept.

Alternatively, Jablensky notes that Essen-Möller had suggested another approach that included a double classification where one focused on etiology and the other focused primarily on syndromes. The difficulty with this is that multiple etiologic factors can give rise to the same syndrome (e.g., psychosis) and one etiological factor (like syphilis) can give rise to multiple syndromes. It is hoped that the relationship between underlying pathophysiology and specific brain functions (e.g., neurocircuitry) and syndromes may be closer than the relationship between etiological (genetic) factors and syndromes.

A major concern in this paper is the continued preoccupation with validity and validators. All of these measures implicitly assume that psychiatric disorders are distinct entities—the possibility that they can merge with one another with no clear boundaries is rarely considered, as was noted in the classic Kendell and Jablensky paper of 2003. Hence, the psychometric theories of construct, concurrent, and predictive validity; Robins and Guze's (1970) clinical validity; Kendler's (1980) antecedent, concurrent, and predictive validity; and the more recent 11 validators raised by Hyman (2010) in the DSM-5 process all share this categorical assumption and problem. However, in the latter example, in which Andrews, Goldberg, Krueger, and colleagues (Andrews et al. 2009) used the 11 validators in a series of papers, they did so to validate larger disorder groupings rather than trying to validate individual disorders currently identified in the DSM or ICD.

In making the distinction between validity and clinical utility, Jablensky leans much more heavily on the value of clinical utility. He quotes Meel, who stated that a diagnosis implies a sufficient amount of prognostic homogeneity among patients in a diagnostic group, such that the assignment of a patient to this group has probability implications that are clinically unsound to ignore. To this I would paraphrase Helen Kraemer, PhD: A dimensional diagnosis is not more useful than a categorical diagnosis only if the categorical diagnosis contains no variation within it (Kraemer et al. 2004). Finally, Hempel in 1961 states that most sciences start with a categorical classification, and they often replace this with dimensions as more accurate measurements become possible.

Certainly as our diagnostic system evolves, we will need to retain many of the categorical conventions to facilitate communication about the "essential functions" that a given disorder implies to clinicians and to patients. The future of our field, however, requires us to move with the science to understand the link between normal psychology and psychopathology as well as the physiology of brain function and pathophysiology, which will be dimensional variations from norms. To the degree that we can begin to incorporate these variations into our understanding of diagnostic syndromes and their dimensional manifestations, the better able we will be to advance the scientific understanding of mental disorders and their treatment. It may not be entirely facetious to focus on examples of organ registration principles to understand the way that different mixtures of independent pipes (genes, personality traits and environmental exposures) can combine to form recognizable registers (symptom/trait domains), which can then be combined even further to form mixtures (syndromes) that are recognizable to the trained ear (experienced clinician/research investigator) (Goode 1964).

Comments References

Andrews, G., Goldberg, D. P., Krueger, R. F., Carpenter, W. T., Hyman, S. E., Sachdev, P., *et al.* (2009). Exploring the feasibility of a meta-structure for DSM-V and ICD-11: Could it improve utility and validity? *Psychological Medicine*, **39**, 1993–2000.

Bleuler, E. (1911). *Dementia praecox oder die Gruppe der Schizophrenien*. In G. Aschaffenburg (ed.), *Handbuch der Psychiatrie*. Leipzig: Deuticke, pp. 124–243. (English translation: *Dementia Praecox, or the Group of Schizophrenias*. New York: International Universities Press (1950).

Goode, J. C. (1964). *Pipe Organ Registration*. New York: Abingdon, pp. 13–38.

Hempel, C. (1961). Introduction to problems of taxonomy. In J. Zubin (ed.) *Field Studies in the Mental Disorders*. New York: Grune & Stratton, pp. 3–32.

Hyman, S. E. (2010). The diagnosis of mental disorders: the problem of reification. *Annual Reviews in Clinical Psychology*, **6**, 155–79.

Kendell, R. E. and Jablensky, A. (2003). Distinguishing between the validity and utility of psychiatric diagnoses. *American Journal of Psychiatry*, **160**, 4–12.

Kendler, K. S. (1980). The nosologic validity of paranoia (simple delusional disorder): a review. *Archives of General Psychiatry*, **37**, 699–706.

Kety, S. S. (1985). Schizotypal personality disorder: an operational definition of Bleuler's latent schizophrenia? *Schizophrenia Bulletin*, **11**, 590–4.

Kraemer, H. C., Noda, A. and O'Hara, R. (2004). Categorical versus dimensional approaches to diagnosis: methodological challenges. *Journal of Psychiatric Research*, **38**, 17–25.

Kraepelin, E. (1920). Die erscheinungsformen des irreseins. (English translation: Patterns of mental disorder. In: S.R. Hirsch and M. Shepherd (eds.) (1974). *Themes and Variations in European Psychiatry*. Charlottesville, VA: University Press of Virginia, pp. 7–30.

Krueger, R. F. (1999). The structure of common mental disorders. *Archives of General Psychiatry*, **56**, 921–6.

Krueger, R. F., Caspi, A., Moffitt, T. E., and Silva, P. E. (1998). The structure and stability of common mental disorders (DSM-III-R): A longitudinal–epidemiological study. *Journal of Abnormal Psychology*, **107**, 216–27.

Robins, E. and Guze, S.B. (1970). Establishment of diagnostic validity in psychiatric illness: its application to schizophrenia. *American Journal of Psychiatry*, **126**, 983–7.

Chapter 6

Introduction

Kenneth S. Kendler

In this very rich essay, full of historical and philosophical insights, Berrios challenges many of the assumptions of the nosologic enterprise as it is now being practiced in early 21st-century psychiatry. Probably the foremost current scholar in the history of psychiatry, Berrios suggests that after the central historical episode of his essay—a debate on the nosology of psychiatric disorders in France in November 1860—"little of substance [on psychiatric nosology] has been written since." I will leave it to the reader to judge the degree to which (if any) this comment is "tongue in cheek."

The most important overarching theme of this essay is the debate about whether psychiatric diagnoses (1) really exist out there in the world and are "discovered" or, (2) are man-made constructions that are "invented." This theme is not unique to psychiatry but rather reflects a long-standing debate within science and the philosophy of science about whether categories in the natural and social sciences (electrons, elements, species and emotions would all be good examples) are "real" versus "socially constructed." Berrios, in contrast to many contributors to this volume, stakes out a claim more toward the socially constructed end of this continuum.

His claim certainly has a priori justification. It does not take a deeply knowledgeable commentator to realize that compared to the harder sciences such as physics, the opportunity for personal, social, cultural and indeed national influences to impact on psychiatric science, in general, and nosology, in particular, are great. Berrios provides several nice examples of how European nosologic processes were influenced by Nationalism, in particular competition between Germans and French for predominance in the world of psychiatry.

It might be helpful to here compare psychiatric nosology with what is often selected as the poster-child for "scientific realism"—the periodic table. If psychiatric disorders were real in the way that atomic elements were real, we would expect that they would be stabile across time and place, and the classification of psychiatric illness should be independent of social, political and cultural influences. Even insurance companies cannot regulate the structure of atomic elements.

Of course, these two positions are not mutually contradictory. Indeed, several philosophers of science (for example Kitcher (1993) and Solomon (2001)) explicitly adopted a hybrid approach, suggesting that scientific constructs—like psychiatric disorders—are typically influenced by both scientific discoveries about the "real" world, and psychological and social processes. The relative influences of these two domains vary. For any readers who want a nice illustration of the intersection of social and scientific influences in psychiatry nosology, they might consult the informative essay on the creation of post-traumatic stress disorder by Scott (1990).

I suspect that if you took most of the psychiatric nosologists active in DSM-5 and ICD-11 and pushed them, they would adopt something like this hybrid approach toward psychiatric illness. They would likely differ, however, in the relative weights attached to the "real" versus "social-cultural" influences. Indeed, I also suspect that they would often adopt different weights for different psychiatric disorders. Most nosologists that I know would believe that autism, schizophrenia and bipolar illness are probably, at least in substantial degree, real things out there in the world. I doubt many would argue so strongly for a similar viewpoint on histrionic personality disorder.

In almost a side-note that I want to emphasize, Berrios provides a critique of the Kraepelinian nosology which remains foundational for a number of aspects of DSM and ICD today. First, he notes that at its broadest level, our approach to psychiatric illness is informed by early faculty psychology which had a tri-partite view of mental functions: intellectual, emotional and volitional. He writes

> In fact, this [typology] constitutes the epistemological basis of our current classifications: schizophrenia and paranoia (first group); mania, depression, anxiety, phobias etc. (second group) and character and personality disorders (third group).

That is, Berrios argues that at a "deep level," the structure of our major nosologies of DSM and ICD reflect one iteration of European faculty psychology. It should also be noted—see his Endnote 6—that Berrios judges the empirical foundation of the Kraepelinian system to be rather more humble than is sometimes claimed.

At the close of his essay, Berrios goes one step further in his critique of psychiatric nosology. He asks whether psychiatric syndromes are, by their very nature, "susceptible to classification." I appreciate the profound philosophical and conceptual issues raised by attempts to classify the highly subjective experiences that form the basis of psychiatric illness. However, I cannot avoid a more "positivistic" response to this deeply challenging conclusion. My thoughts turn to the well-known "miracle" argument of Putnam (1975). In defense of scientific realism (the belief that science studies real things out in the world), he argued that it was "the only philosophy that doesn't make the success of science a miracle." The science of psychiatry is surely in its infancy, and not yet ready for triumphalism about its level of success. However, it has had some solid accomplishments to its name including advances in measurement, psychopharmacology, neurobiology and genetics, many of which were based in part on our diagnostic categories. Although I am hardly one to argue that our current diagnostic systems are more than highly flawed first approximations, would these advances have been possible if all of our attempts at psychiatric classification were, at a fundamental level, deeply flawed?

Introduction References

Kitcher, P. (1993). *The advancement of science: science without legend, objectivity without illusions.* New York: Oxford University Press.

Putnam, H. (1975). *Mathematics, Matter and Method.* New York: Cambridge University Press.

Scott, W. J. (1990). PTSD in DSM-III – A Case in the Politics of Diagnosis and Disease. *Social Problems,* **37**(3), 294–310.

Solomon, M. (2001). *Social Empiricism* Cambridge, MA: A Bradford Book, The MIT Press.

Chapter 6

The 19th-century nosology of alienism: history and epistemology

German E. Berrios

In the technical language of the history of medicine "nosology" refers to the classification and "nosography" to the description of "disease." Given that both disciplines reached their epistemological acme during the 18th and 19th centuries, there is little point in concentrating on any later periods. In regards to madness it would be of course crass anachronism to talk about "psychiatric classifications" during the Enlightenment; however, these started to appear during the first half of the 19th century following the construction of the current concepts of "mental symptom" and "mental disorder" (Berrios 1999).

Within the severe epistemological constraints set by 19th-century philosophy of science and pre-Darwinian taxonomic theory, alienists created the models and frames of current psychiatry. Little has changed since and the classificatory industry they started does not show signs of abating. Important to the academic reputation of alienists and Institutions and to national pride, the dissemination of such classifications has since depended less on "validity" (whatever this term may mean in the context of psychiatry!) than on the political and/or economic power of their creators.

6.1 Matters historiographical

Psychiatric classifications can be conceived of as: (1) chronological catalogues of "achievements" that culminate in a final and definitive grand ordering of mental disorders;[1] (2) enterprises reflecting the social and political needs of a collective[2] or (3) conceptual narratives. According to the third approach mental symptoms or disorders result from the "convergence" (in the work of an author or authors) of words, concepts and associated behaviors which, on further analysis, are often enough found to have participated in earlier convergences. Given that there is no way of telling whether a later one is "truer" or "more valid" than a preceding one, convergences cannot be aligned on a "progressive" series. All that can be meaningfully stated is that each convergence constitutes a self-contained narrative expressing the best that a given historical period can offer. Mental symptoms and disorders are semantically configured cultural objects at the heart of which there is always a neurobiological signal. It follows that they are neither "pure" biology nor "pure" semantics and the challenge to psychiatric modelers is to respect their hybrid nature. This also means that in addition to biological data information is required on the purpose, assumptions and social frames of any classification, on what Lanteri-Laura (1984) felicitously called "*les références non-cliniques.*"

6.2 **Conceptual tools and metalanguage**

Following technical usage, nosology will refer here to the classification of diseases, nosography to their description and taxonomy to the philosophy of classifications. Disambiguating classification is more complicated as it is used to refer to: (1) the principles and rules in terms of which groupings are constituted (what some call taxonomy), (2) the act of grouping (the sortal act) (what in the case of psychiatry partially corresponds to diagnosis), and (3) the groupings themselves (for example, ICD-10 or AMPD).

The main dichotomies of medical taxonomy

The meta-language of taxonomy includes a number of dichotomies. Firstly it differentiates between "system" and "domain": the former refers to the frame, rules and definitions of a classification; the latter to the objects to be classified. Then comes a family of polarities with overlapping referents: "categorical or dimensional"; "monothetic vs polythetic"; "natural versus artificial," "top-to-bottom" versus "bottom-up," "structured versus listing," "hierarchical versus non-hierarchical," "exhaustive versus partial," idiographic versus nomothetic', etc. The first term of the "categorical versus dimensional" polarity can be interpreted as referring to the properties (it is either present or absent: 1 or 0) or to the manner of sorting (an object is or is not a member of a class); and "dimensional" may mean a "quality continuum" or define an object as a cluster of dimensions. Categorical classifications (e.g., species and classes) are popular in biology[3] and depend upon the steady state of their exemplars (at least within a given time frame). Whether in regards to properties (i.e., symptoms) or entities (i.e., diseases), psychiatric objects are far from exhibiting such steady state. "Monothetic versus polythetic" concerns the number and predominance of sorting traits: monothetic definitions are based on the principle that all the objects of a class must share same attributes; polythetic definitions are based on the idea of a "family resemblance" and hence objects within a class do not need to share any attributes.[4]

Since the 18th century, classifications have also been divided into "natural" or "artificial." According to a "weak" version, objects can be classified in terms of "essential" or "man-made features" (e.g., flowers can be grouped according to their sexual organs or simply in terms of their use: funerals, weddings, etc.). According to a "strong" version, "natural" must mean "natural kind" (see Dupré 1981; Granger 1985) and "artificial" man-made (Dagognet 1970).[5] Based on the view that all psychiatric objects are constructs (Ellenberger 1963) it has been argued that psychiatric classifications must be considered as "artificial." This might also explain why since the 19th century "proxy" variables have been persistently used to steady up the ontology of psychiatric objects. "Organic causes," brain inscriptions, neuropathology, electroencephalography, neuropsychological networks, psychophysiological variables, genes, etc., have all been used in their day. Apart from the fact that in psychiatry there is not yet a good theory of proxyhood, there is the danger that the ignorant may confuse it with "naturalization." The "list versus structured" dichotomy refers to the manner in which classes relate to each other. Examples of "listings" are ICD 10 and DSM-IV (Cooper 2005). Social and economic factors are important to listing membership. This is not a problem in itself as long as the classification is not exported from the country in which it was constructed. In "structured" classifications classes constitute a hierarchy and purport to mapping a given universe (e.g., like the periodic table of elements). No one has seriously put forward a structured psychiatric classifications during the 20th century but one could easily concoct one. Hierarchical (multilayered) classifications consist in structures where high-level classes embed lower level ones and can be used as decisional trees (for example, the dichotomous classification that Emil Kraepelin borrowed from Kahlbaum (Berrios 1996) and from his brother Karl, a distinguished classificator of molluscs and scorpions).[6]

"Exhaustive versus partial" refer to the compass of a classification. Exhaustive classifications purport to include all the entities in a given universe, for example, some 19th-century classifications of mental disorders assumed that the entire realm of mental functions could be classified without residuum into intellectual, emotional and volitional. It was further assumed that each of these functional packages could be independently affected by disease leading to intellectual, emotional and volitional "mental disorders." In fact, this constitutes the epistemological basis of our current classifications: schizophrenia and paranoia (first group); mania, depression, anxiety, phobias etc. (second group) and character and personality disorders (third group). To deal with cases where more than one function seemed involved, rules were created to decide on which was primary.[7]

Lastly, idiographic versus nomothetic are occasionally mentioned. Its historical origin has nothing to do with psychology or psychiatry although it concerns efforts made at the turn of the 20th century to differentiate between the natural and social sciences. In his 1894 inaugural lecture as vice-chancellor of Strasburg University, Wilhelm Windelband stated:

> We can therefore say that in approaching reality the empirical sciences search for either of two things: the general in the form of natural laws or the special, as a specific event of history. They thus contemplate the permanent and immutable or the transitory as contained into real life happenings. The former sciences concern laws, the latter events; the former teach what has always been, the latter what has happened once. In the first case, scientific thinking is – if we were allowed to coin new technical terms – nomothetic, in the second case idiographic (Windelband 1949, p. 317).

At the core of any classification there always is a taxonomy, i.e., a theory of sortal concepts. Classifying is the act of sorting natural or man-made entities into pigeonholes themselves provided by nature or invented by man. Pigeonholes are called "classes" and their meaning is given by cognitive devices called "concepts." Now, whilst it is possible for anyone to claim that his classification is theory-free (DSM-IV was once presented as an atheoretical listing) the fact of the matter is that no classificator can avoid assuming a theory of concepts.[8]

What are classifications for?

Of all the potential benefits of a classification the most important is prediction, i.e., a capacity to release additional knowledge about the sorted objects. The fact that this epistemological fruitfulness is rarely present in psychiatry needs to be accounted for. One explanation may be that to start off with, the classification must start from a clear theoretical basis (like the periodic table of elements). There is little hope that this can be achieved in psychiatry. This pessimism led some years ago to resort to the old notions of "prototype" or "ideal type" (the historical origin of these notions is different but they have been handled as related in psychiatry).[9] Hampton (1993, p. 70) has written:

> It is claimed that uncertainty about classification is a result of people's inadequate knowledge of the categories that exist in the real world. The prototype view is directed, however, at a characterization of exactly this inadequate knowledge - it is a model of the beliefs people have. Whether or not the real world is best described with a classical conceptual framework or not is an interesting an important question, but irrelevant to this psychological goal of the prototype model.

Are the notions of "clearest case," "best example," and "procedural criteria" applicable to psychiatry? Can prototypes for all mental disorders be generated? What might their source be? Plausibly, there may be history (i.e., the received view of the disease) and ongoing clinical experience (i.e., the "lived experience" of the maker of the prototype). Which of these epistemic sources should have priority? In psychiatry, the claim that experience (empirical research) necessarily "trims" history is meaningless given that empirical research can only access reality via a preconceived theory. Furthermore, given that (1) as Dilthey would have it history is constituted by episodes of past "lived experience" (*Erlebnisse*) (each of which has generated its own prototype) and (2) that there are no *apriori* rules to decide which prototype should have preference, postulating "prototypes" does not seem to advance psychiatric knowledge. All that we have in our discipline is periodic recalibrations valid within specific time periods. As it is the case with convergences, "prototypes" do not form a progressive series either which may eventually culminate in the identification of a final Platonic idea (the definite phenotype). Prototypes simple capture, as Hampton put it, the extension or our "current beliefs" about the object (disease) in question.

Foucault proposed that the 17th-century drive to catalogue nature resulted from a new way of dealing with *representation*, namely, with the question of linking words to things (so that at a later stage one would only deal with words). For example, the crucial difference between 17th-century animal classifications and Medieval and Chinese bestiaries is that in the latter "everything was said about each animal" whereas in the former old semantic contents were sanitized and new systems of representation created that might apply to a variety of objects. The same shift affected historical narrative which was made to act as a technique to capture the *truth of things*. This change forced history to catalogue and deal with the observed "objects" in a different way (Foucault 1966). This is why during the 18th century, the issue of classifying became linked with the Condillacean concept of science as a "perfect language" (Rousseau 1986) and also with the debate on how sciences related to each other (the problem of the "classification" of the sciences) (Speziale 1973). At the very end of the 18th century, the young

Pinel[10] placed himself at the junction of two traditions. As one of the French transla-
tors of Cullen (who blended the work of various Continental nosologists),[11] Pinel
declared his allegiance to the 18th century; but with his challenge to John Locke (Crane
2003) and in his *Nosographie Philosophique* (Pinel 1813) he tried to step into the new
century. It was only by the division of the 19th century that Bouillaud, still influenced
by Condillac, emphasized the value of a stable nomenclature and of creating a "perfect
language" for science; consequently, he criticized Pinel for not having *defined* any of
his key terms (Bouillaud 1846, p. xxiii). However, in his own definition of classification, Bouillaud was to look back: "a classification of diseases that is truly philosophical
and rational must be based on knowledge on the nature of disease. All nosological
buildings erected on any other foundations will remain fragile and lead to ruin
(Bouillaud 1846, p. xcii). (For a general criticism of this view see Riese (1945)).

6.3 **The beginnings**

The 17th-century classificatory drive mainly involved plants, animals and languages;
during the 18th century it extended to the rest of nature, including diseases. A typical
17th-century definition of classification read something like this:

> ... the universal characters of a plant are extended to every individual of the species; and
> whoever (I speak in the way of illustration) should accurately describe the colour, the
> taste, the smell, the figure, &c. of one single violet, would find that his description held
> good, there or thereabouts, for all the violets of that particular species upon the face of the
> earth (Sydenham 1848, p. 15).[12]

Things became more abstract during the following century: "all [beings] are nuanced
and change by degrees in nature. There is no one being that does not have either above
or below it another that shares with him some features and that differs from him in
other features"; and the 19th century echoed:

> Classification is an operation whereby the mind reduces diverse objects to a small number
> of types ordered hierarchically so that their knowledge can be rendered earlier and more
> exact. Classification can be made not only of the real objects of nature, as it is done in
> geology, zoology or botany but also of ideal objects that only exist in the mind... (Berthelot
> 1889, p. 574).

The 20th century added little: "the identification of the category or group to which
an individual or object belongs on the basis of its observed characteristics. When the
characteristics are a number of numerical measurements, the assignment to groups is
called by some statisticians discrimination, and the combination of measurements
used is called a discriminant function (Anderson 1968, p. 553).

The central debate during the 17th century was whether the taxonomic rules were
inscribed in the human brain,[13] mind[14] or language.[15] Most of these rules concerned
creating taxa in terms of "privileged" features[16] and this is the approach that Linné,
McBride, Sagar, Cullen, Boissier de Sauvages, etc. followed a century later. Against this
tradition the great Adanson (1763) proposed that all features should be taken into
account—insight now considered as a precursor of numerical taxonomy (Vernon
1988).

Given that sortal operations can only be carried out on manifolds already prede-fined, it seems clear that the taxonomic drive in question required a theory of defini-tion and of concepts. Such need was met successively by the logic of the School of Port Royale, Locke, Leibniz, and after the 1780s by Kant. By the late 18th century, the secu-larization of the natural world led to the replacement of God-given rules by evolution-ary principles whose net result by the middle of the 19th century was that taxa should be considered as "natural kinds" reflecting "biological adaptation." Soon enough and with more effort than sense, this principle started to be applied to medical diseases and then to madness.

In the world of psychiatry, classifications (in the manner of catalogues) tell more about the social and aesthetic world in which they have been constructed than about nature. This lecture aims at exploring the myth that psychiatrists are obliged to classify mental disorders because that is the way in which the brain or language works or because the world of psychiatry is populated by natural kinds ready to be classified. There will only be time for discussing one case history in some detail. The 1860–1861 debate on classification at the Paris *Société Médico Psychologique* is arguably the more serious exploration of psychiatric taxonomy that there is no record. Little of substance has been written since.

6.4 **A case history: the 1860–1861 SMP debate**

Introduction

In 1934, Desruelles et al. wrote on the historical formation of French psychiatric classifications:

> In 1843, the year when *Annales Médico-Psychologiques* started their publication, the clas-sification of mental disorders generally accepted included mania, lypemania, monomania, dementia, paralytic insanity, and idiocy; to which some added stupidity. [In fact] this is the classification first put forward by Cullen in 1772 (mania, melancholia and dementia) to which Pinel added idiocy, Esquirol added monomania, and Georget added stupidity (i.e., states of confusional, demented and melancholic stupor which Esquirol had refused to consider as a separate entity). Lastly, Parchappe added paralytic insanity (p. 638).

Corroborated by later historians[17] this account was correct in acknowledging the Cullean origins of the French classification (see López Piñero 1983) indeed, because 20th-century medicine has followed his classification principles, Cullen's ideas remain important in the present. It can even be claimed that the fact that all leading European psychiatric nosologies (e.g., German, French and Italian) were born out of Cullen's nosology suggests that later divergences were due more to the divisive influence of European nationalisms than to any empirical development.[18]

Whilst during the 19th century most alienists believed that classifying was an essen-tial aspect of their work, writers with a deeper social understanding were ambivalent about it. For example, the great Philippe Buchez[19] satirized: "Upon believing that they have completed their studies, rhetoricians will compose a tragedy and alienists a clas-sification" (quoted in Desruelles et al. (1934)). However, he also wrote:

> "in addition to facilitating teaching and helping to remember – by themselves important functions [classifications] have as their most important objective to carry out a diagnosis,

now called differential diagnosis. Now since diagnosis is at the basis of treatment, then it can be said that in the last analysis the objective of classifications is treatment (Buchez 1861, p. 328).

This feeling of confusion about psychiatric classifications continued till the end of the century: "those who debate on psychiatric classifications sound like the workers at the Tower of Babel: the more they talk the less one understands them. If the terms do not mean the same for everyone then they run the risk of being applied to different clinical states." (quoted in Desruelles et al. (1934, p. 638)). This trouble with definitions led Baillarger to suggest that the *Société Médico-Psychologique* should "fix the meaning of the main forms of mental disorder so that their scientific path could, so to speak, be controlled" (Baillarger, quoted in Desruelles et al. (1934); Berrios 2008).

According to Desruelles et al, 19th-century French alienists used at least eight taxonomic criteria to classify mental disorders: *cause* (aetiological); *substratum* (anatomical basis); clinical *outcome* (curable versus incurable); *actuarial* (statistics from main French asylums); *phenomenological* (absence or presence of *délire*); "*natural*" (i.e., correspondence with "real types" as given in nature); *psychological* (i.e., what mental faculty was assumed to be impaired); and *course* of the disease. As all these approaches vied for power, the *Société Médico Psychologique* resorted to a debate[20] on psychiatric classifications.

The debate

The debate was started on November 12, 1860 by Delasiauve[21] who, on the excuse of dealing with Buchez's positive review of Morel's book,[22] reminisced on the classificatory ideas of Esquirol, Ferrus, Falret, Girard de Cailleux, Lasègue and Baillarger. Of Morel's aetiological classification Delasiauve wrote: "Morel is evidently intoxicated by his views. What seems to have seduced him and to certain extent Buchez is the disorders caused by alcohol, lead and epilepsy where the cause is tangible and its effects understandable. Not so with other states where there are multiple factors and influences" (Reports 1861, p. 131). Buchez replied: "Mental illness is characterized by signs and symptoms and these have served always as classificatory principles. Are they sufficient? The answer is not…. it is necessary to search for the pathogenesis of mental disorder… to describe mental illness is not to classify it." (Reports 1861, p. 143).

At the Session of 26 November 1860 Jules Falret[23] offered to identify "the principles that govern, in all sciences, the development of *natural* classifications":

> 1) A class should be defined in terms of a set of features present in all the objects to be encompassed and not in terms of *one* character that might artificially bring together objects which would be different if other features were to be considered; 2) the said feature-set should itself be organized in a hierarchy so that its essential components are clearly identified, 3) the objects that come under one class should not only share the feature set at a given moment in time but show that they have evolved in a similar manner [acquired the features in an order that can be predicted] (Reports 1861, p. 147).

Criteria 1 and 2 addressed the issue of monothetic classifications; criterion 3 reflected the influence of evolution theory and set a task that remains unfulfilled to this day: few psychiatrists will consider *the order in which the symptoms appear* as a classificatory criterion (however, see Fava and Kellner 1993). Falret went on to criticize classifications relying on one feature or character alone: "1) an intellectual faculty or 2) a predominant idea or emotion or 3) act or 4) the features and extension of a *délire*" (Reports 1861, p. 148) and concluded that "mania, monomania, melancholia and dementia are but provisional symptomatic clusters and not true natural species of mental disorders" (Reports 1861, p. 171). Morel replied that "although [he] was not planning to talk... he felt the need to intervene as his ideas had been questioned by Delasiauve and Falret." In a rambly intervention he justified his view that hereditary mental disorders existed although "three elements converge to create them: predisposition, a cause, and a series of transformations of pathological phenomena that... determine the place that a given disorder will occupy in the nosological classification" (Reports, 1861, p. 176).

The session of 10 December was occupied by the debate between Adolphe Garnier[24] and Alfred Maury.[25] Garnier stated that since it was impossible to take all the features of the objects to be classified into account, groupings based on a limited number led to blurred boundaries and to "patients floating between two classes." He explained that this was the reason why alienists tried to complement their classifications with speculation about etiology (what earlier in this chapter was called the proxyhood issue). He believed that such speculation should not be considered as a *feature* of the psychiatric object and concluded, quoting Saint-Hilaire and Cuvier, that this particular issue had no solution. Instead, he suggested a dynamic classification of mental disorders [could be developed] based on mental faculties" (Report 1861, pp. 316–320). Very sensibly, Maury clarified that because in the area of psychological medicine little was known about causes only "artificial" classifications were possible and attacked Garnier for sponsoring a "psychological view," that is for believing that "[mental disorder was just] a consequence of an emotional turmoil present in the heart of man, and which in the event enslaves him and takes his freedom away." Whilst strong emotions might cause insanity there were many cases where the symptoms overcame the patient, for example, those resulting from brain diseases. The question "was not to classify mental disorders from a philosophical viewpoint in terms of which mental faculty seemed involved but in terms of its pathological origins... otherwise it will not be possible to differentiate mental illness from normal behaviour (e.g., monomania from dreaming)": "We must not forget that we are not here in the world of metaphysics but in psychological medicine. We classify mental disorders to cure them and this is why we must try and find out their aetiology" (Report 1861, pp. 320–322). This argument has been repeated ad nauseam every since.

Garnier's rejoinder took most of the session on 24 December. After iterating his view that "looking for efficient causes according to Bacon's principles"[26] was the best way to achieve a classification, he explained why Delasiauve had felt unable to classify insanity according to the received view on the psychology of the intellectual functions:

> It is not possible to create a classification of insanity based on a conventional division of intelligence into judgement, reasoning, etc. because the latter modes are not independent but blend with each other and with attention and memory . . . Hence, it might be better to divide intelligence according to the objects it deals with (Reports, 1861, pp. 323).

Little he knew that this was precisely the way in which classifications were to shape up towards the end of the century. Then, turning on Maury Garnier stated:

> He tells me, you do not take into account physical causes but are only preoccupied with psychological ones . . . I reply, although a spiritualist I am not afraid of matter but when I look for it I cannot find it . . . insanity is a disturbance of the intellectual faculties and requires a specific method of observation . . . there is as little point in listing insanities due to saturnism, alcoholism, etc. as if they were listing due to diseases of the liver. Changes in this organ do not cause the insanity. It is in the brain where the cause must be sought. If that part of the brain that produces hallucinations is affected by a lesion in any way, including by touching it with a finger, it will lead to the same symptom (Reports, 1861, pp. 325)

The issue could not be better argued today.

At the session of 29 January 1861 Buchez summarized the debate thus far: "on the one hand, papers have been read here suggesting that insanity would be just the one disease with diverse manifestations"[27] from which follows that descriptive and classificatory publications only scratch its surface and "on the other hand, papers have been read trying to identify organic aetiology, pathogenesis.". "the Baconian method is used in medicine under the name of 'method of exclusion' but has had little influence on natural history" . . . "Diseases are not independent entities, existing by themselves, with a life of their own, like plants or animals. They fully depend upon a living organism and exist only in it."[28] Because "a classification must be above all a faithful reflection of the science of its time" Buchez felt that he needed to explain to the audience what was the ongoing state of the philosophy of science and proceeded to do so. He concluded by, once again, supporting Morel and his organic classification (Reports, 1861, pp. 326–330).

Garnier retort was conciliatory: "The question then is to know whether there are various insanities or only one. Buchez seemed inclined towards the latter. To determine this we must use the Baconian method… But he is right in saying that the latter is not relevant to natural history" (Reports, 1861, pp. 326–330). Archambault closed the session rather bluntly:[29] "Garnier and Buchez seem to be employing the words madness (*folie*), mental alienation, mental illness etc. as if they meant the same. As far as I am concerned they have different meaning." Stung by this comment Buchez replied: "madness and mental alienation do not mean the same; mental alienation has however a much wider meaning" (Reports, 1861, pp. 332).

The debate went on for three more session: 25 February, 25 March and 29 April. By then it had become repetitive and although various new speakers appeared (e.g., Parchappe and Lisle) no new conceptual points were made.

Desruelles et al. saw in the 1860–61 French debate the reflection of a clash between Traditionalists (defenders of Esquirol's monomania concept) and Innovators (Morel's followers) (Desruelles et al. 1934, p. 648). In fact the debate was more than that: it was the occasion when the taxonomy of psychiatry was constructed. Because the debate was soon taken over by philosophers of science and mind (Maury, Buchez, Garnier, etc) a brilliant opportunity arose to analyze hidden assumptions and set out taxonomic principles and rules. Thus, all participants (including alienists) came to realize that classifying general diseases was not like classifying plants or animals and that classifying madness went well beyond the "unitary psychosis" issue. More to the point, they realized that the classification debate in psychiatry was not to be resolved by the superficial application of some "empirical" method (Berrios and Beer 1994). One wishes that these insights had survived to our own day.

19th-century French alienists were aware of the fact that bad classifications were an obstacle to data collecting and empirical research and this led to a second debate (1889) at the *Société Médico-Psychologique*.[30] At European level, there were also two particularly important meetings. In 1885, The Congress of Mental Medicine at Antwerp appointed a Commission to consider all existing classifications. The results were discussed at the Paris Congress of 1889 and a classification drawn by Dr. Morel from Ghent was adopted. Rather ruefully, Daniel Hack Tuke wrote in 1892: "it has yet to be seen whether asylum physicians will adopt it in their tables" (Tuke 1882, p. 233).

6.5 **Discussion and conclusion**

The psychiatric epistemologist can study classifications in two ways: (1) accept the "received view" that the rules of classifying are inherent to nature and the human mind and that they fit in perfectly into the eternal ontology of all psychiatric objects or (2) consider psychiatric classifications as cultural products. This lecture follows the second approach. After mapping the history of classification and its metalanguage, the first section showed that it is essential to differentiate between taxonomy, classification and its object domain, and that the ontological and epistemological nature of the psychiatric object is far more important to developing a sensical classification than any statistical or empirical procedure that may be applied to objects which are far from understood. It also showed that there is a real danger than proxy variables which originally are chosen as mere handles or correlational terms end up replacing the disease itself by a process that the 20th century has for some obscure reason chosen to call "naturalization."

During the 19th century alienism borrowed from general medicine the so-called "anatomo-clinical" model of disease. To this day, this epistemological device enjoins psychiatrists to anchor both the psychiatric object and its putative classification in neurobiology. Looking for a "biological invariant" responsible for surface events (symptoms) still seems a task worth pursuing. This has led to a neglect of the mechanism of psychogenesis and of the manner in which accepting this principle may lead to an entirely different way of classifying "mental disorders."

During the last few years, the view has been proposed that many "mental disorders" are just episteme-bound clusters of complaints with a low ontological and trans-epistemic index (i.e., they are not natural kinds and hence do not survive well translocation from one historical period to the next) and that "mental symptoms" may in fact be more appropriate units of neurobiological and epistemological analysis (Marková and Berrios 2009). This view has different taxonomic consequences for classifying symptoms becomes a different epistemological enterprise (Marková and Berrios 1995).

In general terms, taxonomy and its associated classificatory activity constitute a self-contained and more or less exhaustive conceptual system. Within a given historical period, thinking about and crafting classifications is like playing a game of chess in that everything will occur within strict boundaries and according to explicit or implicit rules. For example, not all possible moves will be made: some because they are forbidden by the rules, others because they are patently non-sensical and yet others because they are unfashionable. Up to the 19th century most of the classificatory game was played within biology and concerned natural kinds. Within this domain classifications are important for they can generate knowledge. Classifications of artificial objects, common as they may be, have only actuarial function and everyone recognizes that. The issue here is what is the nature of psychiatric classifications. Certainly, it would be rather nonsense to believe that they are like plants and hence one day we will be able to classify mental disorders by using a sort of *per genus et differentia* technique or even worse, creating some sort of neuropsychological periodic table of elements on the basis of which we could predict the existence of some new forms of mental disorder which have not yet been reported!

In summary, 17th-century taxonomic theory was constructed to make possible the classification of plants, animals and minerals, and hopefully be able to predict new information about the nature of the members of a given class (Bowker and Star 1999; Winston 1999). Whether classifications are based on privileged features or countenance the possibility of a numerical taxonomy, they work at their best when the objects to be classified are ontologically stable (e.g., are natural kinds) and epistemologically accessible (defined by capturable attributes). When applied to abstract objects (e.g., virtues), artifacts (e.g., poems) or constructs (e.g., mental symptoms or disorders), such classificatory approaches are no longer on safe territory and require for their functioning of ad hoc epistemological aids. When applied outside of their field of competence and validity, it is not possible to predict what modifications classificatory systems require and much research (both conceptual and empirical) needs to be done to decide which are required by each type of object to be classified. The inchoate nature of our current knowledge on the epistemological and ontological status of psychiatric objects makes it particularly difficult to decide on what modifications within the classificatory system are required and on what expectations should classificators have in respect to the usefulness of classifying mental disorders.

After all, when talking about classifications, one should take the word seriously. Classifications are more than lists, glossaries or inventories; they are structured and (often enough) hierarchical clusters of objects holding a relationship with one another. The more one thinks about their application to mental disorders the more one realizes that the problem here is not only our lack of knowledge about taxonomy but the fact that psychiatric objects may not be susceptible to classification at all.

Endnotes

1 By far this is the most popular method and most historical accounts of classification consist in chronological lists, e.g., Menninger (1964), Faber (1923), Boor (1954).

2 According to this approach, medical classifications reflect more the social and economic variables modulating disease than its biology. Rather surprisingly, no good social history of psychiatric classifications has yet been written.

3 The issue of the "reality" of the concept of species remains unresolved. Darwin himself looked at the term species, as one arbitrarily given for the sake of convenience to a set of individuals closely resembling each other. (Darwin 1970, p. 108). For a discussion of the current state of systematics see Sober (1993).

4 For a proposal for a polythetic classification see Corning and Steffy (1979).

5 For a recent example of a proposal for an artificial classification, i.e., one that emphasizes certain features or "questions" see Mellergård (1987)

6 See Berrios and Hauser (1988). For a retrospective diagnostic ascertainment of a selected cluster of Kraepelin's patients see Jablensky et al. (1993). On the origin of the categories themselves and the small role played by empirical research in Kraepelin's classification see: Weber and Engstrom (1997).

7 In this regard, Jaspers's views are well known: "The principle of medical diagnosis is that all the disease phenomena should be characterized within a single diagnosis. Where a number of different phenomena co-exist the question arises which of them should be preferred for diagnostic purposes so that the remaining phenomena can be considered secondary or accidental" (Jaspers 1963, pp. 611–612).

8 The literature on the philosophical and psychological nature of "concepts" is large, see van Mechelen et al. (1993); Fodor (1998), Peacocke (1992), Palmer (1988), Weitz (1988), Rickert (1986).

9 Prototypes (see Rosch 1978) in the field of psychiatry have also been called "ideal types" (see Schwartz and Wiggins 1987) and "hypothetical construct" (see Morey 1991).

10 Pinel requires no introduction. See Riese (1969) Postel (1981), Garrabé (1994).

11 W. Cullen (1710–1790): born in Scotland, trained in Glasgow, and eventually professor at Edinburgh, Cullen is one of the most important clinicians, classificators and medical philosophers of the 18th century. His emphasis on the role of the central nervous system in the development of all diseases led to his neural-pathology hypothesis. His concept of "neurosis" (a word he coined) is therefore overinclusive and caused much difficulty during the following century.

12 Sydenham's approach has been called more botanico, i.e., "in the fashion of botany" and was firmly held by 18th-century nosologists (see López Piñero 1983, p. 13). In this regard, Linné's epigram is also well known: "Symptomata se habent ad morbum ut folia et fulcra ad plantam". At the beginning of the 19th century, Pinel was still stating: "The revolution brought about by Linné in natural history, together with the introduction of a method to offer descriptions that be short and exact, could not but greatly influence medicine" (see Pinel 1813, p. lxxxiv).

13 Whether such beliefs concern classification or categorization remains unclear. At any rate, the underlying rules and mechanisms are far from being understood (on this see the brilliant Estes (1994)).

14 The "Kantian revolution" was partially about the identification of general categories in terms of which knowledge might be organized.

15 For example, Mill stated that naming something as X is already classifying for two classes follow: X and not X (Mill 1898, p. 76).

16 During the 18th century classifications were also caught up in the issue of whether the mind was capable of penetrating nature or whether divisions were only in the mind of man (see

Jordanova 1984). In regards to the origin of the concept of "privileged features", it is likely that this originated from Locke's view that: "because nature contains only many particulars resembling each other in many ways we must decide which differences between individuals objects, whether grossly salient or barely noticeable, to include in our abstract ideas of them and thus in our definitions of general terms" (Guyer 1994, p. 145).

17 Surprisingly, it is not mentioned in Pichot (1984).

18 It is not often mentioned that men such as Kraepelin and Chaslin went through nationalistic periods and attacked psychiatric developments in rival countries. Kraepelin was a Bismarckian à outrance and wrote a paper comparing his own personality to Bismarck's! (see Kraepelin 1921). Chaslin attacked the use of German nosological categories in France and enjoining his fellow-country men to develop their own nosology (see Berrios and Fuentenebro 1995). There were also efforts to compare French and German psychiatric classifications, e.g., Roubinovitch (1896).

19 Philippe Buchez (1796–1866) physician, publicist and social reformer, for a time associated with the Carbonari and the Saint-Simoniens, he developed a form of Christian socialism and wrote on history, psychology and psychiatry. His parliamentary career came to a holt in 1848 when as President of the Constituent Assembly he showed indecisiveness vis-à-vis the disorderly conduct of pro-Poland protesters (see Biéder 1986; Robaux 1965).

20 The debates of the Société Médico Psychologique brought together the great alienists of the day and often reached important conclusions: themes such as Hallucinations and Classifications were debated more than once.

21 Louis Jean Françoise Delasiauve (1804–1893) was a physician with political and literary interests turned alienist. He researched and wrote on epilepsy, mental retardation and education.

22 Bénédict-Augustin Morel (1809–1873) is well known for his writings on degeneration and démence précoce. However, his output and interests were wider. Morel and Buchez were closed friends. Morel attacked all psychiatric classifications based on symptoms and proposed instead an "aetiological" criterion. Buchez's favourable review appeared as "Rapport sur le Traité des Maladies Mentales de M. Morel". *Annales Médico-Psychologiques* 1860, **6**, 613–35. Morel's classification included six (purportedly aetiological) groups: '1) Hereditary Insanity, 2) Toxic insanity, 3) Insanity Produced by the transformations of other diseases, 4) Idiopathic insanity, 5) Sympathetic insanity, 6) Dementia' (Morel 1860).

23 Jules Falret (1824–1902), son of the alienist Jean Pierre Falret (1794–1870) was a bright and shy academic who grew in the shadow of his authoritarian father. A friend of Lasègue and Morel, he researched into general paralysis of the insane, delusions, epilepsy and folie a deux.

24 Adolphe Garnier (1802–1864), distinguished philosopher of mind, died (it is said of grief after the death of his only son) 4 years after his intervention at the SMP meeting. Trained under Jouffroy, Garnier wrote a thesis on Thomas Reid and can be considered as one of main French expositors of the Scottish Philosophy of Common Sense. A defender of a version of Faculty Psychology (see his *La Psychologie et la Phrénologie Comparées*. Paris: Hachette, 1839), Garnier proposed a new classification of mental faculties in his *Traité des Facultés de l'ame* (Paris: Hachette, 1852). His intervention in the SMP debate is important for it illustrated the interdisciplinary nature of the SMP and because he brought into the debate the tenets of French philosophy of mind: a combination of faculty psychology and spiritualist eclecticism (for an account of Garnier's philosophy see Charles (1875).

25 Alfred Maury (1817–1892) was a polymath trained in mathematics, the law, archaeology and medicine; through his friendship with Baillarger and Moreau de Tours he became interested in psychological medicine. A Republican, he took an anti-Catholic stance and argued always

in favour of an organicist approach to mental illness (on Maury himself see Bowman (1978)). At the debate on hallucinations (particularly as experienced by Roman Catholic saints, Pascal and Socrates) he was on the side of Lélut in believing that these experiences were the result of a disease of the brain (see his *Des hallucinations*, Paris: Bourgogne & Martinet; 1845; for an account of the hallucinations debate see Dowbiggin (1990); James (1995). It is difficult to imagine a wider ideological gap than that separating Maury and Garnier. Hence their debate on psychiatric classification on 10 December 1860 is important.

26 Francis Bacon (1561–1626): Cambridge trained English statesman and philosopher of science whose work underwent a revival during the 19th century. Bacon's principles are contained in the Instauratio Magna (Great Instauration), his grand plan to help man to regain control upon the natural world: a classification of the sciences; new principles to interpret nature (Novum Organon); a guide and catalogue of the phenomena of the universe, i.e., a veritable corpus of empirical data and research methodologies; the Ladder of the intellect; anticipations of the new philosophy; and the new philosophy or active science (see Robertson 1905, p. 248). For a study of Bacon's classification methodology see: Chapters 1–3 of Peltonen (1996). Bacon tried to persuade James I to found "science" chairs at Oxford and Cambridge. His advice went unheeded but there is agreement amongst historians that the later foundation by Charles II of the Royal Society is a late reflection of Baconianism.

27 This concept is currently discussed as the "Unitary Psychosis" hypothesis (see Berrios and Beer 1994).

28 Buchez was here criticizing the 19th-century remnants of the old "ontological" model of disease (see Riese 1953; Vié 1940).

29 Théophile Archambault (1806–1863) was a senior alienist and secretary general of the SMP. He died within 2 years of this intervention. He was a disciple of Esquirol and knew English well. In 1840, he translated into French Ellis's *Treatise on the Nature, Causes Symptoms and Treatment of Insanity* (1838). He did classical work on urinary incontinence in the insane.

30 There is no space in this paper to touch upon this debate (which stretched from the meeting of July 1888 to that of June 1889 [Annales Médico-Psychologiques]) where a new generation of French psychiatrists had a second go at the problem. A conceptual analysis of this debate and a comparison with the 1860–1861 must be part of any future history of psychiatric classifications.

Chapter References

Adanson, M. (1763). Préface Istorike sur l'état ancien et actuel de la Botanike, et une Téorie de cette science. In *Familles des Plantes, First Part*. Paris: Vincent, pp. i–cccxxv.

Anderson, T. W. (1968). *Classification and discrimination*. In Sills, D. L. (ed.), *International Encyclopaedia of the Social Sciences*. London: Macmillan, pp. 553–9.

Berrios, G. E. (1996). The classification of mental disorders: Part III. (K.L. Kahlbaum, trans. and Introduction). *History of Psychiatry*, 7, 167–82.

Berrios, G. E. (1999). Classification in psychiatry: a conceptual history. *Australian and New Zealand Journal of Psychiatry*, 33, 145–60.

Berrios, G. E. (2008). Introduction and Translation of Baillarger "Essay on a Classification of Different Genera of Insanity" Classic Text 75. *History of Psychiatry*, 19, 358–73.

Berrios, G. E. and Beer, D. (1994). The notion of Unitary Psychosis: a conceptual history. *History of Psychiatry*, 5, 13–36.

Berrios, G. E. and Fuentenebro F. (1995). Introduction to, and translation of, Chaslin's 'Is psychiatry a well-made language?' *History of Psychiatry*, 6, 387–406.

Berrios, G. E. and Hauser R. (1988). The early development of Kraepelin's ideas on classification. a conceptual history. *Psychological Medicine*, **18**, 813–21.

Berthelot, A. (1889). *La Grande Encyclopédie Vol 11.* Paris: H. Lamirault.

Biéder, J. (1986). Un précurseur de la démocratie chrétienne et de l'Europe à la Société Médico-Psychologique: Philippe-Joseph-Benjamin Buchcz. *Annales Médico-Psychologiques*, **144**, 109–15.

Boor, W. de (1954). *Psychiatrische Systematik.* Berlin: Springer.

Bouillaud, J. (1846). *Traité de nosographie médicale.* 5 Vols. Paris: Baillière.

Bowker, G. C. and Star, S. L. (1999). *Sorting Things Out.* Cambridge, MA: MIT Press.

Bowman, F. P. (1978). Du romanticisme au positivisme: Alfred Maury. *Romanticisme,* (no volume) 21–22; 35–53.

Buchez, P. (1861). Reports, *Annales Médico-Psychologique*, **7**, 326–30.

Charles, É. (1875). Garnier. In A. Franck (ed.), *Dictionnaire des Sciences Philosophiques* (2nd ed.). Paris: Hachette, pp. 593–94.

Cooper, R. (2005). *Classifying Madness.* Dordrecht: Springer.

Corning, W. C. and Steffy, R. A. (1979). Taximetric strategies applied to psychiatric classification. *Schizophrenic Bulletin*, **5**, 294–305.

Crane, J. K. (2003). Locke's theory of classification. *British Journal for the History of Philosophy*, **11**, 249–59.

Dagognet, F. (1970). *Le catalogue de la vie.* Paris: Presses Universitaires de France.

Darwin, C. (1970). *The origin of species.* Harmonsworth: Penguin (1st edition 1859).

Desruelles, M., Léculier, P. and Gardien, M. P. (1934). Contribution a l'histoire des classifications psychiatriques. *Annales Médico-Psychologiques*, **92**, 637–75.

Dowbiggin, I. (1990). Alfred Maury and the politics of the unconscious in nineteenth century France. *History of Psychiatry*, **1**, 255–87.

Dupré, J (1981). Natural kinds and biological taxa. *Philosophical Review*, **90**, 66–90.

Ellenberger, H. (1963). Les illusions de la classification psychiatrique. *L'Evolution Psychiatrique*, **28**, 221–48.

Estes, W. K. (1994). *Classification and Cognition.* Oxford : Oxford University Press.

Faber, K. (1923). *Nosography in Modern Medicine.* London: Oxford University Press.

Fodor J. S. (1998) *Concepts.* Oxford: Clarendon Press.

Foucault M. (1966). *Les Mots et les Choses.* Paris: Gallimard.

Garrabé, J. (ed.) (1994). *Philippe Pinel.* Paris: Les Empêcheurs de Penser en Rond.

Granger, H. (1985). The Scala Naturae and the Continuity of Kinds. *Phronesis*, **30**, 181–200.

Guyer, P. (1994). Locke's philosophy of language. In Chappell V. (ed.), *The Cambridge Companion to Locke.* Cambridge: Cambridge University Press, pp. 115–45.

Hampton, J. (1993). Prototype models of concept representation. In I. van Mechelen, J. Hampton, R. S. Muchalski and P. Theuns (eds.), *Categories and concepts.* London: Academic Press, pp. 67–95.

Jablensky, A., Hugler, H., von Cranach, M. and Kalinov, K. (1993). Kraepelin revisited: a reassessment and statistical analysis of dementia praecox and manic depressive insanity in 1908. *Psychological Medicine*, **23**, 843–58.

James, T. (1995). *Dream, Creativity and Madness in Nineteenth Century France.* Oxford: Clarendon Press.

Jaspers, K. (1963). *General Psychopathology* (J. Hoenig and M.W. Hamilton trans), Manchester: Manchester University Press.

Jordanova, L. J. (1984). *Lamarck*. Oxford: Oxford University Press.

Kraepelin, E. (1921). Bismarck's Persönlichkeit. Ungedruckte persönliche Erinnerungen. *Süddetische Monatshefte*, **19**, 105–22.

Lanteri-Laura, G. (1984). Classification et Sémiologie. *Confrontations Psychiatriques*, **24**, 57–77.

López Piñero, J. J. (1983). *Historical Origins of the Concept of Neuroses* (D. Berrios trans.). Cambridge: Cambridge University Press.

Marková, I. S. and Berrios, G. E. (1995). Mental symptoms: are they similar phenomena? *Psychopathology*, **28**, 147–57.

Marková, I. S. and Berrios, G. E. (2009). Epistemology of mental symptoms. *Psychopathology*, **42**, 343–49.

Mellergård, M. (1987). Psychiatric classifications as a reflection of uncertainties. *Acta Psychiatrica Scandinavica*, **76**, 106–11.

Menninger, K. (1964). *The vital balance*. New York: The Viking Press.

Mill, J. S. (1898). *A System of Logic*. London: Longmans, Green, and Co.

Morel, B. A. (1860). *Traité des Maladies Mentales*, Paris: Masson, pp. 258–72.

Morey, L. C. (1991). Classification of mental disorder as a collection of hypothetical constructs. *Journal of Abnormal Psychology*, **100**, 289–93.

Palmer, A. (1988). *Concept and Object*. London: Routledge.

Peacocke, C. (1992). *A Study of Concepts*. Cambridge, MA: MIT Press.

Peltonen, M. (ed.) (1996). *The Cambridge Companion to Bacon*. Cambridge: Cambridge University Press.

Pichot P. J. (1984). The French approach to psychiatric classification. *British Journal of Psychiatry*, **144**, 113–18.

Pinel, Ph. (1813). *Nosographie Philosophique* (3 Vols. 5th ed.). Paris: J.A. Brosson.

Postel, J. (1981). *Genèse de la Psychiatrie*. Paris: Le Sycomore.

Rickert, H. (1986). *The limits of concept formation in natural science*. Cambridge: Cambridge University Press (First published in 1902).

Riese, W. (1945). History and principles of classification of nervous diseases. *Bulletin of the History of Medicine*, **25**, 465–512.

Riese, W. (1953). *The Conception of Disease. Its History, its Versions and its Nature*. New York: Philosophical Library.

Riese, W. (1969). *The legacy of Philippe Pinel*. New York: Springer.

Robaux (no initial). (1965). La vie de Buchez. Annales de Thérapeutique Psychiatrique, **4**, 220–34.

Robertson, J. M. (ed.) (1905). *The Philosophical Works of Francis Bacon*. London: George Routledge and Sons.

Rosch, E. (1978). Principles of categorization. In E. Rosch and B. Lloyd (eds.) *Cognition and Categorization*. Hillsdale, NJ: Lawrence Erlbaum, pp. 27–47.

Roubinovitch, J. (1896). *Des variétés cliniques de la folie en France et en Allemagne*. Paris: Doin.

Rousseau, N. (1986). *Connaissance et langage chez Condillac*. Geneva: Droz.

Schwartz, M. A. and Wiggins, O. P. (1987). Diagnosis and ideal types: a contribution to psychiatric classification. *Comprehensive Psychiatry*, **28**, 277–91.

Sober, E. (1993). *Philosophy of biology*. Oxford: Oxford University Press.

Speziale, P. (1973). Classification of the sciences. In P. P. Wiener (ed.), *Dictionary of the History of Ideas, Vol 1*. New York: Charles Scribner's Sons, pp. 462–7.

Sydenham, T. (1848). *The works of Thomas Sydenham MD*. 2 vols. London: Printed for the Sydenham Society.

Tuke, D. H. (1882). Classifications. In D. H. Tuke (ed.), *Dictionary of Psychological Medicine*. 2 vols. London: Churchill, pp. 229–33.

Vernon, K. (1988). The founding of numerical taxonomy. *British Journal for the History of Science*, **21**, 143–59.

Vié, J. (1940). Sur l'existence d'entités morbides en psychiatrie, l'utilité et l'orientation de l'effort nosologique. *Annales Médico-Psychologiques*, **98**, 347–58.

Weber, M. M. and Engstrom, E. J. (1997). Kraepelin's "diagnostic cards": the confluence of clinical research and preconceived categories. *History of Psychiatry*, **8**, 375–85.

Weitz, M. (1988). *Theories of Concepts: a history of the major philosophical tradition*. London: Routledge.

Wilkerson, T. (1993). Species, essences, and the names of natural kinds. *Philosophical Quarterly*, **43**, 1–19.

Windelband, W. (1949). *Historia y Ciencia de la Naturaleza. En Preludios Filosóficos*. Translation of Wenceslao Roces. Buenos Aires: Santiago Rueda, pp. 311–28 (original German edition 1903).

Winston, J. E. (1999). *Describing species*. New York: Columbia University Press.

Chapter 6: Comments

The nature of the psychiatric object and classification

Josef Parnas

In this commentary, I wish to elaborate on some of Berrios's conclusive claims. Berrios offers us his typically erudite and sharp, as well as systematic and instructive, historical and epistemological perspective on the formation of modern psychiatric nosology. One important conclusion from his essay is that psychiatric classification is a cultural, historically situated enterprise, inspired by practical goals, guided not only by empirical knowledge but by conceptual assumptions as well. No classification arises in a conceptual vacuum. None can claim a purely empirical or atheoretical virginity, untainted by thought and ideas. As Jaspers (1963) pointed out, many "main stream" claims rest on unstated, often unexamined, metaphysical assumptions.

Berrios ends with a critical gesture towards our contemporary predicament: "The participants of the French debate all (…) came to realize that classifying (…) diseases was not like classifying plants or animals and that classifying madness went well beyond the 'unitary psychosis' issue (…) They realized that the classification debate in psychiatry was not to be resolved by the superficial application of some 'empirical' method. *One wishes that these insights had survived to our own day*" [my italics].

Berrios is right that the most relevant epistemological discussion in nosology today should concern the nature "psychiatric object": the ontological and epistemological nature of the psychiatric object" is (…) crucial to developing a (…) classification." He believes (and I agree) that this discussion cannot be settled by "any statistical or empirical procedure" (see also Berrios and Merková (2002) for a more detailed account).

Berrios is skeptical of the contemporary mainstream approach ("anatomo-clinical" model of disease) that "anchors both the psychiatric object and its putative classification in neurobiology," often using "proxy variables."

The "psychiatric object" is Berrios' designation for symptomatology of people referred to or seeking psychiatrist or clinical psychologist for help, and it includes what we traditionally call symptoms, signs and syndromes. Berrios claims that "psychiatric object" is a "hybrid," i.e., a culturally constituted entity, carrying within it a "biological signal." This position is sufficiently inclusive that it is impossible to disagree with it. For example, my current interest and reflection on the ongoing political developments in North Africa undoubtedly possess a "biological signal," because this reflection arises in a biological organism (me). This particular "mental object" is also culturally co-constituted and influenced, e.g., by my belief network, geographical and historical knowledge, access to TV and the Internet, etc.—an innumerable host of factors. This interest would be perhaps different (plausibly more intense, engaged, and better informed) if I were born in North Africa. It is not absolutely clear how a "biological signal" inhering in my reflection on North Africa would compare to a hypothetical biological signal inhering in a thematically similar overvalued idea, also concerning North Africa. Were we to venture to study this issue more closely, we would need an a priori examination of whether the "normal" and the "overvalued" thinking are phenomenologically distinguishable, and if so, in what way. In other words, we would like to know if the distinction between "normal" and "overvalued" experience depends on their respective *contents* or on the *structure or form* of experience as well (e.g., in the "overvalued" case, a special dependence on background beliefs such as a general conspiratorial outlook or an extraordinary affective valence). We will most likely come to realize that the issue of *content normality* in this particular case will be heavily dependent on *normativity*, i.e., on common sense and social convention. Perhaps, a clear and sharp distinction between the "biological" and "semantic" components may turn out to be much more difficult than usually anticipated. Perhaps, our useful habitual dichotomies between "internal"/"external," "organism/ environment" (and countless related other) are, in fact, much more fluid or even not quite dissociable (Thompson 2007). Some recent voices from the philosophy of mind and neuroscience deny that we can locate cognition exclusively in the brain (Noë 2009). Rather, their claim is that cognition is always embedded, i.e., truly ecologically distributed.

It is that kind of problems that an informed and non-dogmatic discussion of the "psychiatric object" should include.

So far, several options for linking the "biological signal" and its putative "semantic" expression have been in play, of which I will mention a few, not sharply delimited. A radical but counter-intuitive (and clinically unappealing) philosophical proposal is known as eliminativism (Churchland 1986). Transferred to psychiatry, it would simply claim that the "psychiatric object" *does not exist*. Consciousness needs to be eliminated. It is a misleading illusion, comparable to our earlier, discredited beliefs in, say, phlogiston. A more realistic tendency is to evade, at least initially, the "psychiatric object." The ambitious R-Doc research program of the NIH (First, Chapter 7, this volume) seems in essence to suspend any concern with the psychiatric object and seeks an independent enlightenment through a bottom-up functional study of putatively delimited neural circuits. A similar posture is to replace the "psychiatric object" with "proxy variables," such as the so-called endophenotypes. A tendency to transform the notion of schizophrenia into a cognitive deficit-disorder, i.e., to neurologize schizophrenia into a kind of dementia, is another contemporary example (Urfer-Parnas et al. 2010). When the inner life of the patient cannot be bypassed, then the third-person data-format becomes directly imposed on the exploration of the patients' first person perspective (e.g., through the highly structured interviews, directly producing diagnostic, criteria-compatible information).

From a general epistemological perspective it is not too much to say that the contemporary psychiatric epistemology is strongly behaviorist, favoring "objective signs" ("third-person" features) rather than subjective phenomena ("first person"), as it is metaphysically physicalist (despite its claim of an atheoretical stance). To some extent, both of these attitudes are remnants, fuelled by the still operating, traumatic memories of the era of psychoanalytic domination in the US.

However, the prospects for a physicalist reduction of experiential phenomena remain elusive (Bennet and Hacker 2003; Chalmers 2010). What is at least needed as a preamble is a better understanding of the nature of the "psychiatric object." Phenomena of consciousness are not like the physical *objects* i.e., as *things*, an ancient insight of countless philosophers. The scope of this commentary does not allow to present any alternative in a comprehensive and coherent detail (see Gallagher and Zahavi 2008; Parnas and Sass 2008; Parnas and Zahavi 2002). Yet it is perhaps uncontroversial and acceptable for most people to concur that their conscious life (their personal experiences) is characteristically lived from a "privileged"[1] (radically intimate, private) perspective, "the first-person perspective." The *subjectivity of consciousness is of the essence* (Nagel 1986; see also Searle 1992, pp. 116–118, for a very clear exposition). Foucault (1994), whom Berrios credits with archaeology of links between words and things, stated in his survey of "representation" that "man is a strange empirico-transcendental doublet since he is a being such that knowledge will be attained in him of what renders all knowledge possible" (p. 318). This means, in the epistemic context, that the human being is *both* an empirical object and a transcendental subject, i.e., a condition of possibility for its own study. This essence has implications for the nature of the being of consciousness (and more broadly for the entire "psychiatric object") and on the possible ways of its description, grasping its divisions, internal dynamics and intersubjective dimensions (including the cultural).

I think that it is an empirically unfounded, and conceptually mistaken, view to assume that the empirical, scientific study of consciousness (including its wider connotation as the "psychiatric object") *is precluded* by its subjectivity (first person nature). Rather, I think, the conversion of first person data into the third person format, suitable for empirical use, *is feasible*, but requires a theoretically informed and epistemologically adequate (faithful) and reliable *second person approach*, and a grasp of theoretical complexity of the "psychiatric object." This is basically what the psychiatric phenomenology is all about and why it is relevant for the psychiatric research and practice (Jaspers 1963; Parnas and Zahavi 2002; Sass and Parnas 2006).

It is imperative for any sensical nosological project to adopt an epistemologically *adequate* approach to the nature of its object. Berrios is right in pointing out that a thorough discussion of the epistemological and ontological nature of the "psychiatric object" is an urgently needed, fundamental, and a potentially transformative task at hand, relevant not only for a psychiatric nosology but also, I think, for the entire *metier* of psychiatry. Such a resurrection of psychopathology, a science of the "psychiatric object," should ideally include an interdisciplinary input from philosophy, phenomenology, philosophy of mind and science, biology, linguistics, basic neuroscience, psychology, cognitive sciences and many other relevant disciplines. It would require a space for rigorous theoretical dissent and debate, which is not easy to realize in practice. Berrios's historical reference to Dilthey could be here fruitfully rekindled as a useful preparatory primer for the potential future debaters (Dilthey 2010). And finally, scientific research needs a closer, more intimate contact to the clinical experience.

The debate, in order to stay on track, should be inspired and constrained by the testimonies obtained from our own contemporaneous patients, rather than be predominantly based on the historical narratives collected and communicated by Kraepelin, Bleuler, and their colleagues.

A natural question that imposes itself is whether a nosological debate, which the French alienists held in the 19th century, is repeatable, still possible today, in an "atheoretical" climate, encouraging only a "minimum of inference"?

It is in the nature of science to be conservative (Kuhn 1970). The canonical paradigm always tends to perpetuate itself and eliminates occasional rival novel ideas, which, by the way, often turn out to be false. Probably, certain alternatives never even arise because they are unconceivable under the pressure of the dominating thought (Kyle Stanford 2006).

Yet, on this particular point, there is an immense difference between the 19th-century French debate and the contemporary nosological situation—a difference, quite apart from the obviously striking technological, scientific and sociocultural transformations.

The French debaters, mindful of their intellectual reputation and unaware of their Impact Factors, left the Société Médico-Psychologique and went home to pursue their ideas and treat their patients. Their nosological discussion was a discussion among a few, devoted specialists, with a slow and limited geographical impact. In comparison, the DSM of today has almost a universal biblical status, but unlike the Rosetta Stone, it is readable and used by legion and not only by a handful of initiated scholars.

The DSM-III+ project has been successful beyond any conceivable expectations. The DSM manual and its international counterpart (ICD-10) is being used everywhere and by everyone, by psychiatrists, clinical psychologists, nurses, social workers, bureaucrats of health facilities, insurance companies, legal systems, pharmaceutical industry, and, not least, by the research community, funding agencies, editors, and referees of the scientific journals. One need not to be a sociologist to suspect that the magnitude and the diversity of the vested interests and the extra-scientific influences in today's psychiatric classification is incomparable with what was the case in the 19th-century France (see Kendler's Introduction, this chapter). Reifications of diagnostic categories become inevitable (like in a fashionable expression of "converting" to schizophrenia, from, say, social phobia).

The DSM system as a whole, with its ubiquitous use, creates its own semantic universe, i.e., an adequate vocabulary and tacit and explicit grammar for its use. It secures that whatever is thought and said, is consonant with the canonical descriptions and divisions of the "psychiatric object," and the associated underlying metaphysical axioms. This is what the *contemporary French debaters*, in a slightly different context, designate as "*la pensée unique*"—"the one way thinking" (like in "one way" street). This expression, transposed into psychiatry, signifies a concerted, encompassing drift towards an extreme, global, and ultimately self-defeating *homogenization of ideas*, unmatched by any past experience from earlier historical periods.

So our question of repeatability of the French 19th-century debate is most likely answerable in the negative, not least if we were to expect it to happen in a similarly circumscribed and intellectually elegant form as depicted by Berrios. But the debate never really stopped, it reiterates itself in ever new clothes. It continues today, to which the present volume so forcefully testifies. Kendler (Chapter 15, this volume) will try to convince us that the scientific developments necessarily gravitate towards increasingly truer grasp of the world. I think that in order for that to happen in psychiatry, we need to adopt a conceptually more pluralistic and theoretically more enlightened posture (perhaps allowing for a limited plurality of "tribal classifications," i.e., classifications originating in special purposes), while, at the same time retaining in science a vital clinical contact with the reality of "psychiatric object," i.e., the patients. The increasing interest in the interface between philosophy and psychiatry is certainly reflective of a Zeitgeist change in that direction.

Endnote

1 The term "privileged" refers here to the mode of access and not to the accuracy of self-knowledge.

Comments References

Bennet, M. R. and Hacker, P. M. S. (2003). *Philosophical Foundations of Neuroscience*. Oxford: Blackwell Publishing.

Berrios, G.E., Marková, I.S. (2002). Conceptual issues. *In* H. D'haenen, J. A. den Boer, and P. Willner (eds.). *Biological Psychiatry*. New York: John Wiley & Sons Ltd., pp. 3–24.

Chalmers, D. J. (2010). *The Character of Consciousness*. Oxford: Oxford University Press.

Curchland, P. S. (1986). *Neurophilosophy*. Cambridge, MA: The MIT Press.

Dilthey, W. (2010). *The Understanding of the Human World*. Vol. *II* of *Collected Works* (Makkreel, R.A. and Rodi, F. trans. and eds.). Princeton, NJ: Princeton University Press.

Foulcault, M. (1994). *The Order of Things: An Archaeology of the Human Sciences*. (Tr. *Les mots et les choses*. Paris: Gallimard 1966). New York: Vintage Books.

Gallagher, S. and Zahavi, D. (2008). *The phenomenological Mind: An Introduction to Philosophy of Mind and Cognitive Science*. London: Routledge.

Jaspers, K. (1963). *General Psychopathology*. Chicago, IL: The University of Chicago Press.

Kuhn, T. (1970). *The Structure of Scientific Revolutions* (2nd, enlarged ed.). Chicago, IL: The University of Chicago Press.

Kyle Stanford, P. (2006). *Exceeding Our Grasp. Science, History, and the Problem of Unconceived Alternatives*. Oxford: Oxford University Press.

Nagel, T. (1986). *The View from Nowhere*. Oxford: Oxford University Press.

Noë, A. (2009). *Out of Our Heads: Why You are not Your Brain, and Other Lessons from the Biology of Consciousness*. New York: Hill and Wang.

Parnas, J. and Sass, L. A. (2008). Varieties of 'phenomenology': On description, understanding, and explanation in psychiatry. In K. Kendler and J. Parnas (eds.), *Philosophical Issues in Psychiatry: Explanation, Phenomenology, and Nosology*. Baltimore, MD: Johns Hopkins University Press, pp. 239–77.

Parnas, J. and Zahavi, D. (2002). The role of phenomenology in psychiatric classification and diagnosis. In M. Maj, W. Gaebel, J. J. Lopez- Ibor, and N. Sartorius (eds.) *Psychiatric Diagnosis and Classification* (World Psychiatric Association's series in Evidence and Experience in Psychiatry). Chichester: John Wiley & Sons Ltd., pp. 137–162.

Sass, L. and Parnas, J. (2006). Explaining schizophrenia: The relevance of phenomenology. In M. Chung, W. Fulford, and G. Graham (eds.) *Reconceiving Schizophrenia*. Oxford: Oxford University Press, pp. 63–96.

Searle, J. R. (1992). *The Rediscovery of the Mind*. Cambridge, MA: The MIT Press.

Thompson, E. (2007). *Mind in Life: Biology, Phenomenology, and the Sciences of Mind*. Cambridge, MA: Harvard University Press.

Urfer-Parnas, A., Mortensen, E.L., Parnas, J. (2010). Core of schizophrenia: estrangement, dementia, or neurocognitive disorder? *Psychopathology*, **43**, 300–311.

Chapter 7

Introduction

Kenneth S. Kendler

Michael First provides us with a clear conceptual overview of the development of DSM-III, focusing his essay on the three major changes the manual introduced into psychiatric nosology: (1) the use of operationalized diagnostic criteria, (2) the adoption of a self-consciously descriptive "atheoretical approach" to psychiatric illness, and (3) the inclusion of a multiaxial approach to diagnosis.

I will direct my brief comments here on the first two of these changes. As First reviews, the prime impetus for the adoption of operationalized criteria was to improve reliability. As he notes, conceptual work had suggested three major sources of variation (or unreliability) in diagnosis: (1) information variance, (2) interpretation variance, and (3) criterion variance. The first two were hard to address. Operationalized criteria, theoretically, could substantially reduce the third. As First notes, the widespread adoption of operationalized criteria in DSM-III was based on two prior influential psychiatric diagnostic systems that effectively "field-tested" the use of operationalized diagnoses: the Feighner Criteria (Feighner et al. 1972; Kendler et al. 2010) and the Research Diagnostic Criteria (RDC, Spitzer et al. 1975). The adoption of operationalized criteria in psychiatry had a precedent both from the field of medicine, where there were operationalized criteria for several rheumatologic disorders from the 1940s into the early 1970s (Jones 1944; Ropes et al. 1957), and philosophy, where they were famously recommended to the field of psychiatry by Carl Hempel (1965). Few in the field now question the wisdom of the introduction of operationalized criteria into psychiatric diagnosis.

The second major innovation of DSM-III emphasized by First—the adoption of an atheoretical approach to nosology—has proven much more controversial. As First describes, at the time of the development of DSM-III, a psychoanalytic orientation remained both popular and politically powerful within American psychiatry. Some have thought that the "atheoretical move" in DSM-III, advocated by its chief architect Robert Spitzer, reflected some deep philosophical commitment, for example, to avoid the realism anti-realism debate about the nature of psychiatric illness. In fact, the motivations were more practical. Spitzer saw it as critical to move the official nosology away from the predominant psychoanalytic orientation that had characterized DSM-I and DSM-II. His move toward an atheoretical model was more a statement of what he wanted to avoid than any specific aversion to etiologically-based diagnoses.

Three iterations of the DSM manual later (counting both DSM-IIIR and DSM-IV), the issue about the atheoretical nature of the DSM manual has moved front and center again. The desire to move toward an etiologically based system within the field is palpable. Whether it is practical, now or in the future, is far less clear. One of the "white papers" early in the DSM-5 process asked if any biological markers (from genes, to neuroendocrine tests, to imaging studies) were ready for "prime time"—that is: ready to be included as diagnostic criteria in DSM-5. The answer was "No."

My personal sense is that much of the motivation for etiologically-based diagnoses in psychiatry is unrealistic (Kendler 2011). Given the nature of psychiatric illness, there will not be one, a priori, clear level of explanation on which the field will agree—as might be seen for DNA variation in Mendelian genetic disorders, or the specific microorganism in infectious diseases. Instead, psychiatric disorders are probably highly multifactorial "all the way down." So, the problem may not be that we don't have etiological processes underlying risk for psychiatric disorders, but that we have too many of them. Science will not unambiguously identify one level, so then how do we decide which to emphasize in our etiology?

But that, in part, is an issue for future science to decide. For now, we should be grateful for this clear summary from Dr First of what was surely a paradigm-setting document for psychiatric nosology: DSM-III.

Introduction References

Feighner, J. P., Robins, E., Guze, S. B., Woodruff, R. A., Jr., Winokur, G. ans Munoz, R. (1972). Diagnostic criteria for use in psychiatric research. *Archives of General Psychiatry*, **26**(1), 57–63.

Hempel, C. G. (1965). *Aspects of Scientific Explanation and Other Essays in the Philosophy of Science*. New York: Free Press.

Jones, T. D. (1944). The diagnosis of rheumatic fever. *Journal of the American Medical Association*, **126**(8), 481–4.

Kendler, K. S. (2011). Levels of explanation in psychiatric and substance use disorders: Implications for the development of an etiologically based nosology. *Molecular Psychiatry*, First published online 14 June, 2011, doi:10.1038/mp.2011.70.

Kendler, K. S., Munoz, R. A. and Murphy, G.(2010). The Development of the Feighner Criteria: An historical perspective. *American Journal of Psychiatry*, **167**(2), 134–42

Ropes, M. W., Bennett, G. A., Cobb, S., Jacox, R. and Jessar, R.A.(1957). Proposed Diagnostic Criteria for Rheumatoid Arthritis: Report of a Study Conducted by a Committee of the American Rheumatism Association. *Annals of the Rheumatic Diseases*, **16**, 118–25.

Spitzer, R. L., Endicott, J. and Robins, E. (1975). *Research Diagnostic Criteria for a Selected Group of Functional Disorders* (2nd ed.). New York: New York Psychiatric Institute.

Chapter 7

The development of DSM-III from a historical/conceptual perspective

Michael B. First

It is widely acknowledged that DSM-III represented a paradigm shift in psychiatric classification (Blashfield 1984; Decker 2007; Mayes and Horwitz 2005; Wilson 1993). Klerman (1984 p. 539) called the publication of DSM-III in 1980 "a fateful point in the history of the American psychiatric profession." DSM-III marshaled the use of operationalized diagnostic criteria for the definitions of its mental disorders, removed the influence of untested etiological hypotheses from its organizational structure in favor of a descriptive "atheoretical approach," and reframed the biopsychosocial model in terms of a multiaxial approach to diagnosis. As will be explicated in this paper, none of these innovative ideas arose de novo as a result of the DSM-III developmental process. Instead, the main innovation of DSM-III was its adoption of ideas which had previously been tested and found to be useful in research settings, into a manual of mental disorders designed primarily for clinical use.

7.1 Operationalized criteria

The most significant innovation promulgated by DSM-III is its provision of operationalized diagnostic criteria for virtually every disorder in the mental disorders classification. As explained in the introduction to DSM-III, "since in DSM-I, DSM-II, and ICD-9 explicit criteria are not provided, the clinician is largely on his or her own in defining the content and the boundaries of the diagnostic categories. In contrast, DSM-III provides specific diagnostic criteria as guides for making each diagnosis, since such criteria enhance interjudge diagnostic reliability." (American Psychiatric Association 1980, p. 8). This keen interest in improving diagnostic reliability was largely motivated by the desire to address criticisms of the validity of psychiatric diagnosis which had come under heavy fire in the 1960s and 1970s (Rosenhan 1973; Szasz 1960) Although reliability and validity were understood to be distinct psychometric qualities, given that diagnostic reliability puts an upper limit on diagnostic validity, it was believed that addressing DSM's reliability problems was a necessary step towards ultimately improving its validity. According to Spitzer and Fleiss (1974, p. 341), although "there is no guarantee that a reliable system is valid. . . assuredly an unreliable system must be invalid."

A number of studies conducted from the 1930s through the 1960s supported the suspicion that the reliability of psychiatric diagnosis was problematic (Ash 1949; Beck et al. 1962; Boiseh 1938; Boisen 1938; Foulds 1955; Goldfarb 1959; Masserman and Carmichael 1938; Norris 1959; Sandifer et al. 1964; Schmidt and Fonda 1956; Ward et al. 1962). For example, an early study by Ash (1949) that measured the ability of different clinicians to agree on a diagnosis when seeing the same patient found that three clinicians could agree on a diagnosis only 20% of the time.

In addition to studies demonstrating poor diagnostic reliability, studies conducted in the late 1960s and early 1970s comparing diagnostic practices in clinicians from the UK and the United States (Katz et al. 1969; Kendell et al. 1971; Sandifer et al. 1968) were influential in further establishing the need for operationalized diagnostic definitions. Comparative hospital statistics showed that American clinicians consistently diagnosed a larger percentage of inpatients as having schizophrenia compared to UK clinicians who made the diagnosis of manic depressive psychosis much more frequently (Blashfield 1984). In order to determine whether these diagnostic differences were due to different prevalences of these disorders in the two countries versus clinicians utilizing different definitions of diagnostic terms, most of the studies asked psychiatrists in each country to view the same set of videotaped interviews and to make a psychiatric diagnosis. The 1971 study by Kendell and colleagues (1971), referred to as the "US-UK Study," showed eight videotapes to groups of American and British psychiatrists and found that Americans most frequently assigned a diagnosis of schizophrenia to all eight videotaped cases whereas the British preferred a diagnosis of manic-depressive psychosis for some cases, schizophrenia for others and personality disorder for yet others, indicating that Americans had a relatively broad interpretation of the definition of schizophrenia as compared to those in the UK. Although this study in and of itself does not necessarily support the argument for using operationalized criteria, as reported by Blashfield (1984, p. 95), Kendell believed that the study had a major impact of the thinking of American psychiatrists: "It is my impression that one of the factors that lead to a dramatic change in classification and diagnostic criteria by American psychiatrists earlier in this decade is that they were out of step with the rest of the world."

It is important to understand that there are other factors besides the qualities of the diagnostic nomenclature that might explain why clinicians evaluating the same patient might disagree on the diagnosis. Spitzer and colleagues (1979) proposed that there are three major sources of unreliability in the diagnostic process: (1) information variance, which involves variability in the information elicited by clinicians from the patient during the assessment process (e.g., one clinician elicits a history of hearing voices from the patient whereas another clinician does not); (2) interpretation variance, which involves variability among clinicians in how they interpret the meaning and significance of a sign or symptom (e.g., one clinician interprets the patient's looking around the room as evidence of auditory hallucinations whereas the other clinician sees it as evidence of distractibility); and (3) criterion variance which involves the different definitions that clinicians might associate with a diagnosis (e.g., one clinician considers bizarre delusions pathognomonic of a diagnosis of schizophrenia regardless of the patient's mood state whereas the other clinician considers it a psychotic mood disorder if the bizarre delusions occur only during mood episodes). Accordingly, replacing ambiguous and vague definitions with operationalized criteria improves diagnostic reliability only insofar that the unclear definitions are leading clinicians to differ in their understanding of the definition of disorders. The 1962 study by Ward and colleagues (1962) examined clinicians' own attributions of the reasons for diagnostic disagreement and reported that the clinicians believed that inadequacies in the nosology were the cause of the disagreement in the majority (65%) of cases, thus lending support to the notion that the vague definitions in DSM-I were in large part the cause of poor diagnostic reliability and that improvements in the precision of the definitions would lead to better diagnostic agreement.

DSM-I (American Psychiatric Association 1952), DSM-II (American Psychiatric Association 1968) and ICD-9 (World Health Organization 1978) each provided glossary definitions for disorders included in their classifications. This was a marked improvement over the situation prior to DSM-I in which clinicians seeking guidance on disorder definitions were dependent entirely on textbooks and individual articles in which typical cases were described. Thus, the publication in 1952 of DSM-I was a giant step forward in terms of facilitating standardized data collection and communication, given that it included standardized names, codes, and glossary definitions for each disorder. However, according to Spitzer and colleagues (1975), there were a number of reasons why such glossary definitions were inadequate for achieving high reliability, including: (1) features that are invariably present in the disorder were not distinguished from those that are commonly but not invariably present; (2) there was usually no indication of which features distinguish a disorder from similar conditions; (3) no guidelines were provided regarding which diagnoses were mutually exclusive versus those that could be diagnosed comorbidly; (4) many classificatory principles were a function of tradition or of some hypothesized causal factor with little research evidence; and (5) the lack of clarity in the definitions was often deliberate in order to gain acceptance by groups with widely divergent views.

The inadequacy of using glossary definitions for making psychiatric diagnoses was most evident to psychiatric researchers. The discovery in the 1960s of medications that had some efficacy for treating psychiatric disorders (i.e., chlorpromazine for schizophrenia, lithium for bipolar disorder, imipramine for major depressive disorder) highlighted the need to develop explicit diagnostic criteria in order to gather homogeneous research samples for clinical trials. Researchers responded to this need by developing their own explicit criteria for particular categories of interest (e.g., the New Haven Schizophrenia Index (Astrachan et al. 1972), Carpenter-Strauss criteria for Schizophrenia (Carpenter et al. 1973)). Researchers at Washington University in St. Louis, who had long recognized the importance of reliable psychiatric diagnoses for research developed a set of research diagnostic criteria for those diagnostic conditions which they considered had the most evidence of validity in terms of clear clinical descriptions, consistency over time, and increased familial incidence (Kendler et al. 2010). In 1972, operationalized definitions for 15 conditions, known as the "Feighner criteria," (Feighner et al. 1972, p. 57) were published in the *Archives of General Psychiatry*, with the stated goal of providing a "common ground for different research groups. . . The use of formal diagnostic criteria by a number of groups. . . will result in a resolution of the problem of whether patients described by different groups are comparable." These diagnostic criteria were developed based on an empirical review of over 1000 articles presented at a series of meetings attended by a group of like-minded researchers who were dubbed 'neo-Kraepelinians' by Gerald Klerman (1978) because they shared Kraepelin's emphasis on classifying disorders based on descriptive features and developmental course. The paper concluded with the message that "what we now present is our synthesis of existing information, a synthesis based on data rather than on opinion and tradition" (Feighner et al. 1972, p. 62). Subsequent studies demonstrated high reliability for these criteria (Helzer et al. 1977). It soon became evident that the Feighner criteria met a huge untapped need of the research community at large, as evidenced by the fact that the criteria were cited 1157 times from 1972 through 1980, which was more than 70 times the citation rate of an average article published in the *Archives of General Psychiatry* during that same time interval (Blashfield 1982).

Besides their proximal impact on the conduct of psychiatric research in the 1970s, the Feighner criteria had a major impact on the eventual development of DSM-III, forming as they did the basis for the development of research criteria which were the direct precursor to DSM-III. As part of a collaborative project on the psychobiology of depression sponsored by the Clinical Research Branch of the NIMH, diagnostic criteria and a structured clinical interview were developed to standardize the diagnostic assessments across the various sites in the study (Katz et al. 1979). According to Kendler and colleagues' (2010) detailed account of the history of the development of the Feighner criteria, Robert Spitzer, who was in charge of the assessment component, was asked to collaborate with Eli Robins, one of the coauthors of the Feighner criteria, on the development of Research Diagnostic Criteria (RDC) for the collaborative study. The original 15 criteria sets were modified and diagnostic criteria for ten additional disorders were developed (Spitzer et al. 1978). While many of the specific criteria in the RDC had some research evidence supporting their validity, by necessity many of the criteria were "presented only as an initial attempt to operationalize concepts whose importance for diagnosis is based on a considered amount of clinical wisdom" (Spitzer et al. 1975, p. 1190) thus forming the basis of the expert clinical consensus model used in the development of DSM-III for those categories for which little to no informative empirical data was available.

The RDC were first presented in a conference in June 1974 and first published in 1975 as part of a report of their reliability when applied to psychiatric case records (Spitzer et al. 1975). Shortly thereafter, Spitzer, Endicott and Robins (1975, p. 1190) reported that although "the diagnostic criteria used in the RDC were developed for research purposes...the apparent advantages of this approach have led to a decision by the APA Task Force on Nomenclature and Statistics to recommend that some form of suggested specific criteria for most of the diagnostic categories be included in DSM-III." Purported advantages included: (1) "improving the training of psychiatric residents and other mental health professionals"; (2) improving communication "among mental health professionals;" (3) improving the reliability and validity of routine psychiatric diagnosis; and (4) improving "the value of the nomenclature for all its many uses—clinical, research, and administrative." Of note, the initial thinking of the Task Force was for the operational criteria to be listed under the heading "Suggested Criteria" and that they would "not replace but merely supplement the narrative definitions of the diagnostic categories" and that "any clinician would be free to use them or ignore them as he saw fit" Spitzer et al. 1975, p. 1191). It thus appeared that, at least initially, the main thrust of the DSM-III effort would be to make the "narrative definitions in DSM-III. . . much more elaborate than those in DSM-I and DSM-II" (Spitzer et al. 1975, p. 1190). One member of the DSM-III committee even argued, unsuccessfully, that diagnostic criteria be offered to researchers in a separate manual (Spitzer 2001)

From the outset, it was recognized that adjustments needed to be made to the RDC approach in order to make the criteria more suitable for clinical use. For one thing, because of the researcher's need to identify homogeneous groupings and reduce the risk of false positives with respect to inclusion of inappropriate subjects in research studies, criteria in the RDC often had to be more stringent. (Ironically, the example given by Spitzer, Endicott, and Robins in their 1975 paper of a "more stringent" RDC criterion was the "at least two weeks" duration requirement for the RDC category of major depressive illness which was eventually adopted as the duration requirement in DSM-III; presumably, at the time the DSM-III group was considering a one-week duration for a major depressive episode). Furthermore, the provision in the RDC for indicating whether a diagnosis was "definite" or "probable" would not be offered in DSM-III.

Ultimately, of course, the plan for the DSM-III diagnostic criteria to be considered "suggested" optional elements of the classification was ultimately dropped in favor of having the criteria be included as an integral part of the diagnostic system. Likely this was related to the decision of the DSM-III Task Force to conduct widescale field trials of drafts of the DSM-III diagnostic criteria in clinical settings. The field trials ultimately indicated both their feasibility and acceptability and demonstrated improvements in diagnostic reliability as compared to DSM-II (Spitzer et al. 1979).

7.2 Categorical approach and relationship to the international classification of diseases

Like all medical classifications, the DSM is a categorical system, with each disorder conceptualized as a category that is either present or absent. DSM-II adopted both the classification and text from the mental disorders section of the World Health Organization's International Classification of Diseases—Eighth Edition (ICD-8) with only minor modifications. This was motivated both by a desire for facilitate international communication in psychiatric data collection and research and because clinicians working in the United States are required to use diagnostic codes from the ICD system because of a treaty obligation between the US Government and the World Health Organization.

During the early developmental stages of DSM-III, the first decision the DSM-III committee had to make was whether the follow the DSM-II approach of adopting the ICD system, which was already under development at the time, or whether to go in a different direction and adopt an innovative classification for American use. According to Spitzer (2001), the DSM-III committee believed that despite the value of a single international classification system, it was more important that psychiatric classification benefit from new developments in American psychiatry, such as the development of diagnostic criteria. Although there was still a requirement that clinicians use the diagnostic codes from ICD-9-CM (an American clinical modification of ICD-9), "we were relatively unconcerned by frequently having a different definition of a DSM category than of a corresponding ICD-9-CM category. We believed it was a small price to pay for our ability to be innovative" (Spitzer 2001, p. 353).

Although the DSM system by necessity had to adopt a categorical approach in order to maintain structural compatibility with the ICD, DSM-III explicitly rejected one of the basic tenets of categorical systems, namely that there are distinct diagnostic boundaries separating the categories. In the introduction to the manual, it is emphatically stated that "in DSM-III there is no assumption that each mental disorder is a discrete entity with sharp boundaries (discontinuity) between it and other mental disorders, as well as between it and no mental disorder"(American Psychiatric Association 1980, p. 6). Instead, the manual explains that diagnostic distinctions in the DSM-III are made on the grounds of clinical utility: "for example. . .the inclusion of Major Depression with and without melancholia as separate categories in DSM-III is justified by the clinical usefulness of the distinction. . .[and] does not imply a resolution of the controversy as to whether these two conditions are in fact quantitatively [i.e., a difference on a severity continuum] or qualitatively [i.e., discontinuity between diagnostic entities] different" (American Psychiatric Association 1980, p. 6). Despite this introductory caveat, the DSM system has been widely criticized for being a rigidly categorical system (Helzer et al. 2008; Regier et al. 2009).

7.3 Descriptive "atheoretical approach"

One of the main innovations of the DSM-III was its adoption of a descriptive "atheoretical" approach in which disorders are defined according to their symptomatic presentation, rather than according to unproven theories regarding underlying etiology. It is important to understand that the decision to adopt a descriptive approach was not motivated by some aversion to having a classification system organized around etiology per se, but rather a desire to avoid defining disorders according to unproven and potentially invalid etiological hypotheses. Furthermore, given that one of the main goals of the DSM-III is to facilitate communication among mental health clinicians, defining disorders according to one particular theory would hinder its utility for clinicians who do not subscribe to that theory. For those DSM-III disorders in which the etiology was known (or presumed), the disorders were defined according to etiology (e.g., substance-induced mental disorders which are, by definition, caused by substance use). As explained in the manual's introduction, "the approach taken in DSM-III is atheoretical with regard to etiology or pathophysiological process except for those disorders for which this is well established and they are included in the definition of the disorder. . . The major justification. . . is that the inclusion of etiological theories would be an obstacle to use of the manual by clinicians of varying theoretical orientations" (American Psychiatric Association 1980, pp. 6–7).

This approach harks back to the classifications of Emil Kraepelin which provided exceedingly detailed descriptions of disorders seen in inpatient settings at the turn of the century. Furthermore, Kraepelin strongly advocated that "psychiatrists should avoid postulating etiologies to make a diagnosis and should stick to the course of the illness, attend to the final state, and do follow-up studies where possible (Decker 2007, p. 340). However, psychoanalystic/psychodynamic theories which dominated the practice of psychiatry in the United States in the 1940s, 1950s, and 1960s influenced the structure of both DSM-I and DSM-II. For example, one of the nine major diagnostic groups in DSM-II, the neuroses, was defined in terms of anxiety that was "felt or expressed directly, or. . . may be controlled unconsciously and automatically by conversion, displacement and various other psychological mechanisms" (American Psychiatric Association 1968, p. 39). Such disparate presentations such as depressed mood, obsessive–compulsive symptoms, and dissociative symptoms were all seen as different ways of unconsciously dealing with internal conflict. Consequently, although the adoption of an atheoretical approach hypothetically entailed rejecting the inclusion of any unproven etiological hypotheses in the DSM-III, in practice it was the psychodynamic perspective that was essentially targeted for exclusion.

This decision to develop a DSM-III based on a descriptive approach rather than psychodynamic underpinnings nearly derailed the DSM-III development process were it not for the politically skillful efforts of Robert Spitzer, Chair of the DSM-III Task Force, to placate at least some of the psychoanalysts' concerns. During the initial stages of the process, the DSM-III Task Force was able to establish the atheoretical approach as one of the fundamental principles of the revision process without much fanfare largely because the DSM was of so little interest to psychoanalysts. The almost complete non-relevance of the DSM to clinical practice at the time is illustrated by the following recollection of an interaction that the prominent psychoanalyst Irving Bieber had with a colleague regarding the 1972 decision to remove homosexuality from DSM-II. When the colleague called to say "have you heard the terrible news? They are taking homosexuality out of further printings of DSM-II." Dr. Bieber's reply was "What is DSM-II?" (Spitzer 2001).

By 1978, however, psychoanalytically-oriented clinicians became more aware (and alarmed) about what was happening with the DSM-III revision process and started voicing repeated objections to the loss of psychoanalytic concepts in the DSM-III. In response to such concerns, Spitzer offered a number of compromises that might satisfy their concerns, none of which were eventually adopted. For example, Spitzer suggested the development of an additional axis for etiology that would allow clinicians to express their psychodynamic formulations of their cases (Wilson 1993). Another proposed compromise involved the development of a companion manual for treatment, which would have included chapters for each of the major types of psychotherapeutic techniques, one of which would be psychodynamic treatment. This manual also never materialized in its intended form as a companion to the DSM-III.

Perhaps the biggest concerns raised by psychoanalysts were over the plans to remove the word "neurosis" from DSM, the bread-and-butter of psychoanalysts' practice. Objections concerning its removal had become so strong that, by the spring of 1979,

DSM-III was in serious danger of not being approved by the APA Board of Trustees unless a way was found to appease those who wanted the word "neurosis" to be reinstated in the manual (Wilson 1993). After a series of elaborate negotiations, a compromise was ultimately reached in which a section would be added to the introduction of DSM-III explaining the difference between the concepts of neurotic process ("an etiological notion involving unconscious conflict arousing anxiety and leading to the maladaptive use of defensive mechanisms that result in symptom formation" (American Psychiatric Association 1980, p. 9)) and neurotic disorder ("a mental disorder in which the predominant disturbance is a symptom or group of symptoms that is distressing . . .and recognized by [the individual] as unacceptable and alien. . . [in] which reality testing is grossly intact" (American Psychiatric Association 1980, pp. 9–10)). Furthermore, the word "neurosis" was retained in the body of the manual but in a form that was clearly subsidiary to the new DSM-III terminology, i.e., the name of the neurotic disorder would be included in parenthesis next to the DSM-III term (e.g., phobic neurosis in parentheses alongside "phobic disorder").

7.4 **Multiaxial system**

When DSM-III was introduced, one of the features most heralded was the inclusion of a multiaxial system for assessment. A multiaxial evaluation requires that "every case be assessed on each of several 'axes,' each of which refers to a different class of information" (American Psychiatric Association 1980, p. 23). Five such axes were included in DSM-III. The first three axes "constitute the official diagnostic assessment" and consist of Axis I for the evaluation of clinical syndromes and for conditions not attributable to a mental disorder but that may be a focus of attention or treatment; Axis II for the evaluation of personality disorders and specific developmental disorders, and Axis III for physical disorders and conditions. Axis IV and V were deemed "available for use in special clinical and research settings and provide information supplementing the official DSM-III diagnosis. . .that may be useful for planning treatment and predicting outcomes" (American Psychiatric Association 1980, p. 23). Axis IV allowed for rating the severity of those psychosocial stressors "judged to have been a significant contributor to the development or exacerbation of the current disorder" (DSM-III, p. 14) and Axis V permitted the clinician to "indicate his or her judgment of an individual's highest level of adaptive functioning (for at least a few months) during the past year" (American Psychiatric Association 1980, p. 28). According to DSM-III, use of the system "ensures that attention is given to certain types of disorders, aspects of the environment, and areas of functioning that might be overlooked if the focus were on assessing a single presenting problem" (American Psychiatric Association 1980, p. 23).

The primary stated motivation of including a multiaxial evaluation in DSM-III is to enhance its clinical utility. According to Janet Williams who was centrally involved in the creation of the multixial system, the main advantage of a multiaxial approach over a single axis approach is that it better "reflects the complexity of and interrelationships between the various biopsychosocial aspects of the individual being evaluated" and that "a comprehensive multiaxial evaluation is assumed to be more useful in planning treatment and evaluating prognosis" (Williams 1985, p. 175).

As with many of the DSM-III features, the process by which the multiaxial system was included in DSM-III reflected an effort by the developers of the DSM to adopt and refine ideas previously suggested by others in order to address a problem facing the DSM. The first proposal for the inclusion of a multiaxial system as part of an official psychiatric nomenclature was made by Essen-Moller and Wohlfahrt (1947) who suggested that a two-axial system (one for syndromes and the second axis for the cause of the syndrome) be adopted for the official Swedish classification of mental disorders. Over the next several decades, additional proposals for multiaxial systems appeared in the international literature that generally involved from two to five axes, each focusing on different aspects of the mental disorders themselves, such as phenomenology, etiology, associated features, time frame of the illness (e.g., onset, course and duration), severity and diagnostic certainty (Mezzich 1979).

Specific multiaxial classification schemes for childhood disorders were proposed by Rutter and colleages (1973) based on discussions from a WHO conference (Rutter et al. 1973; Tarjan et al. 1972) for adoption in ICD-9. Dennis Cantwell, a UCLA child psychiatrist who was studying in England with Rutter during this time later became a member of the DSM-III Task Force and suggested that a multiaxial evaluation for childhood disorders be considered for DSM-III and such a proposal was included in a 1976 preliminary draft of DSM-III. Five axes were proposed: Axis I would describe the clinical psychiatric syndrome, Axis II was for current intellectual functioning (IQ); Axis III was for specific developmental disorders; Axis IV would be used for denoting associated biological factors that might be present, and Axis V was for associated psychosocial factors (American Psychiatric Association Task Force on Nomenclature and Statistics 1976). Noting that personality disorders in adults are equivalent to specific developmental disorders in children insofar that they also tend to be stable and relatively enduring and thus are often overlooked, a parallel proposal for recording personality disorders on a separate axis from the rest of the mental disorders was also included in the first draft of DSM-III (Williams 1985). Positive response to these initial proposals during a June 1976 conference entitled "Improvements in Psychiatric Classification and Terminology: A Working Conference To Critically Examine DSM-III in Midstream" ultimately led to the appointment of an Advisory Committee on Multiaxial Diagnosis who developed a five-axis multiaxial system for both adults and children that could be included as a critical part of DSM-III.

Although it might appear that the main reason that the multiaxial system was added to the DSM-III was because "its value for clinical and research work was quickly recognized." (Williams 1985, p. 175), Spitzer (2001) noted that:

> The actual impetus for [the multiaxial system] was to meet the mounting criticism that by developing such a large and seemingly authoritative diagnostic manual, American Psychiatry was giving the impression that the only important part of a psychiatric evaluation was making (or not making) a psychiatric diagnosis. Providing a multiaxial system that included physical disorders (axis III), psychosocial stressors (axis IV) and level of functioning (axis V) enabled DSM-III to be presented as within a broad psychosocial model–rather than the narrow diagnostic model that its critics feared (p. 357).

Thus, the decision to include a multiaxial system was as much about reacting to criticism as it was about innovation.

7.5 **Implications for future revisions**

The DSM-III was far more successful that had ever been anticipated by its creators. Its innovations transformed the American Psychiatric Association's *Diagnostic and Statistical Manual* from a small relatively inconsequential pamphlet used primarily by psychiatrists for coding purposes into one of the most popular medical books ever published, with each edition selling well over a million copies. The DSM is considered the standard reference for the diagnosis of mental disorders not just by psychiatrists, but by non-psychiatric mental health professionals, patients and families, and psychology and medical students, and by government agencies. Several factors contributed to its widespread acceptance. First and foremost, its development coincided with the significant changes that psychiatry as a field was undergoing in the 1960s and 1970s. The successful introduction of psychotropic medications such as lithium carbonate, tricyclic antidepressants and antipsychotics created a need for operationalized diagnostic criteria that could be used to define discrete syndromes that might be a target for pharmacological treatment. Furthermore, growing discontent within the profession with the psychosocial and psychodymanic models of psychopathology (Wilson 1993) coupled with attacks on the legitimacy of psychiatry (Szasz 1960) promoted the embracing of a diagnostic model from medicine where diagnosis is the keystone of medical practice and clinical research (Guze 1974). The DSM-III approach which equated visible and measurable symptoms with the presence of disease allowed researchers to reliably assess symptoms and to legitimize clinicians' claims to be treating real diseases that deserve reimbursement from third-party insurers (Mayes and Horwitz 2005). Moreover, the central element of the DSM-III revolution, namely defining psychiatric disorders in terms of symptom-based operationalized diagnostic criteria, had already been road tested for several years prior to their introduction in DSM-III, establishing both their reliability and utility with regard to the process of psychiatric diagnosis.

The ultimate fate of the DSM-III multiaxial system provides a more cautionary lesson regarding the introduction of innovative features to the DSM. Unlike the decision to introduce operationalized criteria which addressed a widely recognized problem with the DSM (i.e., diagnostic unreliability) with a road-tested solution (i.e., the implementation of operationalized diagnostic criteria widely embraced by the research community), the introduction of the multiaxial system did not occur in response to any identified problem with the diagnostic system. Instead, as discussed above, the multiaxial system was introduced both for political reasons (i.e., to deal with criticisms that the DSM diagnostic process was focused exclusively on the psychiatric diagnosis) and because the creators of DSM-III believed it would be clinically useful without any a priori evidence that it would in fact achieve this goal. In fact, surveys (Bassett and Beiser 1991; Jampala et al. 1986) and anecdotal evidence suggest that clinicians do not find the multiaxial system particularly useful and use the multiaxial system only in situations where its use is required, such as in mental health treatment settings within the Veterans Administration health care system. Indeed, the Assembly of the American Psychiatric Association membership in 2004 passed an "action paper" calling for the elimination of the multiaxial system, noting that "there is no evidence that the most practitioners make use of it when they are free not to" (Peele et al. 2004).

A review of the proposals on the DSM-5 website suggests that the multiaxial system will be eliminated in DSM-5.

Current proposals calling for the inclusion of both cross-cutting and disorder-specific dimensional severity assessments throughout DSM-5 may ultimately suffer a similar fate. Although the many problems with the DSM categorical approach (e.g., high rates of diagnostic comorbidity and excessive use of NOS categories) have been noted (Helzer et al. 2006; Helzer et al. 2008), the addition of dimensional assessments to the categorical system will do little to rectify the problem. Instead, the goal of introducing dimensional assessments into the DSM-5 is to promote the "best practices" goal of measurement-based care (Burke et al. 2010; Regier et al, 2009). Despite some calls for the implementation of measurement-based care in clinical practice (Valenstein et al. 2009), there is as yet no evidence that the use of dimensional assessments actually improves clinical outcomes. Moreover, surveys suggest that clinicians do not routinely use measures in their practice (Zimmerman and McGlinchey 2008) nor do they find them to be clinically useful (Garland et al. 2003). Furthermore, rather than recommending the use of road-tested severity measures, most of the proposed dimensional assessments have been created de novo by the DSM-5 Workgroups and thus have unproven reliability, validity and utility. Without clear and convincing evidence that the implementation of dimensional assessments improves patient care, it is unlikely that clinicians will perceive that the use of such scales is worth the extra time and effort.

Chapter References

American Psychiatric Association (1952). *Diagnostic and Statistical Manual of Mental Disorders*. Washington, DC: American Psychiatric Association.

American Psychiatric Association (1968). *Diagnostic and Statistical Manual of Mental Disorders, 2nd Edition*. Washington, DC: American Psychiatric Association.

American Psychiatric Association (1980). *Diagnostic and Statistical Manual of Mental Disorders, Third Edition*. Washington, DC: American Psychiatric Association.

American Psychiatric Association Task Force on Nomenclature and Statistics (1976). Progress Report on the Preparation of DSM-III, March 1976, unpublished manuscript.

Ash, P. (1949). The reliability of psychiatric diagnosis. *Journal of Abnormal and Social Psychology,* **44**, 272–6.

Astrachan, B., Harrow, M., Adler, D., Brauer, L., Schwartz, A., Schwartz, C., *et al.* (1972). A checklist for the diagnosis of schizophrenia. *British Journal of Psychiatry,* **121**, 529–39.

Bassett, A. and Beiser, M. (1991). DSM-III: Use of the multiaxial diagnostic system in clinical practice. *Canadian Journal of Psychiatry,* **36**(4), 270–74.

Beck, A., Ward, C., Mendelson, M., Mock, J. and Erbaugh, J. (1962). Relability of psychiatric diagnosis: II. A study of the consistency of clinical judgments and ratings. *American Journal of Psychiatry,* **119**, 351–7.

Blashfield, R. (1982). Feignher et al, invisible colleges, and the Matthew Effect. *Schizophrenia Bulletin,* **8**(1), 1–12.

Blashfield, R. (1984). *The Classification of Psychopathology. Neo-Kraepelinian and Quantitative Approaches*. New York: Plenum Press.

Boiseh, A. (1938). Types of dementia praecox: a study in psychiatric classification. *Psychiatry,* **1**, 233–36.

Burke, J., Kraemer, H. and Shaffer, D. (2010). DSM-5 Task Force considers dimensional severity measures. *Psychiatric News,* **45**(17), 6.

Carpenter, W., Strauss, J. and Bartko, J. (1973). Flexible system for the diagnosis of schizophrenia: report from the WHO International Pilot Study of Schizophrenia. *Science,* **182**(118), 1275–8.

Decker, H. (2007). How Kraepelian was Kraepelin? Joe Kraepelinian are the neo-Kraepelinians? – from Emil Kraepelin to DSM-III. *History of Psychiatry,* **18**(3), 337–60.

Essen-Moller, E. and Wohlfahrt, S. (1947). Suggestions for the amendment of the official Swedish classification of mental disorders. *Acta Psychiatrica Scandinavica,* **47**(suppl.), 551.

Feighner, J. P., Robins, E., Guze, S. B., Woodruff, R. A., Jr., Winokur, G. and Munoz, R. (1972). Diagnostic criteria for use in psychiatric research. *Archives of General Psychiatry,* **26**(1), 57–63.

Foulds, G. (1955). The reliability of psychiatric and the validity of psychological diagnosis. *Journal of Mental Science,* **101**, 851–62.

Garland, A. F., Kruse, M. and Aarons, G. A. (2003). Clinicians and outcome measurement: what's the use? *Journal of Behavioral Health Services & Research,* **30**(4), 393–405.

Goldfarb, A. (1959). Reliability of diagnostic judgements by psychologists. *Journal of Clinical Psychology,* **15**, 392–6.

Guze, S. (1974). Psychiatric disorders and the medical model. *Biological Psychiatry,* **5**(3), 221–4.

Helzer, J., Clayton, P., Pambakian, R., Reich, T., Woodruff, R. and Reveley, M. (1977). Reliability of psychiatric diagnosis. II. The test/retest reliability of diagnostic classification. *Archives of General Psychiatry,* **34**(2), 136–41.

Helzer, J., Kraemer, H. and Krueger, R. (2006). The feasibility and need for dimensional psychiatric diagnoses. *Psychological Medicine,* **36**(12), 1671–80.

Helzer, J., Kraemer, H., Krueger, R., Wittchen, H., Sirovatka, P. and Regier, D. (Eds.). (2008). *Dimensional Approaches in Diagnostic Classification: Refining the Research Agenda for DSM-V.* Arlington, VA: American Psychiatric Association.

Jampala, V. C., Sierles, F. S. and Taylor, M. A. (1986). Consumers' views of DSM-III: attitudes and practices of U.S. psychiatrists and 1984 graduating psychiatric residents. *American Journal of Psychiatry,* **143**(2), 148–53.

Katz, M., Cole, J. and Lowery, H. (1969). Studies of the diagnostic process: The influence of symptom perception, past experience, and ethnic background of diagnostic decisions. *American Journal of Psychiatry,* **125**, 937–47.

Katz, M., Secunda, S., Hirschfeld, R. and SH., K. (1979). NIMH clinical research branch collaborative program on the psychobiology of depression. *Archives of General Psychiatry,* **36**(7), 765–71.

Kendell, R., Cooper, J., Gourlay, A., Copeland, J., Sharpe, L. and Gurland, B. (1971). Diagnostic criteria of American and British psychiatrists. *Archives of General Psychiatry,* **25**, 123–30.

Kendler, K., Munoz, R. and Murphy, G. (2010). The development of the Feighner Criteria: A historical perspective. *American Journal of Psychiatry,* **167**, 134–42.

Klerman, G. (1978). The evolution of scientific nosology. In J. Shershow (ed.), *Schizophrenia: Science and Practice.* Cambridge, MA: Harvard University Press, pp. 99–121.

Klerman, G., Vaillant, G., Spitzer, R. and Michels, R. (1984). A debate on DSM-III. *American Journal of Psychiatry,* **141**(4), 539–53.

Masserman, J. and Carmichael, H. (1938). Diagnosis and prognosis in psychiatry: with a follow-up study of the results of short term general hospital therapy in psychiatric cases. *Journal of Mental Science,* **84**, 893–946.

Mayes, R. and Horwitz, A. (2005). DSM-III and the revolution in the classification of mental illness. *Journal of the History of the Behavioral Sciences,* **41**(3), 249–67.

Mezzich, J. (1979). Patterns and issues in multiaxial psychiatric diagnosis. *Psychological Medicine,* **9**, 125–37.

Norris, V. (1959). *Mental illness in London* (Maudsley Monograph #6). London: Oxford University Press.

Peele, R., May, C., Houston, M., Sorel, E., Halpern, A. and Kline, L. (2004). Action Paper: DSM Multiaxial System presented to Assembly of American Psychiatric Association.

Regier, D., Narrow, W., Kuhl, E. and Kupfer, D. (2009). The conceptual development of DSM-V. *American Journal of Psychiatry,* **166**(6), 645–50.

Rosenhan, D. (1973). On being sane in insane places. *Science,* **179**(70), 250–8.

Rutter, M., Shaffer, D. and Shepherd, M. (1973). An evaluation of the proposal for a multi-axial classification of child psychiatric disorders. *Psychological Medicine,* **3**, 244–50.

Sandifer, M., Hordern, A., Timbury, G. and Green, L. (1968). Psychiatric diagnosis: A comparative study in North Carolina, London, and Glasgow. *British Journal of Psychiatry,* **114**, 1–9.

Sandifer, M., Pettus, C. and Quade, D. (1964). A study of psychiatric diagnosis. *Journal of Nervous and Mental Disease,* **139**, 350–6.

Schmidt, H. and Fonda, C. (1956). The reliabiltiy of psychiatric diagnosis. A new look. *Journal of Abnormal and Social Psychology,* **52**, 262–7.

Spitzer, R. (2001). Values and assumptions in the development of DSM-III and DSM-III-R: An insider's perspective and a belated response to Sadler, Hulgus, and Agich's "On Values in Recent American Psychiatric Classification." *Journal of Nervous and Mental Disease,* **189**, 351–9.

Spitzer, R., Endicott, J. and Robins, E. (1975). Clinical criteria for psychiatric diagnosis and DSM-III. *American Journal of Psychiatry,* **132**(11), 1187–92.

Spitzer, R., Endicott, J. and Robins, E. (1978). Research diagnostic criteria:rationale and reliability. *Archives of General Psychiatry,* **35**, 773–82.

Spitzer, R., Endicott, J., Robins, E., Kuriansky, J. and Gurland, B. (1975). Preliminary report on the reliability of research diagnostic criteria applied to psychiatric case records. In A. Sudilovsky, S. Gershon and B. Beer (eds.), *Predictability in Psychopharmacology: Preclinical and Clinical Correlations.* New York: Raven Press, pp. 1–47.

Spitzer, R. and Fleiss, J. (1974). A re-analysis of the reliability of psychiatric diagnosis. *British Journal of Psychiatry,* 125, 341–7.

Spitzer, R., Forman, J. and Nee, J. (1979). DSM-III field trials: I. initial interrater diagnostic reliability. *American Journal of Psychiatry,* **136**, 815–17.

Szasz, T. (1960). The myth of mental illness. *American Psychologist,* **15**, 113–18.

Tarjan, G., Tizard, J., Rutter, M., Begab, M., Brooke, E., De La Cruz, F., *et al.* (1972). Classification and mental retardation: Issues arising in the fifth WHO Seminar on Psychiatric Diagnosis, Classification, and Statistics. *American Journal of Psychiatry,* **128**(suppl), 34–45.

Valenstein, M., Adler, D. A., Berlant, J., Dixon, L. B., Dulit, R. A., Goldman, B., *et al.* (2009). Implementing standardized assessments in clinical care: now's the time. *Psychiatric Services,* **60**(10), 1372–5.

Ward, C., Beck, A., Mendelson, M., Mock, J. and Erbaugh, J. (1962). The psychiatric nomenclature. *Archives of General Psychiatry,* **7**, 198–205.

Williams, J. (1985). The multiaxial system of DSM-III: where did it come from and where did it go? *Archives of General Psychiatry,* **42**, 175–80.

Wilson, M. (1993). DSM-III and the transformation of American psychiatry: a history. *American Journal of Psychiatry,* **150**(3), 399–410.

World Health Organization (1978). *Mental disorders: glossary and guide to their classification, for use in conjunction with the Ninth Revision of the International Classification of Diseases.* Geneva: World Health Organization.

Zimmerman, M. and McGlinchey, J. (2008). Why don't psychiatrists use scales to measure outcome when treating depressed patients? *Journal of Clinical Psychiatry,* **69**(12), 1916–19.

Evaluating DSM-III: structure, process and outcomes

Harold Alan Pincus

Dr First provides a clear, articulate summary of the development of DSM-III, its accomplishments, limitations and caveats for the development of future classifications. But, ultimately, how does one evaluate such an enterprise?

Avedis Donabedian (1980, pp. 653–698) introduced the "Structure–Process–Outcomes" model for evaluating the quality of healthcare. He noted that "structural components have a propensity to influence the process of care... changes in the process of care, including variations in quality, will influence the outcomes of care broadly defined. Hence structural effects on outcomes are mediated through process." In this context, "Structure" incorporates such components as the number and qualifications of personnel and the organization of services and facilities. "Process" refers to how services are actually provided, for example, the degree of fidelity to evidence-based practices. "Outcomes," of course, includes actual results, i.e., clinical improvement or the rise in health status of a population.

I believe that one can adapt and apply the "Structure–Process–Outcomes" model to evaluating the DSM-III. From a structural perspective, DSM-III could be described as organized by a small group of elite, committed, individuals with governance designed to maintain considerable central leadership and control and limited openness or transparency. As Margaret Mead has remarked, "Never doubt that a small group of thoughtful, committed citizens can change the world. Indeed, it is the only thing that ever has." (http://www.quotationspage.com/quote/33522.html [March 23, 2011]). The DSM-III process might be characterized as a BOGSAT process (i.e., a "Bunch of Guys Sitting Around a Table"). In other words, it relied on expert judgment. No formal reviews of the literature were conducted. Meta analysis had not even been invented. There was no formal and open independent review of the products. However, field trials were conducted and these results were made public.

Nonetheless, the outcomes of DSM-III were quite remarkable. It became widely used around the world by multiple disciplines and has served as the primary textbook of psychopathology. The use of DSM-III categories became a virtual requirement for clinical research studies and its use extended to forensic settings and insurance/reimbursement, immigration, disability and other policies. It had huge sales, bringing in enormous revenues. DSM-III became a household word and in the process critics indicted it for "dumbing down" psychiatric diagnosis. Substantively, there were very important content innovations such as operationalized criteria and the multiaxial system. Some of these innovations worked, others didn't. And, overall, there was a sense that the price of enhanced communication and reliability was premature reification of arbitrary categories and criteria and significant misuse of the system. Most importantly, we really don't know whether patient outcomes have improved as a result of DSM-III.

Looking to the future, the bar has been raised considerably with regard to expectations for structure, process and outcomes. The real question is whether future classifications will take on the Bill Gates persona and, like Microsoft, "take over the world." Is there really a sufficient evidence base for a new paradigm? Or, should we be focusing more on serving the goal of clinical utility (First et al. 2004). In other words, perhaps the future belongs to the approach of Steve Jobs as Apple created products that consumers have found more intuitive, reliable and useful.

Comments References

Donabedian, A. (1980). Methods for deriving criteria for assessing the quality of medical care. *Medical Care Review*, **37**(7), 653–98

First, M. B., Pincus, H. A., Levine, J.B., Williams, J. B., Ustun, B., and Peele, R. (2004). Clinical utility as a criterion for revising psychiatric diagnoses. *American Journal of Psychiatry*, **161**, 946–54.

The Quotations Page (1994–2010). Available at: http://www.quotationspage.com/quote/33522. html

Chapter 8

Introduction

Kenneth S. Kendler

Harold Pincus's chapter contains reflections on the process of the development of DSM-IV by one of the key leaders of that effort. His perspective is multifaceted and well displays the range (sometimes bafflingly large) of goals and concerns that go into this strange hybrid enterprise which is the focus of this book—psychiatric nosology. As Dr Pincus emphasizes, such diagnostic manuals have to serve multiple purposes and sometimes it seems very difficult to adequately address them all. Priorities have to be set. One little example is how ease of use and scientific validity may tug against each other. As any psychometrician will tell you, the measurement of any psychological or psychiatric trait nearly always does better with more items than less. But clinicians, by contrast, would, with near uniformity, rather work with simple diagnoses with a small number of salient criteria. Pincus proposes a quite useful framework when he suggests four major goals for a nosologic manual: clinical, research, educational and information management. In this volume, we focus largely on the first two of these goals with relatively modest attention to the latter two.

For readers unfamiliar with this process of nosologic revision, his essay makes clear the mixture of practical and theoretical concerns that need to be addressed. He appropriately emphasizes one major focus of the DSM-IV effort. That is, in line with the increasing emphasis on evidence-based medicine, an important stated goal of DSM-IV was, in so far as possible, to make the changes in DSM-IV evidence based. In this regard, DSM-IV was broadly consistent with an iterative model for psychiatric diagnosis, trying to focus on making "small changes" that improved upon its predecessor.

While keeping changes to those that are evidence based might sound easy, as I know from my substantial personal experience with DSM-IV, implementing this was far from straightforward. Evidence was often lacking to guide key decisions. The interaction between evidence and expert opinion was frequently a moving target. Although one might hope that evidence would always be interpreted in the same way, this was often not the case. The nature of the psychiatric literature is often open to interpretation. Within the nitty-gritty of DSM-IV committee work, discriminating the importance of scientific data versus informed opinion was often difficult. At its basis, such work is inevitably quite a "social process."

A classic and repeated source of disagreement was about the relative value of different validators. Some members of workgroups valued key clinical measures, such as prognosis or treatment prediction. Researchers might value other measures, such as biological correlates or genetic findings. There were sometimes broad disagreements about the relative value of clinical studies of patients in treatment settings versus epidemiological studies. While the latter might study a more representative group of individuals suffering from the disorder, such studies could be charged with being less clinically relevant as a goodly proportion of subjects with some psychiatric disorders never seek treatment. No overarching "criteria for changing criteria" were created in DSM-IV and it is not a surprise that this issue has re-emerged in DSM-5 as a focus of concern.

He also quite usefully reviews the levels of nosologic concern. A great deal of focus is often on the addition of new disorders (and more rarely the deletion of disorders). Also, a good deal of attention often gets focused on the placement of disorders in categories—what in DSM-5, has been called the "meta-structure" problem (Andrews et al. 2009). But as he points out, the "bread and butter" of most nosologic work is the "task of revising the diagnostic criteria."

Dr Pincus concludes his essay with a section on "suggestions for the future." Several points are worthy of brief emphasis. He calls for an improvement of the "data base" allowing more recommendations to be made on empirical grounds. He thoughtfully reviews the differences between "small-picture issues" (e.g. changing diagnostic criteria) with "really big-picture issues" such as criteria for how you place disorders into categories (e.g., clinical resemblance versus etiologic relationship). While initially this might seem counter-intuitive, he is right that the smaller questions are more easily addressed empirically while the larger ones are conceptual and, dare I say, philosophical in nature. He speaks with the voice of experience on one important issue—to test the impact on prevalences of what might seem to be modest changes in criteria. Armchair conclusions that alterations in criteria should produce only "minor" changes in casesness have not proven reliable in the past including with DSM-IV.

Dr Pincus's essay reflects a reasoned and experienced voice with a healthy degree of skepticism about how seriously diagnostic manuals should be taken. He notes particularly that researchers should not be bound by its categories. But as he is also aware, social forces—reimbursement policies, grant review committees and journal editors—sometimes enforce a false hegemony for diagnostic manuals beyond that intended by its creators or warranted by the quality of its often tentative scientific support.

Introduction Reference

Andrews, G., Goldberg, D.P., Krueger, R.F., Carpenter, W. T., Hyman, S. E., Sachdev, P., *et al.* (2009). Exploring the feasibility of a meta-structure for DSM-V and ICD-11: could it improve utility and validity? *Psychological Medicine*, **39**(12), 1993–2000.

Chapter 8

DSM-IV: context, concepts and controversies

Harold Alan Pincus

The intent of this paper is to provide an overview of the circumstances surrounding the development of DSM-IV, the principles and process underlying its development and several especially interesting or controversial issues that were encountered in its development. From the outset, it is worth pointing out that the work on DSM-IV was initiated during a period of burgeoning interest in "evidence-based medicine." Within the leadership of the American Psychiatric Association (APA), most notably Melvin Sabshin, the Medical Director at that time, there was a strong sense that psychiatry must be part of that movement and this intent was inherent in establishing the APA's Office of Research several years prior to initiating the DSM-IV process. In fact, when I established the Office we were given responsibility for spearheading DSM-III-R through the final phases of its process. As such, it was felt that evidence-based approaches to psychiatric classification are essential to assure the credibility of the field and to conform to current scientific standards. They do, however, have important limitations and are not without their own explicit and implicit set of values. More on this later.

8.1 Context

Why classify? Goals of a classification

The goals of the DSM-IV can be divided into four main categories: clinical, research, educational and information management. The clinical goals of the DSM-IV were paramount because the book is used primarily by clinicians.

Clinical

In our view, the highest priorities in developing the DSM-IV were the clinical application of criteria to define specific mental disorders and the enhancement of the reliability of communication and assessment among clinicians. The definitions and subclassifications of the DSM-IV should be of use to them as they conceptualize their treatment planning and in predicting the future course of the patient's illness. However, as stated in the DSM-IV introduction, a DSM-IV diagnosis by itself should in no way constitute the full spectrum of the knowledge needed to develop a treatment plan. It is simply a start. Also, the text in the DSM-IV also provides some useful collateral information that is helpful for clinicians in their work with patients.

Research

An important research goal of the DSM-IV was to define reasonably homogeneous groups for study. Especially in a research setting, with the capacity and expectation of careful training and tuning of assessors, the criteria can also enhance the reliability of assessment. We encouraged researchers, however, not to be limited by the DSM criteria, since we are rapidly learning more about psychiatric disorders and the classification should be continually evolving. We felt it was important to encourage research in this regard by considering alternative definitions and to promote further hypothesis testing. As the field moves forward with increasing capacity in neuroscience, imaging, genetics, etc. it is expected that purely descriptive approaches will become less relevant; however that time is not approaching nearly as fast as we would want (or had anticipated).

Educational

The DSM-IV has served, with both good and bad effects, as a textbook of psychopathology. It has been used to teach residents in psychiatry as well as students in psychology, social work, nursing and other disciplines. To some extent, it has been used as a teaching tool in medicine in general. In 1995, a primary care version of the DSM-IV was developed to provide a better link to the educational needs of primary care physicians and to aid them in making a clinical diagnosis in mental health (it was a failure). There are also a number of important appendices in the DSM-IV which are particularly useful for educational purposes. Among these are decision trees, a conceptual framework for cultural assessment of individuals with a mental disorder, and a glossary of culturally related conditions. Importantly, the educational applications of DSM-IV extend beyond clinicians, to patients, family members, attorneys, the media and policymakers.

Information management

The DSM-IV categorizes information derived from many different clinical sources and clinical practitioners for use in information management. The book was designed to be completely compatible with the codes and short glossary definitions of the International Classification of Diseases, 10th edition (ICD-10) which is, by treaty, the international standard for reporting mortality and morbidity. At the time of initiating DSM-IV, the World Health Organization (WHO) had already begun development of the ICD-10 and the need to coordinate efforts was a key reason for developing DSM-IV. As it turned out, while DSM-IV was published at roughly the same time as ICD-10, the United States is one of very few countries in the world that has not yet officially adopted the ICD-10. The DSM-IV was also designed to be fully compatible with the Clinical Modification of the ICD-9, the ICD-9-CM, which is the classification system used in the United States for coding. The ICD-9-CM, as the official reimbursement classification in the United States, adapted from the WHO ICD-9 and developed and maintained by the federal government, is required for reimbursement from Medicare, Medicaid and most third-party payers. It is also used routinely in formulating payment categories for hospitals and in compiling quality indicators that hospitals and doctors are increasingly being required to report. At the same time, however, the DSM-IV is not and was not developed to be a reimbursement manual for psychiatry. The DSM-IV simply selects the appropriate codes from the ICD-9-CM and attaches them to DSM definitions.

The DSM-IV introductory chapters were designed to be essential reading for all users. They clarify the intent of the manual, provide detailed guidance in its use and lay out a detailed elaboration of its limitations and a strong self-critique of the manual. Ultimately, the DSM-IV is simply a convention for communication; that is, the primary purpose of the DSM-IV is as a communication tool for use among clinicians and between clinicians and researchers.

8.2 **Historical context**

Efforts to classify mental illness have existed for thousands of years, and multiple other presenters will discuss the broader and more distant historical context. This paper will discuss our perceptions of the role, context, advantages and disadvantages of DSMs generally and especially DSM-III and DSM-III-R.

Early history of DSM classifications

Long before the DSM-IV was published, during the early days of the US census, the very first attempt at classifying mental disorders in the United States occurred. In 1840 there was a single classification in the census for people who were hospitalized in mental institutions. Current classifications have their roots in data collection purposes of the census. Today, the ICD-9-CM and the DSM-IV are still used for data collection, and these data are used for statistical and epidemiological reporting purposes.

The first international classification system, the ICD-6, was developed by WHO in 1948. In the United States, the APA developed an alternative classification, the DSM-I (American Psychiatric Association 1952), which had short glossary definitions for the different disorders. The ICD-8 and the DSM-II (American Psychiatric Association 1968) were, for the most part, very similar and consisted of a paragraph of general description of the different conditions. Both were fairly short volumes and did not receive the broad public and clinical attention of DSM-III and DSM-IV.

DSM-III paradigm shift

The DSM-III represented a major shift in psychiatric diagnosis. It was intended to be descriptive and have, by and large, an "atheoretical" perspective (or at least a non-etiologic focus). It introduced diagnostic criteria to define disorders more clearly and to provide a way of improving reliability through these explicit definitions.

The DSM-III also introduced a multiaxial system, which acknowledged that simply having a single name attached to a diagnosis was not sufficient information to assess the treatment needs of a particular individual. In addition, it introduced the concept of multiple diagnoses, which held that there was not necessarily a single diagnostic class in which a patient might fit.

DSM advantages

The DSM-III had important advantages. It improved reliability and facilitated communication between clinicians and researchers. It enabled a clinician to make a reasonable judgment as to how an article in, for example, the *American Journal of Psychiatry* or the *Archives of General Psychiatry* that used DSM criteria for describing the clinical population of subjects in a study might relate to one's own patients. The DSM-III was widely used by clinicians, researchers, educators and trainees. It included important methodological and content innovations such as diagnostic criteria and the multiaxial system. The DSM-III was a success far beyond expectations, and it promoted an emphasis on empirical data.

DSM disadvantages

There were, however, some important disadvantages to the DSM-III. Users took the manual very seriously—much more seriously than the developers intended. Many categories were long, complex and user-unfriendly. In some instances, the criteria were made very specific (e.g. that the symptoms had to occur within 1 month or within 60 days, five out of 10 symptoms had to be present) in an attempt to become more precise. This "pseudoprecision" of the diagnostic criteria was often arbitrary because of limitations in the available empirical data. It introduced communication problems among DSM-III users and international users of the ICD 9 because of the substantial differences between the two classification systems. In addition, there were a number of specific disputes, for example, the elimination of neurosis and the controversies over homosexuality, which became embarrassing political conflicts.

DMS III-R

Seven years later, in 1987, the DSM-III-R was published. Like the DSM-III before it, the DSM-III-R had important advantages and disadvantages. By and large, this revision followed the same model and the same architecture of the DSM-III, but it was intended to identify and correct inconsistencies. It also demonstrated that the DSM system was self-correcting—that it was not a static process but a system that responds to new empirical data and information. The DSM-III-R introduced several diagnostic categories, modified criteria, reduced diagnostic hierarchies and heightened the issue of comorbidity as a way to describe the clinical picture for a given individual.

Many perceived this as being too much change too soon. It was seen as going too far beyond simply correcting inconsistencies by changing criteria and was therefore a disruption to researchers and educators. Researchers had to redevelop their instruments, and many studies already under way had to be changed. An important disadvantage of the DSM-III-R (and the DSM-III, for that matter) was that for many of the changes no consistent rationale was provided. In some cases there was clear empirical support, but in others there may not have been empirical support, or if it existed, it was not specified or documented. In developing the DSM-IV, we took into consideration the lessons learned during both the DSM-III and the DSM-III-R processes.

Principles and processes for the DSM-IV

DSM-III/DSM-III-R/ICD-10 processes

The DSM-III and DSM-III-R were developed by "expert consensus" groups, or what some have termed the "bogsat" method (i.e., "a bunch of guys sitting around a table"). The expert consensus or "bogsat" method involves bringing together individuals who, in an informal way and, using their knowledge of the literature and professional experiences, make determinations about the issues at hand.

This approach has limitations. The decisions made by the consensus group are not necessarily generalizable to a broad population. The decisions reflect the group's own experience and views of the literature. The range of specialty interests may not be fully represented on the panel, and the individuals chosen may not represent all the interests in their specialty. In addition, the consensus group decision may not reflect a balanced and comprehensive review of the literature if a systematic search has not been conducted. Finally, documentation of the process and the rationale for the decisions may not occur.

When the DSM-II and DSM-II-R were developed, the available literature had enormous gaps and limitations, and the tools to conduct systematic and comprehensive searches of the peer-reviewed literature were not as readily available as they are today. Review and revision by expert consensus was the most viable option for DSM-III and DSM-III-R. In fact, the major contribution of DSM-III was that it did lead to the availability of a large amount of relevant evidence and information that would later be applied in the DSM-IV process.

There was a major difference in the research environment at the time the DSM-III and DSM-III-R were being developed, as compared with the DSM-IV development period, when a great deal more data and more research funding were available. For example, in 1984, departments of psychiatry received approximately $82 million in National Institute of Health (NIH) research support. In comparison, by 1998, the NIH provided more than $400 million in research support. Psychiatry went from being the tenth-ranked department in medical schools in research funding support to the second-ranked. While, obviously not all this research was relevant to DSM-IV, empirically derived information that was not previously available could now be applied to inform the DSM decision-making process.

Evidence-based medicine

During the years between the DSM-III-R and the DSM-IV a sea change was going on throughout medicine, with increased calls for accountability, increased expectations for the application of evidence and empirical data in clinical decision-making, and the increased availability of data. Sackett (1997, p. 3) and proponents of evidence-based medicine, which extended from England and Canada to the United States, define evidence-based medicine as "the conscientious, explicit, and judicious use of the current best evidence in making decisions about the care of individual patients." For the DSM-IV that definition was taken beyond individual patients and applied systematically in a broader clinical/policymaking process.

The principles of evidence-based medicine have been described by Sackett and others. A critical component of evidence-based medicine is the understanding of the rules of evidence, what are called "critical appraisal skills for the evaluation of published studies." Another important component of evidence-based medicine is that there is a comprehensive and systematic searching, extracting, arraying, documenting, assessing and integrating of all the published literature. This process must be stewarded in an unbiased, systematic manner. Such stewardship is enabled by the availability of new information technologies, the growth of electronic search techniques and the development of more extensive library systems. The methodologies used to conduct the literature review (e.g., the specific search terms, databases searched, criteria used to extract the literature, arraying the information) should be documented in a fashion similar to the methods used in research studies to allow for replication. The decision-making process for inclusion/exclusion of studies should be explicit and documented as well.

The stepwise process that was applied in DSM-IV began with applying systematic methods for searching the published literature, extracting the data from the literature, synthesizing and arraying the information, assessing the data and using and integrating the data into the consideration of the options being developed. Multiple, diverse, clinical and research perspectives must also be solicited and integrated in an open manner. Finally, this is a feedback process in which the process and outcomes are transparent and continually monitored and fully documented.

Principles of the DSM-IV process

One of the principles of the DSM-IV process was to involve the leaders in the field, as well as regular clinicians, from a broad array of disciplines and specialties. It was important to represent as wide a breadth and diversity of people and expertise as possible. Literally thousands of individuals participated in the DSM-IV process in one form or another. A second principle was to decentralize, so that the task force was informed by the field rather than the field being informed by the task force. To that end, for each work group, an expert from that area was appointed as chairperson. The work group members were experts in that field representing multiple disciplines and perspectives. In order to avoid individual bias, each member was asked to function as a "consensus scholar" rather than promote their own proposals. Fostering a completely open and transparent process with complete documentation was the third principle. Every piece of information about the process was made available so that one would know what decisions were being made and understand why they were made since this was well before the Internet, to encourage the sharing of information, the DSM-IV Task Force published a large number of articles about the process as it developed. In addition, a newsletter about the DSM-IV development and process and progress was sent to more than three thousand individuals worldwide as well as an options book midway in the process. Many of the individuals involved in the process (i.e., work groups and members) published articles and presented papers at meetings on the progress of the work groups. Finally, the four-volume DSM-IV Sourcebook documented the entire process. There was also a great deal of international collaboration, especially with those developing the ICD 10.

The most important principle of the DSM-IV process was that all changes should be based on systematic data collection and review by potential critics. This basic principle undergirded the entire project and the functioning of each work group. At the very beginning of the project a methods workshop, attended by the major participants in the process, was held. The workshop, a seminar on how to implement evidence-based medicine, laid out very explicit instructions on what the work groups were supposed to do and how they were to do it. The specific steps and the process each work group had to follow to come to a decision were explained in detail and with examples (Frances et al. 1989). This process included the following steps:

+ Identify issues.
+ Prioritize issues.
+ Formulate approach for "working up" each prioritized issue and establish evidentiary hierarchy.
+ Systematically gather evidence from published literature.
+ Draft literature review and circulate among advisors.
+ Formulate proposed options for change.
+ Consider and delineate risks and benefits for each option.
+ Solicit relevant data sets.
+ Reanalyze data sets.
+ Solicit wide response to options from the field.
+ Conduct field trials to examine relative merit of proposed options.
+ Formulate "final" criteria set.
+ Solicit additional responses from field.
+ Final approval and publication.

Types of changes

The work groups were asked to resolve five types of issues: adding and deleting categories, subtyping disorders, revising criteria sets, considering the placement of disorders in the classification and updating the text. It is important to note that the DSM-IV consists of several different elements. One is the classification itself, which lists the names and disorders and their ICD-9-CM codes; another is the diagnostic criteria. In addition to the diagnostic criteria, text information about prevalence, course, familial patterns, age, gender and cultural issues of the disorders is provided to help clinicians and students understand how to apply the criteria.

The *addition and deletion of disorders* was one of the high-profile issues for the DSM-IV process, but it was not the "meat and potatoes" of the revision. More than 150 different proposals were received for adding categories to the DSM-IV. These proposals ranged from off-hand ideas to very serious recommendations with a rich tradition of clinical literature and empirical support. A number of arguments were made for adding and deleting categories. The most common argument in support of adding a new category (or not deleting an old one) was that if the category was not included, there would be a large number of individuals whose treatment needs would go unmet and whose conditions would not be researchable; clinicians might also have problems communicating about the nature of the treatment for these individuals (Pincus et al. 1992). For many proposals, the generalizability of the supporting data for the proposed condition was problematic. Oftentimes the suggested additions were proposed by individuals, groups, or centers that had a great deal of experience in assessing a particular class of individuals, but it was unknown if the components of the condition they assessed would translate more broadly to the full range of persons whose disorders were diagnosed using the DSM-IV. Therefore, one of the questions asked with regard to a proposed condition was, Is there a generalizable set of information in support of including this new disorder? Another problem with some of the suggested additions was the potential for misuse. Would the condition be appropriately used once it was disseminated more broadly? Do the data support the fact that it can be reliably assessed by average clinicians? Yet another concern was the added complexity of the system. Ultimately, there had to be a substantial amount of evidence—from peer-reviewed literature—to add something new to the DSM-IV.

Unlike the DSM-III and DSM-III-R, which included many categories intended to stimulate research, the DSM-IV was intended to be led by research. Nevertheless, to encourage research, the DSM-IV had an appendix that included certain conditions with a substantial research literature behind them but which are not formally included in the DSM-IV. This appendix offered a common language to encourage research on those conditions. Conditions that were considered for addition, such as mixed anxiety-depression and other subthreshold conditions, binge-eating disorder, and premenstrual dysphoric disorder, were included in the appendix. Only 13 new disorders were added to the DSM-IV (e.g. acute stress disorder, bipolar II, Asperger's disorder). Most of these additions were simple oversights that had not been added to the DSM-III-R, such as substance-induced sexual dysfunction. Several conditions were deleted from the classification because there was no evidence base to support their continued inclusion and no literature showing ongoing research into the conditions (e.g. identity disorder). In addition, the childhood anxiety disorders were reformulated and incorporated within the adult disorders.

The *subtyping of disorders* was another area that was tackled by the work groups. The inclusion of subtypes was similarly based on a comprehensive review of the research and clinical utility. For example, in anorexia nervosa, two subtypes—a binge-eating subtype and a restricting subtype—were added because in the past individuals with binge eating in addition to anorexia nervosa had been given two different diagnoses, bulimia nervosa and anorexia nervosa. By adding these subtypes only one diagnosis need be given. Another example of the addition of subtypes is specific phobia. There was good evidence that the blood injection/injury-type phobias were different from the other phobias, both from a family history perspective and physiologically, resulting in different treatment implications. Subtypes for depression and dementia were also added. A thorough review of the literature for the melancholic features of depression was conducted, and the condition remained in the DSM with some changes in the criteria. Dementia with behavioral disturbance as a subcategory of dementia was added because it is an important issue in nursing homes for treatment planning.

The task of *revising the diagnostic criteria* was the bulk of the work for the work groups, and it became a balancing act for them. For each set of criteria the work group had to weigh a number of different issues. One issue was whether to increase the relevance and the importance of core features of a particular condition in a prototypical way versus improving the capacity to discriminate features of the disorder from those of other disorders ("near neighbors") in a differential diagnosis. Another issue was balancing the complexity or simplicity criteria sets and considering how that would affect the validity and reliability. A great deal more reliability could be gained by very complex criteria sets. On the other hand, the criteria could be made so complex that they would not be used. Other questions of balance concerned how specific and detailed each criterion should be in terms of its operationalization versus the level of inference that could be expected (which also affects the reliability and validity of the category) and how one balances operational rules versus clinical judgment. Finally, there was the issue of thresholds. Where should a fixed threshold be established, when should a threshold be changed, and on what sort of evidence should these decisions be based?

These questions, when applied to the criteria sets, resulted in some of the following investigations. One was an attempt to have somatization disorder defined by a much less complex set of criteria. The issue for somatoform disorder was that the DSM-III-R criteria set was rarely applied because there were 35 different items and the clinician had to decide whether 13 of them would be endorsed. The literature review documented the high reliability and validity of the condition, and through an analysis of data pooled from a number of different sites, a much simpler criteria set was defined, one that identified the same group of patients. A five-site field trial of this reformulated criteria set examined the proposed criteria, assessed the set's ease of use, reliability and generalizability, and used semistructured interviews comparing the simplified set with the DSM-III, DSM-III-R, ICD 10 and original Briquet syndrome. The field trial results found that there was virtually no change in caseness and excellent reliability for the revised criteria set (Yutzy et al. 1995).

The issue of adding more inference to antisocial personality disorder (i.e., attempting to incorporate notions of a lack of conscience) was reviewed and evaluated. Although some minor changes were made, there were insufficient data to implement this proposal. The potential for operationalizing bulimic episodes, defined as eating a large amount of food in a very short period of time, was also considered. Could the amount of food and the time period be specified? These particulars could not be operationalized in a reliable and valid manner and therefore were not added to the criteria set.

For schizophrenia, the issue of duration was examined because the ICD 10 required a 1-month duration of active symptoms and the DSM-III-R used a 2-week duration. A field trial conducted to examine this issue empirically demonstrated little change in caseness if the DSM-IV moved to a duration of 1 month, to be compatible with the ICD-10 (Flaum et al. 1998).

The *issues of placement* deal with both the overall organization of the DSM-IV and the conceptual framework for the various groupings—that is, what level of abstraction should be applied, under what name a disorder should be categorized, and finally, what the location of each specific disorder should be. Typical questions were 'should hypochondriasis be an anxiety disorder or a somatoform disorder?' and 'should we have a section on stress-related conditions?'

Each work group formulated each of these issues as a question and established hierarchy of evidence that could be relevant for answering the question. A literature search was conducted to gather evidence, which was ordered from most important to least important according to this a priori hierarchy. Once the literature review had been completed and the data compiled and summarized, the summary was circulated to between 50 and 100 international and national advisors/experts in the field to determine if the work group had missed any pertinent literature of if the data had been misinterpreted. These summaries of the literature review were formulated as options for solutions to resolve the questions. Across all work groups, these options were collated into the DSM-IV Options Book, which was made widely available for review and comment. A second version, the DSM-IV Craft Criteria, developed from responses to the Options Book, as well as additional reviews, data analyses and field trials, was disseminated to another 4000 individuals. This version was then slightly modified and approved by the APA before publication.

To assist in the DSM-IV process, the work groups solicited relevant data sets that may not have been analyzed with regard to specific issues for the DSM-IV but which could be reanalyzed and which could be funded under a grant from the MacArthur Foundation. Many of the work groups formulated options for making changes which were researched through the MacArthur Data Reanalysis Studies. The National Institute of Mental Health/NIDA/NIAAA (NIMH) funded trials for the DSM-IV projects. This was, in fact, one of the most complex grants that the NIH ever evaluated through extensive, independent peer review. It involved 12 different projects with 88 sites internationally and more than 7000 patients.

Throughout the process an atmosphere of conservatism prevailed to avoid the disruption of clinical and research efforts begun with the DSM-III and DSM-III-R. Compatibility between the DSM system and the ICD-10 system was also important. Most important, the changes that resulted in the DSM-IV were driven by the data available, balanced with clinical judgment, and the liberal application of common sense. Small changes supported by substantial data that fixed big problems were favored over big changes with limited data for little problems. In addition, a clear risk:benefit analysis was applied to evaluating potential unintended consequences of changes. By far the most important change in the DSM-IV was the use of a methodical, evidence-based process to develop the manual. As we will discuss, all of this effort did not protect against several serious problems that negatively impacted psychiatric care as a result of DSM-IV changes.

Limits of an evidence-based classification

Although the DSM-IV represented a successful use of an evidence-based process, there are some problems in applying evidence-based approaches, as Ken Kendler (1990) discussed in his article "Toward a scientific psychiatric nosology."

Kendler discussed these issues from the framework of an evidence-deterministic approach in contrast to the other extreme of a more advocacy-driven model. With an evidence-deterministic model (in which there must be direct empirical testing of all nosological hypotheses), historical tradition, clinical evidence, clinical experience and common sense have very limited roles. Some areas that are less accessible to scientific investigation (e.g. the requirement of a multiaxial system) cannot be included. There are also clinical and educational needs that may not necessarily be served by a purely evidence-based process, because it could create a degree of complexity which might not be realistic or practical in application to the real world. Issues that need to be resolved should also be covered completely and thoroughly. If a very, very high standard of evidence is applied, only a very small number of conditions would be validated, and these would not meet administrative or clinical needs.

Applying strict empirical approaches also presents a variety of specific problems. Disagreement can arise over the construct of a disorder. For example, is depression a mood disorder, a cognitive disorder or a motor disorder? (E.g., how would a Martian observer categorize a group of depressed people?) Depression can be conceptualized in any one of those three ways, and how it is conceptualized will change how it is assessed and what kind of criteria are used. There may be disagreement about the importance of different validators. For example, is family history more important for determining the criteria for schizoaffective disorder, or is clinical course more important? The importance of varying data in forming different goals (e.g., reliability versus validity) can also be a source of disagreement. Obviously, in all of science there can be disagreements about the interpretation of data. The non-generalizability of data is another problem. Most of the data collected in the empirical literature are from tertiary care medical centers. How well that translates to the average patient of the average practitioner (especially in primary care or in community-based epidemiological studies) is not always clear. Data may also be insufficient. Little or no data may be available for many areas, and many of the studies that do exist may not have been conducted with an ideal level of rigor.

DSM-IV controversies/disasters

Inevitably, the profile of DSM-IV, the political climate of the US and the importance of social and economic forces in the use of psychiatric diagnosis led to a number of well publicized controversies which continue to this day. The fact that the evidence base was highly imperfect and often conflicting or absent made resolution of these controversies difficult. Time and additional research have demonstrated that a number of the issues dealt within DSM-IV did not turn out well. In particular, we did not fully anticipate how limited the generalizability of much of the research that was done in the context of the much larger social and economic forces that took over once the book was published. Most notable are the "epidemics" of bipolar II disorder, attention deficit hyper-activity disorder, autism and the misapplication of certain conditions in forensic settings.

8.3 **Suggestions for the future**

There are a number of recommendations for improving the DSM developmental process. First, the database needs to be improved. More evidence, better evidence and more relevant evidence are needed. It is unclear, however (especially given the short time frame), the extent to which the initial work done in the series of DSM-5 conferences conducted with NIMH support actually resulted in timely new studies that have provided data directly applicable to the questions being addressed. In particular, more information on the application and performance of alternative options in non-specialty and non-clinical (i.e., community based) populations is essential (White 1961) to reflect the actual "ecology" of healthcare.

Truth in advertising is also necessary. All people using the DSM-IV should read its introduction because it contains an extensive critique of the manual. We knew our process and product were not perfect and wanted to convey a sense of humility and display the limitations and risks as comprehensively and transparently as possible from the outset. It also outlines the process for the development of the DSM-IV— what was done, how it was done and why it was done. This description and documentation was greatly extended in the DSM-IV Sourcebook. Importantly, the introduction points out that the DSM-IV is not to be taken too literally. This is an important message. Somebody once said during the DSM-IV development process that subliminally emblazoned on every page of the DSM-IV should be the word "THINK!"

Although the DSM-IV process was explicit, open and documented, the DSM process could be improved in a number of ways. More could be done to involve patients and families. The link with clinicians could also be made stronger by informing them early and continuously of the issues so that they can participate more fully, perhaps establishing a formal multidisciplinary clinical advisory group. A more effective dialogue and collaboration internationally, and specifically with the ICD-11, are needed. In fact, there is little justification in having two different systems.

The evidence-based process can be further delineated by being more explicit about how we think about the evidence-based issues, separating out the "big-picture" and "small-picture" issues. As Kendler said, when working on the small-picture issues, evidence plays a larger role than when working on medium- and big-picture issues. For both sizes of issues the subsets of these issues must be separated out. Then, in an a priori manner, the basis for making determinations on each issue can be further explicated.

From the start, the "really big-picture issue" of clarifying the primary purpose and evidence of the classification is not an evidence-based decision. It is no longer possible to ignore all the multiple ways in which DSM is used and the social, economic and policy forces in the environment that affect that use. "Use cases" for different applications need to be worked up and need to be considered in determining approaches and strategies. For example, in the overall ICD-11 process a "use case" Technical Advisory Group on Quality and Patient Safety has been established to consider how to make the classification more useful in gathering data for populating numerators and denominators of performance indicators.

In addition, a number of "big-picture" issues affect both the development of the DSM and, more importantly, the future of psychiatric classification and nosology. For most of these issues some amount and types of evidence are useful, but do not play a major role. Some of these issues relate to the basic nosological approach that is applied: categorical versus dimensional approaches (in particular, in the personality disorders) or cross-sectional versus longitudinal approaches. Other issues involve varying consideration of what might be termed "dependent variables and independent variables" in diagnosis (i.e., should measures of neuropathology or structural or functional imaging be the independent variables for a classification and descriptive data be the dependent variable, rather than the reverse, which is the way we do it now), the role of symptoms versus impairments in criteria, whether to incorporate both descriptive and biological measurement into the diagnostic criteria, integration of phenotype and genotype data, and how information on internal and external experiences, behavior, treatment response, and biological mechanisms should be addressed.

"Medium-picture" issues are more specific and affect more directly the clinical practice of psychiatrists both diagnostically and for treatment planning. Included in this set of issues is the question of which multiaxial approaches to assessment should be included. And should there be distinct axes for syndrome, pathology/pathophysiology, genetics, course of a disorder, the level of impairment/disability and the patient's personality and adaptive mechanisms?

For both "medium-picture" and "big-picture" issues, the ways of defining mental disorders involve more than evidence. The information for responding to these issues is drawn from sources that might not be clearly labeled "evidence" but may relate to different evidentiary bases such as logic, common sense, tradition, the elegance, clarity and utility of an idea, administrative requirements, practicality and time. But "evidence" remains highly relevant as well—more on this later.

Psychiatric classification also has an array of specific issues (i.e., "small-picture" issues) related to the actual content of the DSM which were discussed earlier. Among these are decisions about what disorders are added or deleted, revisions to the criteria sets, subtyping of disorders, the organization and placement of disorders in the DSM and, finally, text revisions. Here is where evidence can make an enormous difference. In particular, is the need to test the impact of potential changes in DSM in population-based samples. There is simply no other way to assess the impact of changes in shifting caseness across the boundary of pathology and normality or across different categories. Simply using convenience samples in specialty mental health or even primary care settings is no longer sufficient. Given that the extremely conservative and evidence-based changes in DSM IV resulted in highly significant unintended consequences, such data should represent a minimum threshold for change.

There are many issues to address, studies to conduct and evidence to gather, but not all of these can be done. Priorities need to be set. In addition, some "non-evidence" items can be subject to a kind of evidentiary evaluation. For example, there are approaches to assess "clinical utility" in an empirical manner (First et al. 2004). In short, the role and type of evidence shifts depending on the size and level of abstraction of the kinds of issues being addressed.

In fact, I would contend that given the current lack of understanding of the etiopathogenesis of the vast majority of psychiatric conditions, the continued revision of a descriptive classification has little utility. Ultimately, I believe that DSM is simply a "convention for communication" that can serve as a kind of "Rosetta Stone" for communication among and across the multiple "tribes" of mental health disciplines, investigative groups and cultures (i.e., researchers, clinicians, educators). In fact, the most important effort for classifying mental disorders with a focus on etiologic mechanisms, NIMH's RDoC project, is being conducted independently of the DSM and ICD processes.

Allen Frances, Michael First and I wrote about the epistemologic perspective of three baseball umpires:

◆ Umpire 1: there are balls and there are strikes and I call them as they are.

◆ Umpire 2: there are no balls and no strikes until I call them.

◆ Umpire 3: there are balls and there are strikes and I call them as I see them.

We explained that Umpire 3 represented our perspective. At this point, I would add a fourth umpire:

◆ Umpire 4: there are balls and there are strikes and I call them as I use them (with DSM/ICD serving as an ontology/"Rosetta Stone" to anchor communication and assure interoperability).

From my perspective the world has changed and the management of information has become the pre-eminent task of a classification system, overshadowing (but also enhancing), the clinical, research and educational goals of a classification.

The information management goal intersects with multiple user groups in terms of:

◆ Health policy

◆ Clinical decision-making

◆ Quality measurement

◆ Epidemiology

◆ Educational certification/accreditation

◆ Multiple areas of research from genetics to psychopharmacology to cognitive science, etc.

The way this would work is that the DSM/ICD classification (they would need to be combined into a single system) would remain relatively stable. Each individual user "tribe" (or individual scientist) would be free to identify various alternative classifications. However, all journals or other public reporting mechanisms would require that any clinical population also be described in the ICD/DSM classification in addition to whatever tribal classification is being used. (i.e., "Of the subjects meeting criteria for the 'Pincus syndrome', 70% met ICD/DSM criteria for GAD, 40% OCD, and 30% Anxiety Disorder, NOS"). This approach is similar to the concept of different types of alloys in Rachel Cooper's chapter (Chapter 4, this volume).

Changes in future (descriptive) classifications should be infrequent and guided by a highly conservative process that would only incorporate changes with strong evidence that they:

1. Enhance overall communication among the "tribes."

2. Enhance clinical decision-making.

3. Enhance patient outcomes (First et al. 2004).

However, ICD/DSM would have a section describing the relationships among the various tribal concepts that could be updated on a more frequent basis.

Note that this approach gives up the ideal (or even a focus) on validity, per se. Maintaining effective communication (most notably, effective use, reliability and understandability) and clinical utility (either the more limited improvement of clinical and organizational decision-making processes or the ideal of outcomes improvement) become the principal goals of the classification. In other words, while a psychiatric classification must be useful for a variety of purposes, it cannot be expected to be simultaneously at the forefront of, for example, neurobiology and genetics, psychoanalysis, and the education of mental health counselors, primary care providers and psychologists.

However, multiple groups can continue their work on epistemic iteration using genetic approaches and others can develop ways to better measure quality or costs of care and yet others can study dimensional ratings of personality. However, each tribal group would need to be able to communicate across the commons using the "Rosetta Stone". Thus, we would not be wobbling toward the asymptote of true validity, but, instead, be very slowly, but continually rising toward the goal of better outcomes for patients.

Endnote

1 These remarks are adapted and much extended from several previous publications: Pincus and McQueen (2002), Frances et al. (1989, 1990, 1991) and Pincus et al. (1992).

Chapter References

First, M. B., Pincus, H. A., Levine, J. B., Williams, J. B., Ustun, B., and Peele, R. (2004). Clinical utility as a criterion for revising psychiatric diagnoses. *American Journal of Psychiatry*, **161**, 946–54.

Flaum, M., Amador, X., Gorman, J., Bracha, H. S., Edell, W. S., McGlashan, T. *et al.* (1998). Field trial for schizophrenia and other psychotic disorders. In T.A. Widiger and A.J. Frances (eds.), *The Importance of What We Care About*. New York: Cambridge University Press.

Frances, A. J., Widiger, T. A., and Pincus, H. A. (1989). The development of DSM-IV. *Archives of General Psychiatry*, **4**, 373–5.

Frances, A. J., Pincus, H. A., Widiger, T. A., and Davis, W. W. (1990). DSM-IV: work in progress. *American Journal of Psychiatry*, **147**, 11.

Frances, A. J., First, M. S., Widiger, T. A., Miele, G. M., Tilly, S. M., Davis, W.W. *et al.* (1991). An A to Z guide to DSM-IV conundrums. *Journal of Abnormal Psychology*, **3**, 407–12.

Kendler, K. (1990). Toward a scientific psychiatric nosology. *Archives of General Psychiatry*, **47**, 969–73.

Pincus, H. A., Frances, A., Davis, W. W., First, M. B., and Widiger, T. A. (1992). DSM-IV and new diagnostic categories: holding the line on proliferation. *American Journal of Psychiatry*, **149**, 112–17.

Pincus, H. A. and McQueen, L. E. (2002). The limits of an evidence-based classification of mental disorders. In J. Z. Sadler (ed.), *Descriptions and prescriptions: Values, mental disorders, and the DSMs*. Baltimore, MD: The Johns Hopkins University Press, pp. 9–24.

Sackett, D. L. (1997). *Evidence-Based Medicine: How to Practice and Teach EBM*. New York: Churchill Livingstone.

Yutzy, S. H., Cloninger, C.R. and Guze, S. B. (1995). DSM-IV field trial: Testing a new proposal for somatization disorder. *American Journal of Psychiatry*, **152**, 97–101.

DSM-IV: some critical remarks

Mario Maj

The DSM-IV is a text put together with a lot of competence, accuracy and wisdom. This has become even clearer to me now that I am a member of one of the workgroups for the DSM-5. It is obvious that most of the issues we are now debating had been already identified in the development of the DSM-IV, and addressed in a reasonable way, based on the evidence which was available at that time.

I have produced along the years several editorials and research papers analysing in a critical way various aspects of the manual, but my criticism mostly applied to the DSM-III and its successors in general, rather than to the DSM-IV specifically. This was also the case for several other commentators, not to mention the many critical positions reflecting a more general negative attitude towards the use of classification systems in psychiatry or the psychiatric profession in itself.

Harold Pincus opens his piece by outlining the "context" in which the DSM-IV was developed, dominated by a strong motivation to apply the principles of evidence-based medicine to psychiatry and by the confidence that an evidence-based refinement of the diagnostic criteria would facilitate the elucidation of the etiopathogenesis of mental disorders. Only a couple of decades have passed, but those already seem "good old days." Much of that enthusiasm and faith has now vanished, whereas critical positions have become even more vocal, with the very bad news that they are now increasingly shared by users and their carers, and given a lot of visibility through the Internet. It is symptomatic, in this respect, that the questions I am now receiving from journalists in my country (Italy) about the revision of the DSM-IV focus not so much on "new developments in the manual" (the most common question when the DSM-IV was launched) as on "why we issue a new version of the manual, since nothing new has been discovered meanwhile", or "why we produce this classification at all, since we do not have a solid ground on which to base it." My argument, of course, is that a diagnostic manual such as the DSM is essential for us and our patients exactly because we do not have laboratory or instrumental tools on which to base our diagnoses. Clinical interview and observation are all that we have, and it is therefore essential for us to make them as precise and reliable as possible. However, the parallel disenchantment about the effectiveness of our treatments, fueled by several colleagues whose positions are biased by ideological prejudice (see Maj 2008), does not help us in our attempt to convince the public opinion that a precise and reliable psychiatric diagnosis is really important.

In the current climate, the priority is no more to point out the limitations of our diagnostic tools and treatments, in order to stimulate further progress, but to emphasize the strengths of those diagnostic tools and treatments, in the interest of our patients and our profession. Nevertheless, in the specific context of this conference, it is part of my task to make a few critical points about the DSM-IV and its immediate predecessors, in order to contribute to the general discussion. This is what I will do now.

One of the main problems of the DSM-IV (and of its immediate predecessors) is the oversimplification of psychopathology. This starts from the decision to assign, in a volume of 886 pages, only nine pages to the definition of the symptoms which are supposed to be the building blocks of all the disorders described so precisely in the manual. Are we really sure that the problem of unreliability of psychiatric diagnosis only occurs at the level of the identification of syndromes as opposed to symptoms? Are we sure that the passivity experiences of people with schizophrenia are "delusions" (i.e., "false beliefs based on incorrect inference about external reality") or that the DSM-IV definition of anxiety ("the apprehensive anticipation of future danger or misfortune") applies to the anxiety experienced by a patient with mania as well as to that of people with generalized anxiety disorder?

Indeed, it has been argued that the opportunity offered by the DSM-IV to diagnose, for instance, "panic disorder" in "comorbidity" with schizophrenia or mania represents a useful development, because it allows a more complete characterization of the individual case, which may be important for its management. But, are we really sure that the panic of a patient with schizophrenia, with mania, with depression or with agoraphobia is exactly the same psychopathological entity, which simply "coexists" with each of the others and always requires the same management? Would you really treat the panic of a patient with mania or with schizophrenia with the same selective serotonin reuptake inhibitor you use for the panic of people with agoraphobia?

The list of symptoms provided in the diagnostic criteria for schizophrenia (22 words in total) may be seen as a further example of this oversimplification of psychopathology. In my 1998 editorial published in the *British Journal of Psychiatry* (Maj 1998), I pointed out that the diagnosis of schizophrenia proposed by the DSM-IV is essentially one "by exclusion." In fact, the symptomatological, functional and chronological criteria can be simultaneously fulfilled by several patients with major depression, mania or dementia, so that what is really decisive for the diagnosis is the final exclusion criterion. Schizophrenia is defined by what it is not rather than by what it is. However, the 22 words composing the DSM-IV symptomatological criterion for schizophrenia are also an indication of another general problem: the same version of the manual may be not suitable for such different purposes as the clinical diagnosis of patients seen in a busy practice, the education of a resident in psychiatry, the selection of a homogeneous patient sample for biological research, and the assessment of an individual in a forensic setting. Indeed, those 22 words may represent a useful algorithm, easy to memorize and to recall, for the experienced clinician who already has a clear idea of what schizophrenia is, having read Kraepelin and Bleuler several years before. But this may not be the case for the student or resident who has the first contact with the concept of schizophrenia through those 22 words, getting the message, which may remain

in his mind forever, that a clinical picture consisting of any delusion plus any hallucination qualifies for the diagnosis of schizophrenia.

The DSM-IV criteria do not convey the "essence" of schizophrenia as a qualitatively
distinct psychosis, as they do not convey the "essence" of depression as opposed to
ordinary sadness. This may reflect the intrinsic limitations of the operational approach
(arguing for a reformulation of "prototypes" of mental disorders as an alternative to
the refinement of operational criteria), or an imperfect application of that approach
(for instance, in the case of schizophrenia, the core disturbance of intersubjectivity
may be currently missed), or the illusory and volatile nature of that "essence", that the
operational approach, being more precise, has revealed (e.g., there is a continuum
between ordinary sadness and clinical depression; schizophrenia is nothing more than
any non-affective, non-organic psychosis with an enduring cognitive and functional
impairment). Future research will probably shed light on this.

An important point made by Harold Pincus in his paper is that the involvement of
practicing clinicians in the development of the DSM-IV could have been much more
substantial. I totally agree that a continuing feedback from an independent, representative network of clinicians throughout the process of development of a diagnostic
manual is essential. There are assumptions made by academicians on the basis of their
own experience which may be clearly identified as flawed by clinicians who see several
hundred patients per month in a non-university clinical setting. A good example is the
assumption that "cutting the diagnostic pie into small slices" (Pincus et al. 2004), i.e.,
including a number of narrowly defined diagnostic entities and encouraging multiple
diagnoses in the same patient, would increase the amount of information collected in
ordinary clinical practice. There is now substantial evidence that this assumption was
wrong. What happens in clinical practice is that, for various reasons, only one diagnosis is usually made in each patient, corresponding to just one of the slices of the "diagnostic pie," and this slice is often not the same when the patient is seen by different
clinicians, which represents a new powerful source of diagnostic unreliability (Maj
2005). For example, a patient who in the past would have received a diagnosis of, say,
"neurotic depression," and is supposed now to receive the multiple diagnoses of major
depression + panic disorder + social phobia + obsessive–compulsive disorder, will
actually receive just one of those diagnoses, and this diagnosis will often not be the
same if he is seen by different clinicians. This outcome would have probably been
foreseen if an independent, representative network of clinicians had been asked to
provide its feedback on the idea, when it was formulated.

My final comment is about the notion that the DSM should be regarded as a mere
convention for communication among the multiple "tribes" of mental health professionals. I fully understand the rationale for this statement, but I would submit that,
exactly because the world has changed and the management of information has
become a priority, we should not forget that there are several further "tribes" to be
considered in the mental health context: patients, families, journalists, colleagues of
other medical disciplines and the public at large. All these "tribes" may have difficulties in understanding the difference between balls and strikes as they are, as we see
them and as we use them, and may be finally reinforced in their opinion that there is
nothing really solid in our discipline and that mental health issues are a matter for

philosophers more than for physicians. I would feel more confident in communicating to these "tribes" that there are balls and strikes and that we call them as they seem to be at the current state of knowledge. If we convey the message that our classification system does not reflect anymore the state of the art of our discipline, that the state of the art is somewhere else, it will only be a matter of a few years before the system will fall into disrepute and nobody will use it anymore.

Comments References

Maj, M. (1998). Critique of the DSM-IV operational diagnostic criteria for schizophrenia. *British Journal of Psychiatry*, **172**, 458–60.

Maj, M. (2005). "Psychiatric comorbidity": an artefact of current diagnostic systems? *British Journal of Psychiatry*, **186**, 182–4.

Maj, M. (2008). Non-financial conflicts of interests in psychiatric research and practice. *British Journal of Psychiatry*, **193**, 91–2.

Pincus, H. A., Tew, J. D., Jr., and First, M. B. (2004). Psychiatric comorbidity: is more less? *World Psychiatry*, **3**, 18–23.

Part III

The problem of validity

Chapter 9

Introduction

Josef Parnas

Kenneth Schaffner's chapter and the subsequent commentary by Peter Zachar give much food for thought. These are important philosophical sections of this volume. Schaffner's piece spans a great range of issues, from the purely conceptual and philosophical to more empirically anchored reflections on the psychiatric nosology, drawing on his expertise and knowledge of science and philosophy and history of science. Very briefly, Schaffner declares himself as a "pragmatist" or "conditional realist," with a view of science as providing us with actionable information about the world, but he distances him from the belief that we can have an absolute knowledge of reality as it is "truly" and essentially in itself. He entertains a "multilevel" view of reality. A lesson that transpires from the biological research, says Schaffner, is that the segmentations of different reality levels of a given entity need not to map perfectly to each other (see especially Figure 9.2). Thus Schaffner (and Zachar) are both skeptical of the neo-Kraepelinian goal of point-to-point reductions to the biological substrate, "naturally articulated at its joints." Schaffner finds similarity of his own "conditional realism" to Arthur Fine's (1984) "natural ontological attitude." This is an old and central concept in phenomenology. We live in a realistic attitude, taking the existence of the independent world for granted. This tacit conviction is at the basis of all our commerce with the world. This attitude may be shattered in certain cases of psychiatric illness or intentionally suspended in a philosophical reflection.

Schaffner resuscitates the notion of prototype, as being adequate for psychiatric nosology (see also Chapter 12 by Parnas). Two additional remarks can be perhaps inserted here. First that the notions of prototype, ideal type, type, typology, typification, etc. have their roots in phenomenological tradition and phenomenology-oriented psychiatry. Second, I wish specifically to refer the reader to two seminal American papers, jointly written by a psychiatrist and a philosopher, who, with unmatched clarity and clinical accessibility, describe the role of prototypes in the psychiatric diagnostic process and classification (Schwartz and Wiggins 1987a, 1987b).

I will end this introduction with a short lexicon, explaining a few terms of the chapter, which a reader with no philosophical background may find difficult to understand. Philosophy has been sometimes divided into *ontology* (philosophy of being), *epistemology* (philosophy of knowledge and knowledge acquisition) and ethics or moral philosophy. There are today many more divisions and one may question a neat separation of ontology and epistemology.

The term "*metaphysics*" is roughly equal to ontology. However, sometimes in today's lay parlance, "metaphysical" may signify especially dogmatic and "speculative" ontological considerations. The ontological questions ask about the manner and the nature of being in general or of some particular entity (e.g., what is the nature of bipolar illness?). The prime and general ontological question, which probably can only be settled religiously, is "why there is something rather than nothing?" Epistemology is closely linked to ontology: e.g., if we believe that all ontology is exhausted by quantum physics, we would of course consider physical methods as a privileged and adequate epistemological approach. But it is not a necessary relation: e.g., one can claim that consciousness is entirely physical but at the same time insist that the (subjective) first person perspective has to be included in any sensical investigation of consciousness. Ontology deals with "reality." "*Realism*" (from Latin "res"=thing) was originally opposed to "*idealism*" (or as Bishop Berkeley called it, "immaterialism"), the latter claiming that whatever exists is the product of our mind. Realism claims a reality existing ("out there") independently of the human mind. There are multiple subdivisions, emphases or different "isms" here: e.g., *materialism*=only matter exists; *physicalism*=only microphysical entities and physical laws *truly* exist, etc. Physicalism entails sometimes a position of *eliminativism*, relevant for the psychiatric, nosological context. Eliminativism considers consciousness (mental phenomena) as spurious and illusory, and best substituted by references to brain states and processes. Yet for most of those involved in the field, reality may seem difficult to reduce exhaustively through a reference to physics. It does not seem feasible to re-describe the US presidential elections (that are quite real) with the equations from quantum physics. This is one of the reasons behind our talking about "*multiple levels of reality.*" An important question is how we approach the level of reality which Berrios (Chapter 6, this volume) terms as "psychiatric object."

Introduction References

Fine, A. (1984). The natural ontological attitude. In: Leplin, J. (ed.), *Scientific Realism*. Berkeley, CA: University of California Press, pp. 84–107.

Schwartz, M. A., and Wiggins, O. P. (1987a). Typifications. The first step for clinical diagnosis in psychiatry. *Journal of Nervous and Mental Disease*, **175**, 65–77.

Schwartz, M. A., and Wiggins, O. P. (1987b). Diagnosis and ideal types: A contribution to psychiatric classification. *Comprehensive Psychiatry*, **28**, 277–91.

Chapter 9

A philosophical overview of the problems of validity for psychiatric disorders

Kenneth F. Schaffner

9.1 Introduction

This paper defines and briefly summarizes several concepts of validity, including diagnostic validity and etiopathogenic validity. It then begins to introduce the notion of "clinical validity" via a critique of the work of Kendell and Jablensky, noting that molecular biological investigations find no clear points of rarity in molecular mechanisms that might be relevant to psychiatry. Instead, a Rosch-like prototype form of analysis is proposed, which identifies the most robust categories as prototypes, related to other prototypes by similarity. These prototypes are typically interlevel, and *not* unilevel and simply reductionistic, a view which it is argued is applicable more generally to psychiatry. For the foreseeable future, such prototypes can also best be confirmed via the clinical validity approach, viewed largely as predictive validity (and utility). Predictive validity can be embedded in a larger philosophical "pragmatic" framework that is a compromise way of addressing the realism–instrumentalism dichotomy—a position I term "conditionalized realism." With this framework as a backdrop, I look speculatively at how some forms of "structural realism" might assist in facilitating progress in psychiatry, as well as raise the question whether the current constellation of psychiatric disorders might be replaceable by a molecular-based classification system, and how this could possibly occur.

9.2 Concepts of validity, including diagnostic validity and etiopathogenic validity

The validity notion is clearest in deductive logic where it refers to truth preserving inference. In empirical science the validity concept is typically involved with the notion of capturing an objective external "reality." In philosophy, the view that scientific concepts point toward an attempt to mirror such an external reality is termed "realism," and a contrary position, which contends that scientific ideas are only useful ways of predicting events, is termed "instrumentalism." In psychology, the validity issue historically arguably arises out of the psychological testing literature, where a classical source is Cronbach and Meehl's 1955 article "Construct validity in psychological tests" (Cronbach and Meehl 1955). There, "construct validity" assessed whether a test is a good measure of some quality that is not "operationally defined."[1] In psychiatry, the validity issue was first explicitly addressed by Robins and Guze (1970), but independently at that time of the psychological literature.[2]

The traditional concepts of psychiatric validity, however, include a version of construct (or external) validity, for example, that diagnosis correlates with expected external validators, such as family history, and neurobiological markers. On this point, see First et al. (2004), who follow in the tradition of Robins and Guze's (1970) classic article, about which more will be said shortly. Additionally, psychiatrists refer to the notion of "face validity," which is prima facie, first impression validity (and in my view at best heuristic). Psychiatrists also consider "descriptive validity," where some define this as whether the features of a category are unique to that category relative to other mental disorders, as well as the very important notion of predictive validity, where a diagnosis predicts future course, complication and treatment response. Other validity concepts have also been discussed in many literatures, including: content, internal, interpretive, theoretical, etc. validities. The definitions of the different types of validity are not always fully identical; on this variation compare Blacker (2008) and Jablensky (2002).

For our purposes, the notion of "diagnostic validity" is of special importance. This concept comes from Robins and Guze's classic and extraordinarily influential 1970 article noted earlier. In a way, this article adapted the construct validity notion to psychiatric diagnosis by using the term "diagnostic validity" (Robins and Guze 1970), though there is no reference to the term "construct validity" nor to Cronbach and Meehl's (1955) article in their 1970 paper. Robins and Guze proposed a "method" consisting of five phases: clinical description, laboratory studies, exclusion criteria (to distinguish a diagnosis from other disorders), follow-up studies and family studies. These phases were not necessarily a linear sequence, but were expected to be an interactive process. These five approaches to obtaining a valid classification in psychiatry were expected to triangulate on or converge on the same diagnostic groups, though as we shall see later, this has turned out not always to be the case. In a series of papers in the 1980s, Kendler refined and amplified on these notions to specify additional criteria, such as antecedent validators (familial aggregation, precipitating factors) and predictive validators (relapse and recovery rates, response to treatment). Importantly, Kendler pointed out that many types of nosological questions, such as conflicts among validators, cannot be answered empirically, but will involve *value* judgments (Kendler 1990), an issue further developed recently by Fulford and Sadler—see Fulford (2005) and Sadler (2005).

Nancy Andreasen has also stressed a "newer program," complementary to Robins and Guze's, involving genetic and neuroimaging studies, as well as other neurobiological markers (Andreasen 1995), and subsequently Stephen Hyman suggested a similar approach (Hyman 2002). Andreasen's and Hyman's proposals hope for strong diagnostic validity based on a neurobiological approach, which can be thought of as a search for what Mezzich has termed "etiopathogenic validity": looking for validators that point to the cause of a disorder, or that clarify the pathogenetic process involved in a disorder. This approach typically involves a search for neuroanatomical, neurophysiological and especially molecular genetic factors, and thus tends to be reductive or reductionistic. In addition, this type of research often involves a search for endophenotypes (Gottesman and Gould 2003). Thus far, however, in spite of the hopes of the last 15 years for breakthroughs in classification clarification, this type of approach is more speculative than empirically validated. Recent genome-wide association studies (GWAS), as well as genome-wide searches for copy number variants (CNVs), are suggestive, but both continue to have very low odds ratios, as well as replication problems. In the present article, that etiological approach to validity is supplemented with what I term a clinical approach to validity. In the course of this discussion, I will further suggest that "reality" is multilevel, and includes subjective and intersubjective mental life, and what might be termed "clinical reality," among its levels. The general philosophical orientation in this article is pragmatic, in the tradition of James, Pierce, and Dewey, but also relates to more recent pragmatic approaches in philosophy as well to analytic philosophical aspects.

9.3 **Clinical validity**

Etiologic-based or etiopathogenic validity, as the term is often used in the psychiatric literature, will continue to grow in importance as the molecular biological revolution penetrates deeper into neurobiology, and later in this paper I will mention some relevant developments and also the National Institute of Mental Health's (NIMH's) Research Domain Criteria (RDoC) project in this area. For the in-progress revisions of ICD-11 (International Classification of Diseases, 11th edition) of mental disorders, as well as the national DSM-5 (Diagnostic and Statistical Manual, 5th edition) revision scheduled for 2013, however, I believe the major work that will be done will involve *clinical validity*, a notion that I shall re-examine further later in this chapter, and one that was given that name by Kendell (1989). This clinical validity concept carries forward both the Robins and Guze and the Kendler multifaceted and multilevel approaches, more than it does the reductive Andreasen and Hyman etiopathogenic programs, which may achieve success for future ICD-12 and DSM-6 versions, an admittedly optimistic prediction.

To assess the extent, as well as the limitations, of how reductive etiopathogenic validity may figure in diagnostic classification, and also to motivate the notion of clinical validity, I want to begin from a provocative 2003 article by Kendell and Jablensky (2003). Kendell and Jablensky proposed two very strong conditions for validity. First they wrote: "We suggest . . . that a diagnostic category should be described as valid only if one of two conditions has been met. If the defining characteristic of the category is a syndrome, this syndrome must be demonstrated to be an entity, separated from neighboring syndromes and normality by a zone of rarity. . . .[i.e., interforms would be very rare]." (p. 8). They also proposed another condition, writing: "Alternatively, if the category's defining characteristics are more fundamental—that is, if the category is defined by a physiological, anatomical, histological, chromosomal, or molecular abnormality—clear, qualitative differences must exist between these defining characteristics and those of other conditions with a similar syndrome." (p. 8).

Though Kendell and Jablensky argue persuasively for their position, I want to take a different approach. In my view, studies of simpler organisms such as regulatory mechanisms in bacteria and behavioral traits in the worm (*Caenorhabditis elegans*) and the fly (*Drosophila*), suggest that such traits will *not* resolve into simple discrete forms at the molecular level. This view seems supported by similar considerations regarding lessons for behavioral studies from simpler organisms (see Kendler and Greenspan 2006; Schaffner 2008). The evidence from such organisms demonstrates that there are numerous interforms and *quantitative* traits: *this is dimensionality all the way down*. A good example of this is found in the operon model of gene regulation in an even simpler organism, *Escherichia coli* bacteria, where there are many interforms. Lewin, the author of a major textbook on molecular genetics, called this broad diversity of subtly varying mechanisms "a panoply of operons" (Lewin 1994).[3] Expecting discreteness because of fundamentality is, I think, a "Platonic" prejudice. It can be satisfied in chemistry, as in the periodic chart, but it is rare, and for evolutionary reasons should be expected to be rare, in biology.[4] The main evolutionary issue here is the extensive variation among the models and mechanisms which is a natural consequence of the result of how evolution operates: by replicating entities with many small variations, and assembling odds and ends—thus "tinkering," as François Jacob has written about evolution (Jacob 1977).

9.4 **A prototype approach**

In spite of the complexities created for categorization by variation and dimensionality, I believe that classification can still be made tractable, by using an approach which identifies the most robust categories as prototypes, related to other prototypes by similarity. There are other models that model dimensionality, which will be remarked on further below, but for various reasons I believe that a prototype approach has the strongest case. Relatedly, some, such as Mezzich—see Cantor et al. (1980)—think that a related fuzzy set, grade of membership (GoM), analysis will also assist a prototype approach representation schema, a point to be developed in a moment.[5] I would argue that the prototype approach is supported by the deep structure of biology, and I develop such a prototype approach to biology, including genetics and the neurosciences, in my 1993 book (Schaffner 1993). In that book, I contrasted the structure of the physical sciences, such as in mechanics, electromagnetic theory and quantum mechanics, with an alternative theoretical structure for biology.

In my view, we do not have what Cronbach and Meehl in their 1955 validity article called a simple "network of [universal] laws" that constitutes a theory, either in biology, psychology or psychiatry, though we do find such networks frequently in physics, and occasionally in chemistry.[6] Rather in biology, and I would argue eventually in psychiatry, we have families of models or mechanisms with, in any given subdiscipline, a few prototypes. These prototypes are typically interlevel: in biology they *intermingle* ions, molecules, cells, cell–cell circuits and organs, in the same causal/temporal process—an issue I shall return to in a moment. The prototype models are related to each other by dimensional similarity, and there are many interforms. The prototypes in this view are narrow classes, but do allow for law-like/causal predictions, and explanations, sometimes just for individuals. Extensive variation among the models and mechanisms is a natural consequence of the result of how evolution operates: by replicating entities with many small variations, and assembling odds and ends—thus Jacob's "tinkering," noted previously.

But a prototype/GoM approach has other independent arguments in its support in addition to consistency with the way that relationships among biomolecular models seem to behave. Psychologists, beginning with the pioneering work of Rosch in 1975, have argued that prototype representations are closer to the way that humans think naturally than are other more logically strict approaches to concepts. Rosch's work was initially grounded in psychological anthropology. In her investigation, Rosch found to both her and others' surprise, that primitive peoples as well as advanced societies do not represent concepts or categories as collections of necessary and sufficient properties. Rather a category is built around a central member or a prototype which is a representative member that shares the most attributes with other members of that category and which shares the fewest with members of the contrasting category (Rosch and Mervis 1975). Thus a robin would be a more prototypical bird than either a penguin or a chicken. Rosch wrote:

> Categories are coded in cognition in terms of prototypes of the most characteristic members of the category. That is, many experiments have shown that categories are coded in the mind neither by means of lists of each individual member of the category nor by means of a list of formal criteria necessary and sufficient for category membership, but, rather, in terms of a prototypical category member. The most cognitively economic code for a category is, in fact, a concrete image of an average category member (Rosch 1976, p. 212).

Rosch went on to extend her views to learning in children and to question the sharpness of boundaries between concepts. Her contributions are viewed as major advances in our understanding of memory and knowledge representation, though her account has been construed by some as needing supplementation for complex category representation (Osherson and Smith 1981) but also defended by others (Cohen 1982; Cohen and Murphy 1984; Fuhrmann 1991). The Roschean view of concepts as being built around prototypes shares certain similarities with Putnam's urging we consider meanings as "stereotypes." In the more recent psychiatric literature on disorders as prototypes see Lilienfeld and Marino (1995 and 1999) and Wakefield's (1999) critique.

In their 1980 paper, Cantor et al. (1980) argued that psychiatrists model psychiatric disorders using prototype constructions, and that they also diagnose by making use of an implicit GoM reasoning strategy. They also point out that standard DSM categorical disorders are, in an important sense, prototypes (p. 190). A prototype approach—again see Cantor et al. (1980) for an early discussion of this approach in psychiatry by Mezzich's group—can conform well to a polythetic categorical approach in the limiting case. But a prototype approach can also permit a dimensional representation as well. A GoM model has been applied to several different psychiatric disorders including depression and a range of personality disorders, and relatively recently was coupled with genomic search strategy to identify a new subclass phenotype of schizophrenia, and present reasonably strong evidence of a linkage of that subtype to chromosome 6p22–24 (Hallmayer et al. 2005).

It is apparently in the area of the personality disorders that the most developed case has been made for the need for a dimensional approach in contrast with or as a supplement to a traditional DSM categorical approach. Researchers in that field seem to prefer alternatives to GoM strategies, including models that are known as Latent Class and Latent Trait (also known as item response) types. Recently, there has been an increased interest in even more general taxometric approaches, of the sort pioneered by Meehl (Trull and Durrett 2005). But the jury is still out on the best way to approach such modeling even in the area of personality disorders, and there are strong indications that this topic is receiving considerable additional discussion as DSM-5 and ICD-11 develop. We may see a dimensional approach as a parallel analysis to a standard categorical definition—see First et al. (2002)—or we may see some hybrid approaches, (personal communication, Pilkonis, 2004). Such an approach, whether it be dimensional or hybrid, will have to be carefully developed and rigorously tested for clinical validity and user friendliness. An evidence-based psychiatry is key for ensuring clinical validity. Finally, the prototype-dimensional approach may also be more consistent with etiopathogenic validations to come in the future, perhaps in DSM-6 and ICD-12.

9.5 Reductive versus interlevel approaches to neurobiology: reiterating a theme

As argued repeatedly elsewhere (Schaffner 1993, 2008), I believe a close inspection of the disciplines of molecular genetics and neuroscience, including their research articles and textbooks, will indicate that the prototypes which are used in these sciences are actually and typically interlevel, and *not* unilevel and simply reductionistic: i.e., one does not *only* use molecules in describing the results of studies in these area. These levels include atoms and molecules at the smallest level, but can range up through organisms, social groups, and also include internal (subjective) monologue and inter-subjective dialogue, as well as values, at the upper levels.

Recall that recent work on how molecular geneticists explain the difference between social and solitary feeding in the worm, C. *elegans*, shows an interlevel example of a circuit in the worm controlling social feeding—see de Bono et al. (2002) and Schaffner 2008) for details and Schaffner (1998a, 1998b) also, for background on the worm. That work from simpler organisms suggests that important information, and generalizations, might be obtained at *any* level of aggregation—in fact, the molecular level may not be the best place to identify such information, intervene and predict. Paying attention to interrelations and possible integrations among different levels of aggregation, often in the "same process," is an important feature of the biomedical sciences, and also for any science that depends on the basic biomedical sciences.

A useful way to depict diagrammatically how progress in molecular and imaging research may affect psychiatric disorder definition, and diagnostic strategies, is represented in Figure 9.1.

In this perspective, two prototypes, of which one initially involves no molecular correlates and the second which has some molecular markers, evolve so that in a later stage both are more molecular, as well as more integrated with each other. However, behavioral, including subjective, features of both disorders continue to be retained, and may actually increase in terms of scope and complexity, as well as specificity and

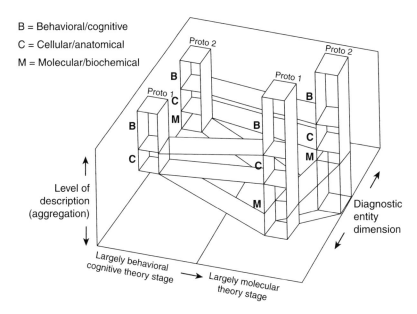

B = Behavioral/cognitive
C = Cellular/anatomical
M = Molecular/biochemical

Figure 9.1 Evolving diagnostic entity changes. Examples for the prototypes might be Proto 1 as bipolar illness (BPI) and Proto 2 as schizophrenia (SZ). Behavioral components could include a manic type of psychosis in Proto 1 and auditory hallucinations in Proto 2; cellular/anatomical descriptors might refer to different brain volume studies in both prototypes. In the older SZ prototype, M may indicate dopamine dysregulation. In the later stage towers, M may also include abnormalities of serotonin receptor gene HTR2A in both BPI and SZ, as well as a much more developed molecular picture, some elements common to both disorders, and some differentiating molecular elements and circuits.

sensitivity. Recent work in schizophrenia suggests this is in the early stages of development (Meyer-Lindenberg 2010).

9.6 Clinical utility and clinical validity

With these considerations as background, let us again return to Kendell and Jablensky's important 2003 paper to consider what type of validity might be feasible in the area of psychiatry. In that seminal paper, Kendell and Jablensky also sharply distinguish diagnostic *validity* from diagnostic *utility*, and write: "In our view, it is crucial to maintain a clear distinction between validity and utility, and at present these two terms are often used as if they were synonyms." At this point in their article they (disapprovingly) cite Spitzer's classic writings in connection with DSM-III, which does use the terms as synonyms. Kendell and Jablensky then add: "We propose that a diagnostic rubric may be said to possess utility if it provides nontrivial information about prognosis and likely treatment outcomes, and/or testable propositions about biological and social correlates." (p. 9).

Though the Kendall and Jablensky definition of utility is excellent, *it is also what has traditionally been called "predictive validity,"* as has been noted by First et al. (2004).

First et al. (2004) also state that Kendall and Jablensky represent the opposite extreme from Spitzer's approach, which perhaps inappropriately largely identified validity with utility. First et al. themselves prefer what they term a "middle ground," noting that though they "view validity and utility as separate constructs, there is considerable overlap between them." They recognize that "diagnostic validity is a complex multi-faceted construct . . ." and add "since many of these elements of diagnostic validity are inherently useful in the care of patients (e.g., in predicting treatment response or course of illness), it is not surprising that improving diagnostic validity often improves clinical utility as well." (pp. 947–948).

And to philosophical pragmatists, among which I include myself, such *utility* is constitutive of what we think of as *reality*, and thus such utility is an indicator of an appropriate form of validity (clearly here as predictive validity; less certainly construct validity) in the realm of clinical reality. The next few sections try to develop this idea.

9.7 **Conditionalized realism and direct evidence**

How might we best try to think further about this very complicated notion of "reality" in an attempt to grasp this multifaceted notion of diagnostic validity? Can a straight-forward and defensible realist (or realism) approach be developed that might assist with the problem of psychiatric validity? In part, the problem arises because we are mainly interested in the validity of behavioral and psychiatric *constructs*. And as Cronbach and Meehl noted over 50 years ago, "Construct validity is ordinarily studied when the tester has no definite criterion measure of the quality with which he is concerned, and must use *indirect* measures. Here the trait or quality underlying the test is of central importance, rather than either the test behavior or the scores on the criteria" (Cronbach and Meehl 1955, quoting Committee on Test Standards 1954, no page given, my emphasis). Absent ultimate standard or gold standard criteria, these authors also noted that "When an investigator believes that no criterion available to him is fully valid, he perforce becomes interested in construct validity because this is the only way to avoid the 'infinite frustration' of relating every criterion to some more ultimate standard" (Cronbach and Meehl 1955, p. 176). A philosophical pragmatist does not think we can directly access an independent reality: there is no simple "gold standard" waiting "out there." And, as the article on validity in the American Psychiatric Association's *Handbook of Psychiatric Measures* reminds us, "assessing validity in areas in which there are few established measures and for which a gold standard or criterion of accuracy cannot be established is difficult" (Blacker 2008, p. 13). In the absence of such a gold standard, we can only "triangulate" or perhaps better "converge" on it through multiple useful indicators and interventions in the world. In psychiatry, these are often called *external validators*.

It was these external validators that Robins and Guze (1970) seemed to put the greatest trust in to establish the validity of nosological constructs. Again, the concept of an external validator involves testing a diagnostic hypothesis by using data not related to the diagnostic process. External validators have included "family history, demographic correlates, biological and psychological tests, environmental risk factors, concurrent symptoms (that are not part of the diagnostic criteria being assessed), treatment response, diagnostic stability, and course of illness" (Kendler 1990, p. 970). But work in the 1980s and 1990s, much of it by Kendler and his colleagues, indicated that external validators may not agree. Examples where there is a divergence are in familial and clinical constructs of schizotypal personality disorder (SPD) and also in validating the subtypes of schizophrenia (see Kendler 1985, and also Kendler 1990, p. 971 for details). Also many of these (hopefully) triangulating or converging indicators and interventions that help us towards a pragmatic reality do involve sophisticated technologies and long chains of inference, e.g., gene action and functional magnetic resonance imaging (fMRI) results. But information from all levels, including high levels such as interpersonal experience—which may be "more real" for many purposes for a pragmatist than molecular pathways—will continue to be key for psychiatry, as depicted in Figure 9.1.

I do not think any critical scientist actually believes we can always knowingly and directly access a gold standard of truth. A believer in scientific intuitionism, perhaps of a Kantian type whereby a scientist could directly intuit the truth or falsity of a scientific hypothesis,[7] might not be in such a position of uncertainty, but it is difficult to find recent scientific or philosophical proponents of such an intuitionist view who have offered convincing arguments for their positions. The great American pragmatist, Charles Saunders Peirce, proposed a weak form of realism when he suggested we would only get to true reality at the end of time, or when we had a completed science. But this type of Peircean realism, in which scientific theories only achieve consensus belief at the end of time, is utopian and at best a regulative ideal (compare Laudan 1973 and Sellars 1977). The question thus arises whether there is any defensible "realism" position one can take in the present day. It seems to me that the two "extreme" or "idealized" positions of realism and instrumentalism actually each contain important elements, which, when recognized, lead to a view that may best be expressed by the phrase *conditionalized realism*. This view has analogs with previous and current philosophers' suggestions,[8] and also is arguably the position that is most in accord with scientists' attitudes as revealed in the history of science and in contemporary science.

Possibly the closest analog to "conditionalized realism" in the recent philosophical literature is that of Arthur Fine's "natural ontological attitude" or NOA (pronounced "Noah.") In his paper (Fine 1984) he disarms the critic who worries that acceptance of this view would lead to an anti-scientific relativism writing that "it seems to me that both the realist and the antirealist [instrumentalist] must toe what I have been calling 'the homely line.' That is, they must both accept the certified results of science as on a par with the more homely and familiarly supported claims," (p. 96) such as "the existence and features of everyday objects" (p. 95). Fine proposes to "call this acceptance of scientific truths the 'core position.'" He then suggests that the realists' so-called addition to the core amounts to little more than "a desk-thumping, foot stamping shout of 'Really!'" (p. 97). Fine's positive suggestion, NOA, "is the core position itself, *and all by itself*" (p. 97). From this perspective any invoking of "the external world" is just another shout-out to an inscrutable and inaccessible "something out there." Appeal to something that is "out there" cannot and will not justify any legitimate form of realism (see p. 97).

I see this NOA view as salutary and as clearing up a lot of muddy thinking that is based on strong habits and metaphysical confusion, though whether it "marks a revolutionary approach to understanding science," as Fine writes (p. 101), might be too strong a claim.[9] I approach the NOA-like position that I favor, and what I term "conditionalized realism," in the following way. If one analyzes the notion of scientific "truth" involved in the realistic position from the perspective of a critical empiricist position, the notion soon becomes suspect. As already indicated, the empiricist denies any direct intuitive experience of the certitude of scientific hypotheses or theories. Hypotheses and theories are universal and thus cover (infinitely) many more cases than have been examined in tested situations. Furthermore, theories (or constructs) generally have observationally inaccessible or latent variable aspects to them, and these cannot be completely verified via "direct" observation. If one accepts a kind of generalized empiricist position of the sort held by the typical working scientist, then the most that one can assert regarding the adequacy of a hypothesis is that there is (relatively) *direct* evidence in its favor. But any close analysis of the expression "direct evidence" will show that such testimony or proof is always *conditioned* by the acceptance of both (1) auxiliary assumptions, which describe how instruments used to observe the entity of interest work, and (2) the non-availability of plausible, alternative incompatible theories that account for the same "direct" evidence.[10] An examination of the realistic position within the framework of the epistemological tenets sketched earlier (and presented in more detail in Schaffner's 1993 book, see especially pp. 197–199), leads, then, to a *conditionalized realism* at most.

A similar critical examination of the prima facie quite opposed instrumentalist position will disclose a convergence of instrumentalism toward the seemingly very different position of realism. For example, an instrumentalist will not deny the importance of deductive consequences of a hypothesis or a theory, especially insofar as those consequences lead to further observable predictions. One subclass of those implications will be tests that scientists characterize as "direct evidence" for a hypothesis. Scientists, moreover, will view such direct evidence as crucial for an estimation of their confidence in further predictions of the hypothesis in new domains and its likely "elaborability" and fertility in scientific inquiry. Consider, for example, what the "falsification" of a hypothesis by a generally agreed upon "direct test" of the hypothesis would mean even to a scientist who asserted (verbally) that he or she was an instrumentalist. It is exceedingly likely that such a negative outcome would engender serious qualms on his or her part about the future reliability and heuristic character of such a hypothesis. As far as the *behavior* of all scientists is concerned, then, the two positions converge, and it therefore seems permissible to attribute, at least behavioristically, a conditionalized realism to all scientists. It is this conditionalized realism, along with its correlative relativized notion of truth and falsity, which my earlier analysis seems to lead us to. But further, I see this conditionalized realism both as consistent with Fine's NOA view, and as extending it to indicate how we have strong scientific beliefs in those entities for which we have, albeit conditionalized, direct evidence.

This explicit reference to the *conditionalization* of realism allows for an important aspect of the provisional "acceptance" of hypotheses and theories. There have been many theories that have had a most important impact on the historical development of science but have turned out to be false. The conditions cited concerning the limits of direct evidence would seem to rationalize the provisional and tentative "acceptance" in the sense of high probability of hypotheses. When, however, the conditions regarding auxiliary assumptions and the availability of plausible alternative, incompatible hypotheses or theories change, one is likely to see a change in the "acceptance" status of a hypothesis or theory by the scientific community. An analysis of evaluation and "acceptance" from the perspective of conditionalized realism will accordingly importantly depend on the precise articulation of these conditions in specific cases. With the possibility of a conditionalized realism it becomes unnecessary to subscribe to the (naive) instrumentalist's conception of scientific theories because of the existence of many false but "accepted" theories in the history of science, an issue often termed the "pessimistic induction" argument (Laudan 1981).[11]

9.8 **Relations of truth, validity and utility**

I have noted different views about the relations of utility and validity expressed by Spitzer, First, and Kendell and Jablensky, the first two recognizing some overlap between the concepts and the last two authors proposing the notions be sharply distinguished. As also noted, from the philosophical pragmatist position, utility is constitutive of truth, and a fortiori of validity. But the classical pragmatists differed among themselves about the strength of the utility–truth relation, and it will be helpful to clarify what I take to be the better of their views. This then will allow a more subtle distinction of the notions of utility and validity in psychiatry.

Perhaps the boldest claim of the relation of truth and utility was made by Dewey, who wrote in his *Reconstruction in Philosophy* that ". . . truth is defined as utility. . ." (Dewey 1920, p. 157). But Dewey articulated this view as "a corollary from the nature of thinking and ideas." Approaching thinking from an adaptive evolutionary point of view, he wrote:

> [If] ideas, meanings, conceptions, notions, theories, systems are instrumental to an active reorganization of the given environment, to a removal of some specific trouble and perplexity, then the test of their validity and value lies in accomplishing this work. If they succeed in their office, they are reliable, sound, valid, good, true. If they fail to clear up confusion, to eliminate defects, if they increase confusion, uncertainty and evil when they are acted upon, then are they false. Confirmation, corroboration, verification lie in works, consequences (p. 156).

Furthermore, Dewey cautioned that we view this notion of utility not as personal or idiosyncratic, but as "public and objective," writing:

> Too often, for example, when truth has been thought of as satisfaction, it has been thought of as merely emotional satisfaction, a private comfort, a meeting of purely personal need. But the satisfaction in question means a satisfaction of the needs and conditions of the problem out of which the idea, the purpose and method of action, arises. It includes public and objective conditions. It is not to be manipulated by whim or personal idiosyncrasy (p. 157).

James has been construed, probably unfairly, as permitting a loose version of pragmatism, and viewing truth as whatever works in any context. This is not the place to further analyze and defend James' more subtle analysis that can be found in his *Pragmatism* and other publications but it should be noted that Peirce himself felt that the term "pragmatism" had been hijacked by "literary journals," though other evidence suggests Peirce had concerns both with James and Schiller. Probably for all these reasons in 1905 Peirce proposed a new locution for the approach he had developed in his earlier essays of 1877–1878 ("The Fixation of Belief" (1877) and especially "How to Make Our Ideas Clear" (1878)). Peirce named this rehabilitated notion "pragmaticism," a word he thought was "ugly enough to be safe from kidnappers" (Peirce et al. 1994, CP 5.414).

The use of Peirce's account of the pragmatic approach to truth allows a clearer account of the general pragmatic doctrines and permits a more satisfactory application to the senses of validity and utility in psychiatry. The gist of Peirce's analysis can be summed up in his 1905 reformulation:

> In order to ascertain the meaning of an intellectual conception one should consider what practical consequences might conceivably result by necessity from the truth of that conception; and the sum of these consequences will constitute the entire meaning of the conception (Peirce, CP 5.9).

The words "practical" and "truth" in this claim, often called the "pragmatic maxim," need urgent unpacking. First, "practical" in this sense for Peirce means no more than what can be experienced—it is not equivalent to "useful" in any simple sense, though some consequences may turn out to be "useful" in the colloquial sense. Peirce himself made this clear by writing in the same place: "Such reasonings and all reasonings turn upon the idea that if one exerts certain kinds of volition, one will undergo in return certain compulsory perceptions. Now this sort of consideration, namely, that certain lines of conduct will entail certain kinds of inevitable experiences is what is called a 'practical consideration'" (Peirce, CP 5.9). Second, "truth" here for Peirce is purely hypothetical and inferential, as in an "if—then" expression.

I want to purse this Peircean line but to further interpret it in the following ways. I want to start by proposing, like Peirce, that a truth claim for a concept, in general, and which could include a psychiatric disorder concept, is an elliptical statement which needs to be unpacked in terms of all conceivable consequences. But an appropriate sample of the consequences needs to be verified to "establish truth." However that is all that can be done, other than "foot stamping"—to echo Fine's comments noted earlier.

I elaborate. The consequences of a claim or concept are (in principle) infinite, but in that kind of "long run," we shall, as Keynes noted, "all be dead." So some sampling is needed, and better defined and tougher tests (as Popper recommended) increase credibility in the "truth." We sample naively in everyday life (just look!—or better look again!); and in a more sophisticated way in more scientific contexts—we choose alphas, betas, likely effect sizes and compute Ns—then go on to use t-tests, F-tests, etc. (unless we are Bayesians, in which case we identify/estimate priors, conditionalize, etc.—on these issues (see Schaffner 1993, pp. 252–260).

All "practical" consequences have utility, *in the broadest sense of potential experiences* that may relate to both applications and testing. (In "testing," I would include tests for consistency with other well-established principles, statements and theories, and even consistency with broadly accepted "metaphysics" (e.g., no ghosts), as well as methodological tests for "simplicity").[12] A *subset* of a claim's broadly "practical" consequences has more *direct applicability*, as in the clinical sciences, or in engineering. Clinical utility can be defined further developing subsets of this narrower notion, as in Michael First's recent paper on clinical utility. First is expansive on the notion of clinical utility, noting the purposes of psychiatric classification comprise the "practical needs including helping clinicians diagnose and treat patients, assisting researchers in selecting populations for study, facilitating administrators in their collection of health statistics, and teaching students how to recognize presentations of mental disorders" (First 2010, p. 465). Other consequences of a truth claim are less directly useful, though they could be strong tests, e.g., Einstein's general relativity predictions of light ray bending. Think of these less directly useful consequences as falling more into the "basic sciences" rather than the "clinical sciences." These consequences traditionally have been seen as testing for "validity." As with narrower utility, one can define subsets of validity consequences as well, but even these have utility in the broad sense, and may eventually translate into narrower utility, when, for example, an etiology permits better patient prevention and management.

In general, truth, as Schiller says, is contingent on purpose. Specifically he says, "The making of an assertation, the application of an alleged truth to the experience that tests it, can only occur in the context of and in connection with some purpose, which defines the nature of the whole ideal experiment" (Schiller et al. 2008 p. 50). Schiller is also supposed to have said that "truth is what works," but I have not been able to confirm an exact quote as yet. However I see this view as consistent with what Kendler has written: "From a biomedical perspective, the validity of a diagnostic category has traditionally meant, in its most basic sense, that the category 'does some work in the world' – that it tells us something useful about the individuals so classified" (Kendler, personal communication in "Draft Comments on Validity").

9.9 Changing classifications and the role of clinical validity

That all said—"all" here referring both to the discussion of conditionalized realism and the pragmatism background—there remains an issue related to the provisional acceptance of theories and constructs that has been discussed both in the philosophical and the psychiatric literature. This is whether, as we go forward with our more sophisticated understanding of molecular genetics and neuroscience, what we take to be settled reality—especially involving the standard set of mental disorders such as schizophrenia and depression—might *radically* change. The multilevel "reality" that we commit to as a result of this ongoing (scientific) process is, as argued above, always provisional or conditioned. Thus it *could* be subject to *major* modifications via scientific revolutions of a Kuhnian sort, as described by Kuhn in his extraordinary book, *The Structure of Scientific Revolutions*. It is thus *possible* that our current classification categories will radically change and be replaced as a result of advancing genetics and neuroscience, a thesis that I have speculated on in print as long as two decades ago

(Harris and Schaffner 1992). In such a view, the towers shown in Figure 9.1 would not persist and grow, both in up and down directions, but would crumble, and rise anew with very different looks and interrelations.

Philosophically, one suggestive way to retain the results of earlier scientific advances, even during a fundamental change in the ontology of science, is to adopt a position of structural realism. The core idea of this view is that the mathematical structures of theories (= basic and applied equations) can be retained as one shifts from an earlier discarded theory to a newer one. Retained, only in a way however, by de-interpreting the theoretical terms so they become variables, limiting them, then roughly identifying the *old variables* with the *new* theory's *ontology* or fundamental entities. So using John Worrall's favorite example (Worrall 1989), Fresnel's optical aether displacement vector V becomes a generalized or ontically neutralized vector that is then approximately identified with Maxwell's electrical displacement vector D in the well-known equations of electromagnetic theory. The idea in this example is that Fresnel was able to obtain highly detailed equations for the intensity of reflected polarized light on the basis of a luminiferous aether theory. And the same equations were subsequently obtained in an aetherless Maxwellian theory of electrodynamics, so the structure of the equations was preserved, though the terms pointed at different entities: in Fresnel's case to a very strange kind of a wave in a mechanical elastic solid; in Maxwell's case to varying electrical and magnetic field intensities and the related D vector.

This approach *may* work to some degree outside of physics, but not so obviously, because the structures are not as clear—and the theories are not axiomatized and put into relatively simple equation form as in Fresnel's and Maxwell's theories. But genetics might be a biological case, where the gene was once viewed as a protein (until about 1950) but was subsequently identified with a stretch of DNA. And the Mendelian "laws" (the old structural relations) can be carried over, albeit in a limited way (e.g., genes are no longer inherited independently even by Morgan's work in 1910–1915, so the classical Mendelian 9:3:3:1 ratio for the inheritance of two independent traits is retained only in the limit where the genes are on different chromosomes, but becomes modified due to linkage when the genes governing the traits are on the same chromosome).

But what about psychiatry? In some recent correspondence (and in his article for this conference) Krueger seems to suggest that DSM disorders (e.g., schizophrenia) are structures that might be preserved as ideal types (or the mean of a distribution/spectrum) if the relations among the defining elements of the structure (say hallucinations and delusions) also are found to co-occur in a similar way in populations tested for the disorder. If that is the core idea, for me structural validity does not seem to add much to the notion of plain old empirical confirmation (call this POEC).

But perhaps a focus on an instrument that can be analyzed to evaluate the co-occurrence of test items adds something more to the discussion? It is here that my intuitions begin to run out on exactly what the "more" is beyond POEC. Krueger, however, has made this suggestion for what "more" may be involved, writing: "So the idea is: a model of human individual differences [ID] (psychopathology being one type of ID) is structurally valid if (a) there exists a formally articulated statistical model of those IDs and (b) that model fits data suited to evaluating the model" (personal communication, October, 2010). For more details on this idea, see the essay by Krueger and Eaton, in Chapter 10 in this volume.

There is another possible difference between structural validity and structural realism: the latter was proposed to account for the "success" of earlier discarded theories, i.e., that the old science, and even current successful science, seems to be more than a miracle). Secondly, structural realism answers the progress argument, insofar as one can, in contrast with Kuhn's view (see the following discussion), retain something of the earlier discarded *theory* by recognizing the persistence of its structure, if not its entities, in the newer theory. It is not evident to me that Krueger's account does that.

But does psychiatry even need to account for its earlier successes with patients, and does it need to hold onto elements of an earlier structure? If so, and arguments could be made it does, then some of the ideas behind structural realism might be useful in accounts of structural validity.

One further thought here is that independently of a pre-existing classification, clusters of distressing (reported) symptoms and (behavioral) signs may travel together. Perhaps paranoiac delusions and auditory hallucinations travel together, as Krueger has suggested. These clusters of symptoms and signs might have the status of a constraint on any new classification and theoretical explanation, which would be required to account for the clustering. Much as a new theory of optics was required to account for the clustering of refraction phenomena, and separately for various interference and diffraction phenomenal classes. I discuss how latent class analysis (LCA) might apply this intuition in my comments on Kendler in this volume (see Chapter 15).

Several other writers in psychiatry have also speculated on something like this type of radical change, particularly in the area of personality disorders. Widiger, for example, has suggested that DSM-5 might replace the traditional categorical disorders with a version of the well-known five-factor model from personality research (Widiger 2011). First writes that "transitioning from a categorical to a dimensional DSM would involve radical changes in the diagnostic groupings, individual diagnostic entities, and in diagnostic assessment procedures" (First 2005). Krueger and his colleagues have proposed a reconstrual of personality disorder categories under a new rubric that emphasizes a new category of externalizing behaviors (Walton et al. 2011). However, it is the role of genetics and the use of endophenotypes that perhaps pose the most radical realignment of psychiatric disorders, both in terms of definition and interrelations. Recent findings regarding the neuregulin gene, for example, suggest that it may be etiologically involved both in schizophrenia and in bipolar disorder, provoking some to speculate that the area of psychosis may be reordered in a significant manner (Walker et al. 2011).

However, my best guess at present is that current ICD-10 and DSM-IV-TR categories will *slowly* evolve etiopathogenically, and at the margins, rather than suffer a catastrophic collapse and replacement with some as yet unforeseeable psychiatric classification system. This guess so far seems to be supported by the preliminary postings regarding DSM-5 on the website dsm5.org. But we should also keep in mind yet another possibility—that what we could call our "Ptolemaic" ICD-10/DSM-IV classification system may continue as mainly *clinically valid*, while an etiopathogenic, but horrendously complex and *clinically promising* but *problematic* "Copernican-like" more valid system slowly emerges.

It is worth elaborating on how this possibly might happen in general terms, and what types of validity such a development would support. Philosophers of biology and psychology have investigated how sciences at two different levels of aggregation might describe the basic entities of the world and their interactions. One intriguing position developed independently by Fodor in psychology (Fodor 1975) and by Hull in genetics (Hull 1974), is that there may be no simple systematic connections between the way things are grouped and relate at a macroscopic level (psychology or Mendelian genetics) and the way microscopic entities (in neuroscience and molecular biology) are categorized and interact.[13] A similar point has been made by Wimsatt regarding how closely things and their interrelations will track as one examines ever smaller units (Wimsatt 1974). For Wimsatt, simple (physical) science such as geology will cohere during this process of level deepening, whereas complex systems such as are found in biology may not track uniformly in such a process. In some important sense, this disaggregation and realignment of entities and relations may be what psychiatrists are encountering as they attempt to find the underling genetic and neuronal structure for psychiatric disorders. A diagram similar to ones that Fodor has published, but here with significant additions, is shown in Figure 9.2, and may make this position clearer.

Should such disaggregation and reassembly be what molecular biology and neuroscience are in the process of imposing on psychiatry, it may be many years before enough is known to be able to approach mental disorders in a non-research context molecular manner that permits clinically useful diagnosis and treatment to occur, though the relatively straightforward decomposition shown earlier is promising. The developing RDoC project of the NIMH seems to be moving in this direction and recent studies on the molecular genetics and neuroscience of schizophrenia suggests vast complexity (see Lewis and Sweet 2009 and Meyer-Lindenberg 2010 for complexity; see Sanislow et al. 2010 for RDoC information). But it is also possible, that in the face of molecular complexity, psychiatry may have to accept the Fodor–Hull position, but continue to work to refine such disorders at higher levels of aggregation, while at the same time attempting to sort out the many-many relations emerging in the course of an Andreasen–Hyman type of future. The only partially developed "heuristics" for such a project have been sketched in my article (Schaffner 2008). For clinicians, such a view would privilege predictive validity, and reliability, over etiopathogenic validity in the near term. Such a view is not disagreed with by Hyman, who wrote that "Given the fact that the science of mental disorder is in its early stages, we must recognize that near term revisions to the DSM or ICD will perforce remain a provisional diagnostic system. The problem of validity will not yet be solved for most diagnoses" (Hyman 2002). Hyman added that "progress in genetics, neuroscience, cognitive science, and epidemiology will markedly improve the validity of diagnosis, but the stories will almost certainly not yet be complete." But this may actually be too optimistic an assessment given what we have seen in more recent analyses by Hyman (2007, 2010).

In summary, I think that "reality,"—interpreted in the minimalist NOA way described earlier—and attempts to validate our constructs in this "reality," will take the form of provisional multilevel prototypes that interrelate dimensionally. I believe we will encounter these both in the clinical validity area, as well as ultimately, i.e., but perhaps not for many years to come, in any full sense in the etiopathogenic area, since

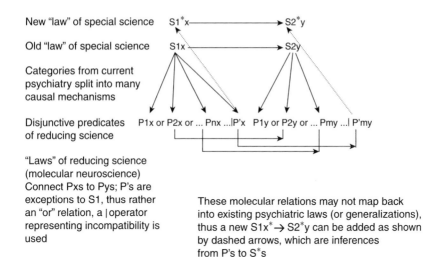

New "law" of special science   S1*x————————▶ S2*y

Old "law" of special science   S1x————————▶ S2y

Categories from current
psychiatry split into many
causal mechanisms

Disjunctive predicates   P1x or P2x or ... Pnx ...|P'x   P1y or P2y or ... Pmy ...| P'my
of reducing science

"Laws" of reducing science
(molecular neuroscience)
Connect Pxs to Pys; P's are
exceptions to S1, thus rather   These molecular relations may not map back
an "or" relation, a | operator   into existing psychiatric laws (or generalizations),
representing incompatibility is   thus a new S1x* → S2*y can be added as shown
used   by dashed arrows, which are inferences
     from P's to S*s

Figure 9.2 Molar and micro relations in a partial reduction; modified from Fodor (1975) with additions. Fodor talks of a "law" or "laws" but "generalization(s)" is a better term to use in biology and in psychiatry. Here S level generalizations are clinical interventions and observations, P level predicates represent connections (here interventions) at the neuroscience level. A more specific illustration of the schema might take S1 as schizophrenia (SZ) generally with S1x being an intervention of an atypical antipsychotic drug such as risperidone, with amelioration of auditory hallucinations S2y. S1 may then be "reduced to" several different etiological disorders at the neuroscience level, where P1x could be an intervention into that form of SZ due to dopamine dysregulation, P2x the intervention in neural circuitry underlying delusions, and Pnx an alteration of the pathology in the AI auditory cortex neural circuitry triggering auditory hallucinations. Here P′ is a hitherto unrecognized exception to the standard the DSM-IV characterization of SZ of S1—say an intervention in the pathology in the dorsolateral prefrontal cortex (DFLPC) affecting the cognitive function of short-term memory (P'my), perhaps due to chandelier and basket cells misfiring and affecting Purkinge cells. Further investigation of the pathology in the DFLPC may yield a new therapy, such as Lewis's experimental drug MK-0777 or some other GABA-related agonist, thus here a new S1*x intervention representing P′ at the molar level. This may address newer cognitive deficits (S*) in schizophrenia via correcting the GABA circuitry represented by P'my. Improvement can be tested at the psychological clinical level among other ways by the n-back short-term memory test, with n-back improvement being signified by S2*y. For a discussion of some of the background to this illustration see (Lewis and Sweet 2009) as well as (Wallace et al. 2011); this illustration is also based on a lecture by David Lewis, March 22, 2011, University of Pittsburgh.

we do not have sound etiopathogenic reductionist prototypes, even in such well plumbed areas as schizophrenia, as yet. For reasons for this concern, see, for example Harrison and Weinberger (2005), Lewis and Sweet (2009) and Meyer-Lindenberg (2010), where any promising advances are cautioned by the extensive speculations and caveats about the current state of affairs in applied genetics and neuroscience.

Endnotes

1 More precisely, Cronbach and Meehl stated that "*Construct validation* is involved whenever a test is to be interpreted as a measure of some attribute or quality which is not 'operationally defined'" (Cronbach and Meehl 1955, p. 175). This statement needs to be contextualized within their article as a whole, which does not subscribe to any kind of simple operationalist philosophy of science. The 1955 article was also reprinted in Volume 1 of the famous *Minnesota Series in the Philosophy of Science*, where Meehl was actively involved in the Minnesota Center for Philosophy of Science. Thanks to both Irving Gottesman and Peter Machamer for referring me to this article.

2 I thank Bob Krueger for pointing this disciplinary independence out to me.

3 This expression was used in Lewin's (1994) edition (*Genes V*). In a later edition (*Genes VIII*), Lewin described the notion of gene regulation as "an extremely flexible idea with many ramifications" (Lewin 2004, p. 301).

4 I will say more on this evolutionary rationale further later in this chapter.

5 Biologists seem to think in terms of GoM, as when they compare operons to the *lac* regulatory systems, though they do not consciously use GoM statistical techniques. I suspect this is because informal modeling suffices for such comparison. Possibly when sequence comparisons are made to simple systems DNA sequences, this also reflects GoM similarity thinking.

6 Later I will qualify on this claim, since as psychiatry increasingly involves genetic and neuroscientific entities and features, these will be interrelated among themselves and to behavioral constructs by complex networks of inference, that often assume auxiliary theories of how an instrument, e.g., magnetic resonance imaging scans, work. On this issue see Logothetis (2008).

7 I use the notion of a Kantian type of intuition here in the sense that Kant believed that certain scientific truths such as Euclidean space were synthetic a priori and given as "certain" forms of our knowledge.

8 See Nagel (1961), pp. 129–152 and also Fine (1984, p. 98) in which Fine develops a notion of a "natural ontological attitude" (NOA) which is "neither realist nor antirealist."

9 Fine himself remarked in a recent lecture (March, 2011) that a scientist's position on realism or instrumentalism may ultimately come down not to argument but to the scientist's temperament.

10 I provide such arguments in my book (1993, pp. 156–165), along with an extended example involving how "direct evidence" for the *lac* repressor was developed.

11 It might be wise to point out, however, that the significance of "direct evidence" in connection with evaluation and "acceptance" should not be overemphasized, since occasionally one encounters less directly empirical factors that are important in both an individual's and a scientific community's decision to (conditionally) accept a hypothesis or theory, such as consistency with well-entrenched theories or well-founded methodological assumptions.

12 For a further discussion of, and references to, these "tests," or to use another term, "criteria of theory choice," see my comments on Kendler's paper in this volume (Chapter 15).

13 I think that this thesis makes more sense in psychology than it does in genetics, and have criticized Hull's views in my (1993) book; also see (Schaffner 2002).

Chapter References

Andreasen, N. C. (1995). The validation of psychiatric diagnosis: new models and approaches. *American Journal of Psychiatry, 152*(2), 161–2.

Blacker, D., and Endicott, J. (2008). Psychometric properties: Concepts of reliability and validity. In: Rush, A. J., First, M. and Blacker, D. (eds.), *Handbook of psychiatric measures*, 2nd ed. Washington, DC: American Psychiatric Association, pp. 7–13.

Cantor, N., Smith, E. E., French, R. S. and Mezzich, J. (1980). Psychiatric diagnosis as prototype categorization, *Journal of Abnormal Psychology, 89*(2), 181–93.

Cohen, B. (1982). Understanding Natural Kinds. Unpublished Ph.D. Dissertation, Stanford University.

Cohen, B. and Murphy, G. L. (1984). Models of concepts. *Cognitive Science, 8*, 27–58.

Committee on Test Standards, (1954). Technical recommendations for psychological tests and diagnostic techniques: preliminary proposal. *Psychological Bulletin (Supplement), 51*(2, part 2).

Cronbach, L. J. and Meehl, P. E. (1955). Construct validity in psychological tests. *Psychological Bulletin, 52*, 281–302.

de Bono, M., Tobin, D. M., Davis, M. W., Avery, L. and Bargmann, C. I. (2002). Social feeding in Caenorhabditis elegans is induced by neurons that detect aversive stimuli. *Nature, 419*(6910), 899–903.

Dewey, J. (1920), *Reconstruction in philosophy*. New York: H. Holt and Company.

Fine, A. (1984). The natural ontological attitude. *In:* Leplin, J. (ed.), *Scientific Realism*. Berkeley, CA: University of California Press, pp. 84–107.

First, M. B. (2005). Clinical utility: a prerequisite for the adoption of a dimensional approach in DSM. *Journal of Abnormal Psychology, 114*(4), 560–4.

First, M. B. (2010). Clinical utility in the revision of the Diagnostic and Statistical Manual of Mental Disorders (DSM). *Professional Psychology: Research and Practice, 41*(6), 465–73.

First, M. B., Bell, C. C., Cuthbert, B., Krystal, J. H., Malison, R., Offord, D. R., *et al.* (2002). Personality disorders and relational disorders: A research agenda for addressing crucial gaps in DSM. In: Kupfer, D. J., First, M. B. and Regier, D.A. (eds.), *APA Research Agenda for DSM-V*. Washington, DC: American Psychiatric Association, pp. 123–99.

First, M. B., Pincus, H. A., Levine, J. B., Williams, J. B., Ustun, B. and Peele, R. (2004). Clinical utility as a criterion for revising psychiatric diagnoses, *American Journal of Psychiatry, 161*(6), 946–54.

Fodor, J. (1975). *The Language of Thought*. New York: Crowell.

Fuhrmann, G. (1991). Note on the integration of prototype theory and fuzzy-set theory. *Synthese, 86*, 1–27.

Fulford, K. W. M., Broome, M., Stanghellini, G. and Thornton, T. (2005). Looking with both eyes open: Fact and value in psychiatric diagnosis? *World Psychiatry, 4*, 78–86.

Gottesman, I. I. and Gould, T. D. (2003). The endophenotype concept in psychiatry: etymology and strategic intentions. *American Journal of Psychiatry, 160*(4), 636–45.

Hallmayer, J. F., Kalaydjieva, L., Badcock, J. *et al.* (2005), Genetic evidence for a distinct subtype of schizophrenia characterized by pervasive cognitive deficit. *American Journal of Human Genetics, 77*(3), 468–76.

Harris, H. W. and Schaffner, K. F. (1992). Molecular genetics, reductionism, and disease concepts in psychiatry. *Journal of Medicine and Philosophy, 17*(2), 127–53.

Harrison, P. J. and Weinberger, D. R. (2005). Schizophrenia genes, gene expression, and neuropathology: on the matter of their convergence. *Molecular Psychiatry,* **10**(1), 40–68.

Hull, D. L. (1974). *Philosophy of biological science.* Englewood Cliffs, NJ: Prentice-Hall.

Hyman, S. E. (2002). Neuroscience, genetics, and the future of psychiatric diagnosis, *Psychopathology,* **35**(2–3), 139–44.

Hyman, S. E (2007). Can neuroscience be integrated into the DSM-V?, *Nature Reviews. Neuroscience,* **8**(9), 725–32.

Hyman, S. E (2010). The diagnosis of mental disorders: the problem of reification. *Annual Review of Clinical Psychology,* **6**, 155–79.

Jablensky, A. and Kendell, R. E. (2002). Criteria for assessing a classification in psychiatry. *In:* Maj, M., Gaebel, W., Lopez-Ibor, J. J. and Sartorius, N. (eds.), *Psychiatric diagnosis and classification.* New York: John Wiley, pp. 1–24.

Jacob, F. (1977). Evolution and tinkering. *Science,* **196**(4295), 1161–6.

Kendell, R. (1989). Clinical validity. *Psychological Medicine,* **19**(1), 45–55.

Kendell, R. and Jablensky, A. (2003), Distinguishing between the validity and utility of psychiatric diagnoses. *American Journal of Psychiatry,* **160**(1), 4–12.

Kendler, K. S. (1985). Diagnostic approaches to schizotypal personality disorder: a historical perspective, *Schizophrenia Bulletin,* **11**(4), 538–53.

Kendler, K. S. (1990). Toward a scientific psychiatric nosology. Strengths and limitations. *Archives of General Psychiatry,* **47**(10), 969–73.

Kendler, K. S. and Greenspan, R. J. (2006). The nature of genetic influences on behavior: lessons from "simpler" organisms. *American Journal of Psychiatry,* **163**(10), 1683–94.

Laudan, L. (1973), C.S. Peirce and the trivialization of the self-corrective thesis. In: Westfall, S. and Giere, R. (eds.), *Foundations of Scientific Method in the 19th Century.* Bloomington, IN: Indiana University Press, pp. 275–306.

Laudan, L. (1981). A confutation of convergent realism. *Philosophy of Science,* **48**(1), 19–49.

Lewin, B. (1994). *Genes V.* New York: Oxford University Press.

Lewin, B. (2004). *Genes VIII.* Upper Saddle River, NJ: Pearson Prentice Hall.

Lewis, D. A. and Sweet, R. A. (2009). Schizophrenia from a neural circuitry perspective: advancing toward rational pharmacological therapies. *Journal of Clinical Investigation,* **119**(4), 706–16.

Lilienfeld, S. O. and Marino, L. (1995). Mental disorder as a Roschian concept: a critique of Wakefield's "harmful dysfunction" analysis. *Journal of Abnormal Psychology,* **104**(3), 411–20.

Lilienfeld, S. O. and Marino, L. (1999). Essentialism revisited: evolutionary theory and the concept of mental disorder. *Journal of Abnormal Psychology,* **108**(3), 374–99.

Logothetis, N. K. (2008). What we can do and what we cannot do with fMRI. *Nature,* **453**(7197), 869–78.

Meyer-Lindenberg, A. (2010). From maps to mechanisms through neuroimaging of schizophrenia. *Nature,* **468**(7321), 194–202.

Nagel, E. (1961). *The structure of science; problems in the logic of scientific explanation.* New York: Harcourt.

Osherson, D. and Smith, E. (1981). On the adequacy of prototype theory as a theory of concepts. *Cognition,* **9**, 35–58.

Peirce, C. S. (1994). *Collected papers of Charles Sanders Peirce. Vol. 5, pragmatism and pragmaticism.* Charlotteville, VA: Intelex.

Robins, E. and Guze, S. B. (1970). Establishment of diagnostic validity in psychiatric illness: its application to schizophrenia. *American Journal of Psychiatry,* **126**(7), 983–7.

Rosch, E. (1976). Classification of Real-World Objects: Origins and Representations in Cognition. In: Johnsen-Laird, P. N. and Wason, P. C. (eds.), *Thinking: Readings in Cognitive Science.* Cambridge: Cambridge University Press.

Rosch, E. and Mervis, C. B. (1975). Family resemblances: Studies in the internal structure of categories. *Cognitive Psychology,* **7**(4), 573–605.

Sadler, J. Z. (2005), *Values and psychiatric diagnosis* (International perspectives in philosophy and psychiatry). New York: Oxford University Press.

Sanislow, C. A., Pine, D. S., Quinn, K. J. *et al.* (2010). Developing constructs for psychopathology research: research domain criteria. *Journal of Abnormal Psychology,* **119** (4), 631–9.

Schaffner, K. F. (1993). *Discovery and Explanation in Biology and Medicine.* Chicago, IL: University of Chicago Press.

Schaffner, K. F. (1998a). Genes, behavior, and developmental emergentism: One process, indivisible? *Philosophy of Science,* **65**(June), 209–52.

Schaffner, K. F. (1998b). Model organisms and behavioral genetics: A rejoinder. *Philosophy of Science,* **65**, 276–88.

Schaffner, K. F. (2002). Reductionism, complexity and molecular medicine: genetic chips and the "globalization' of the genome. In: Regenmortel, M. and Hull, D. (eds.), *Promises & Limits of Reductionism in the Biomedical Sciences.* Somerset, NJ: John Wylie, pp. 323–47.

Schaffner, K. F. (2008). Etiological models in psychiatry: reductive and nonreductive. In: Kendler, K. S. and Parnas, J. (eds.), *Philosophical Issues in Psychiatry.* Baltimore, MD: Johns Hopkins University Press, pp. 48–90.

Schiller, F. C. S., Shook, J. R., and McDonald, H. P. (2008). *F.C.S. Schiller on pragmatism and humanism: selected writings, 1891–1939.* Amherst, NY: Humanity Books.

Sellars, W. (1977). Is scientific realism tenable? In: Asquith, P. and Suppe, F. (eds.), *PSA 1976: Proceedings of the 1976 Biennial Meeting Philosophy of Science Association.* East Lansing, MI: Philosophy of Science Association, pp. 307–34.

Trull, T. J. and Durrett, C. A. (2005). Categorical and dimensional models of personality disorder. *Annual Review of Clinical Psychology,* **1**, 355–80.

Walker, R. M., Christoforou, A., Thomson, P. A., *et al.* (2011). Association analysis of Neuregulin 1 candidate regions in schizophrenia and bipolar disorder, *Neuroscience Letters,* **478**(1), 913.

Wallace, T. L., Ballard, T. M., Pouzet, B., Riedel, W. J. and Wettstein, J. G. (2011). Drug targets for cognitive enhancement in neuropsychiatric disorders. *Pharmacology, Biochemistry, and Behavior,* **99**(2), 130–45.

Walton, K. E., Ormel, J. and Krueger, R. F. (2011). The dimensional nature of externalizing behaviors in adolescence: evidence from a direct comparison of categorical, dimensional, and hybrid models. *Journal of Abnormal Child Psychology,* **39**(4), 553–61.

Wakefield, J. C. (1999). Evolutionary versus prototype analyses of the concept of disorder. *Journal of Abnormal Psychology,* **108**(3), 400–11.

Widiger, T. A. (2011). The DSM-5 dimensional model of personality disorder: rationale and empirical support. *Journal of Personality Disorders,* **25**(2), 222–34.

Wimsatt, W. (1974). Complexity and organization. In: Schaffner K. F., and Cohen R. S. (eds.), *PSA-1972: Proceedings of the 1972 Biennial Meeting Philosophy of Science Association.* Dordrecht: Reidel, pp. 67–86.

Worrall, J. (1989). Structural realism: The best of both worlds? *Dialectica,* **43**, 99–124.

Validity, utility and reality: explicating Schaffner's pragmatism

Peter Zachar

9.10 Introduction

Distinguishing between the meanings of technical terms is important to an academic discipline. Examples of such distinctions in psychiatry include those between reliability and validity and between validity and utility. Although conceptual definitions of abstract terms have an inherent fluidity, it is crucial to not use this fluidity to obscure distinctions, as might be done in claiming that reliability is a type of validity or that clinical utility is validity.

As I have argued elsewhere in this volume, reliability can be a consideration in assessing *comparative validity*, but it is only one factor. The various kinds of reliability (e.g., inter-rater or test-retest) are asking whether the measurement of a construct is consistent and stable. The various small "v" validities (predictive, explanatory, content, etc.) are asking different and distinct questions about constructs.

One effective way to keep the reliability versus validity distinction clear is to focus on the meaning of reliability—which is well demarcated. Validity is not as well demarcated. It is both a conceptual abstraction (a big "V" notion of validity such as "the disorder really exists") and a composite of more or less explicit definitions (the little "v's"). Because utility is relative to goals, purposes and values, it is also not well demarcated. Because the two constructs overlap where some fuzziness occurs, the validity versus utility distinction, although important, is not clear cut across the board.

In this commentary I will explore the complicated validity and utility relationship from the standpoint of Schaffner's claim that *utility constitutes what we think of as reality*. I also talk about the very difficult philosophical issue of reality, and how Schaffner's pragmatism skirts the line between instrumentalism and scientific realism. Finally, I round out Schaffner's pragmatism by exploring his notions of prototype models and multiple levels of reality.

9.11 Pragmatism and utility

What can Ken Schaffner mean in claiming that utility constitutes what we think of as reality? To begin, let me note that the concept of utility in the philosophical pragmatist's sense should not be confused with the more common sense notion associated with the utilitarian who is interested in an economic bottom line. The utility of the pragmatists is not "expedience" or "profit." To illustrate the distinction, let me review a famous but probably apocryphal story about Michael Faraday.

Faraday was a 19th-century experimentalist who did groundbreaking work on electricity and magnetism. For example, he discovered both electric and magnetic fields. He also performed work that led to the development of electrical generators. According to scientific legend, a governmental minister visiting Faraday's lab one day asked him "Of what utility, Mr. Faraday, is this thing called electricity?" In response, Faraday is said to have replied. "Well minister, one day you will be able to tax it."

The utility that would be of appeal to our hypothetical government official is not the kind of utility emphasized by philosophical pragmatists. The utility of Faraday's experiments leading to the generation of electricity was in all the new things we learned to do. This includes lighting and heating homes, refrigerating food, storing information on magnetized tapes and keeping human hearts beating at a regular pace. For pragmatists, utility is about interaction, experiment and the craft of making things happen.

When considering the well-known Kendell and Jablensky (2003) distinction between validity and utility, a pragmatist such as Schaffner is going to have qualms. Kendell and Jablensky construed valid disorders as natural groupings. They claimed that members of such groups are qualitatively distinct from non-members with respect to the defining characteristics of the group. They considered this categorical validity to be an invariant property that is present or absent. It is similar to Meehl's (1995) notion of a taxon. In contrast, Kendell and Jablensky claimed that utility refers to whether a diagnosis provides non-trivial information about prognosis, treatment response or testable hypotheses about etiology. Because there is a plurality of utilities, they claim that utility is graded. According to Kendell and Jablensky, many diagnostic constructs can have some utility without being valid natural groups. For example, whether schizophrenia is a homogeneous syndrome with clear boundaries separating true cases from non-cases is different conceptually from whether the diagnosis allows us to predict treatment response.

A pragmatist might step back, however, and inquire about why we would set ourselves the goal of discovering categories that demonstrate the kind of qualitative distinctions between cases and non-cases that Kendell and Jablensky emphasize. The pragmatist's answer is that such diagnostic groups are not valuable in themselves, but valuable because they seem to make it more likely that we can reliably predict prognosis, treatment response, etc.—so utility is still relevant even for Kendell and Jablensky's well-demarcated notion of validity.

More trenchantly, Schaffner also questions the scientific plausibility of the Kendell and Jablensky distinction by noting that evolution is not the kind of process that produces neat and tidy categories (or natural kinds) that conform to the Kendell and Jablensky's notion of valid diagnostic category. This amounts to the strong claim that the conceptual distinction they draw is, for most cases, an empirically inadequate fiction, although I suspect both he and Assen Jablensky would agree that the taxon versus family resemblance-cluster-graded category issue is amenable to empirical testing.

9.12 **Pragmatism and reality**

In broaching the topic of reality, we encounter very difficult philosophical issues. I begin by exploring more familiar territory. For the sake of argument, let's say that in the 1960s many psychoanalytic therapists were able to successfully treat cases of depression, i.e., psychoanalysis possessed clinical utility. Can we then conclude that the psychoanalytic theory of depression was a valid representation of reality? A parallel question can be asked about the early treatment of schizophrenia with Thorazine. Because it worked better than competing treatments, were its users justified in concluding that the dopamine theory of schizophrenia was a correct representation of reality? Many scientific psychiatrists and psychologists would argue that the answer is to both questions is "No." For example, the kinds of case studies favored by psychoanalysts as bedrock data have come to be seen as scientifically inadequate and provisional at best (Meehl 1972), whereas the dopamine hypothesis has been proven to be oversimplified and arguably false (Kendler and Schaffner 2011).

As Ken Schaffner notes, there are two exemplary philosophical views about the relationship between scientific theories and reality. The first is called instrumentalism. The instrumentalist says that valid theories, constructs and models are tools that allow us to make reliable predictions about what to expect and that allow us to intervene and change things, but they do not have to be literally true representations of external reality. B. F. Skinner (1953) was a prominent advocate of this perspective. In contrast, the scientific realist says that the aim of science is to propose theories that accurately represent or correspond to external reality. Successful theories are successful, they say, because they at least approximate reality. The great clinical psychologist Paul Meehl (1978) advocated this perspective.

Going on common sense, most readers are probably inclined to throw their lot in with the scientific realist. So what motivates the instrumentalist? As shown by Larry Laudan (1981), throughout history, communities of scientists have been convinced that their best extant theories correspond to reality, but subsequent discoveries showed that those theories were not correct. Examples include the caloric theory of heat, vital force models in physiology and just recently, the molecular model of "the gene." Laudan argues that these theories were successful and productive according to the accepted criteria of the day, but that success did not legitimate inferences about approximating reality. The notion that, for all we know, the same may be true of our best current theories is called *the pessimistic induction*. An analogy in psychiatry would be the psychoanalysts asserting that their theory of depression as anger turned inward must correspond to what depression really is because so many psychoanalytic therapists can successfully treat depression.

Schaffner can be numbered among those philosophical pragmatists who occupy a middle-ground position between instrumentalism and scientific realism. They agree with the basic arguments of the instrumentalists: scientists develop networks of concepts, theories and models whose adoption is very much tied to their contribution to making connections between things, predictions about things and successful interventions to change things. Being successful does not guarantee that one's theory corresponds to an external reality. But these pragmatists are reluctant to just give up on such a useful concept like "reality." The pragmatists' notion of intervention and interaction highlights the role of both successes and failure. The combination of being able do things that were previously unimaginable (like refrigerating food) and also trying and failing (like not discovering "the gene" for schizophrenia) fits with the notion that we are bumping up against the world in some way. As Schaffner says, utility constitutes what we think of as reality. This is, however, a somewhat deflated and minimalist notion of reality.

Schaffner makes it clear that the basic assumption of scientific realism, i.e., that the goal of science is to develop theories and models that we know correspond to external reality, is not one that he considers philosophically justified.[1] A crucial argument to keep in mind is this: you cannot prove that your favored theory corresponds to reality by pointing to its successes because theories that clearly do not accurately represent reality have also produced successful predictions and interventions (e.g., the phlogiston theory). There must be some argument/evidence in addition to "success" to confirm the existence of an additional relation called "corresponding to the external world," and that something is just not there.

Defenders of this species of pragmatism generally contend that we need to be clear on the reasons we have for accepting that a construct, theory or model is "valid," "true," or "correct." For example, we might agree that a valid diagnostic construct/model allows us to predict treatment response or is consistent with what is known about genetics or allows us to understand the relationships between the observed symptoms. Following Arthur Fine (1986), Schaffner suggests that both instrumentalists and scientific realists can potentially agree on the reasons for taking a particular theory to be validated. One of Fine's interesting claims here is that there are criteria, tests and standard conditions for accepting the truth of assertions such as "This umbrella is green." These include looking at the umbrella in sunlight or asking someone with normal color vision what color they see. Assertions about electrons and quarks work the same way. There are epistemological norms for deciding if such claims are legitimate, and (ignoring hidden agendas and ideologies) finding agreement on these claims works somewhat like agreement on the color of umbrellas. This is called "the core position." These norms tend to be local and historical, rather than general and universal—one of the ideas behind Schaffner's term *conditionalized realism*.

Schaffner and Fine both say that nothing much is gained in terms of advancing knowledge by adding philosophical inferences in addition to these reasons for acceptance. Fine has a humorous construal of what it is that the scientific realist adds on to the core position. For example (following Fine's construal), in addition to agreeing with all the reasons for accepting that bipolar disorder really does run in families and really does involve episodes of mania and depression, the scientific realist stomps his foot and shouts out—"Bipolar disorder really does run in families, *REALLY*!" When imagining this scenario it is helpful to think of a stubborn kid with a shaking head and clenched fist engaged in an exaggerated stomping of the floor. Were we doing philosophical therapy, we might ask him to sit down and then calmly note that we agree on the various reasons for saying that this construct is valid, including the conceptual integration of the experimental evidence, the correlational evidence and the clinical evidence. We accept the claims made about bipolar disorder as true, we consider the bipolar construct to be valid, etc.—what more do you need? If he were a hard case, he might sit up, thump his desk and blurt out: "And it is valid, REALLY!"[2] Here "really" denotes some additional notion of correspondence with the external world on top of all the reasons for accepting the results of the scientific study of bipolar disorder.[3]

What Fine calls "the homely line" involves agreeing on the criteria for what counts as scientifically valid, but eschewing metaphysical inferences about correspondence to an external world out there. Rather than validity being a sign of approximating reality, the scientific realists' appeal to "approximating reality" could just as well be seen as a fringe benefit that they believe they can claim once they have developed valid constructs.

One potential criticism of this position is that realism is being belittled, in an almost anti-intellectual manner, largely because the philosophical issues seem so unresolvable. Being a hard problem, says Fine's critic, does not make something a bad problem. Trying to explain why science succeeds in addition to accepting that it does succeed, says the scientific realist, is a worthwhile task. The non-realist might agree that it is a worthwhile task, but holds that using "approximates reality" to explain the success of science begs the question and is therefore is not up to the task.

9.13 **Pragmatism, prototypes and pluralism**

I round out Schaffner's pragmatism by briefly exploring his pluralism. To do so let me return to our previous supposition about psychoanalytically-oriented therapy successfully treating many cases of depression. Once we can successfully intervene and make things happen, is that all there is for the pragmatist? The answer is "*no.*" Unlike a hard-core instrumentalist such as B. F. Skinner, a pragmatist such as Schaffner believes that it is worthwhile to figure out why the therapy worked, and included in this would be understanding why the symptoms of depression occur. These "why questions" however, cannot be construed according to the narrow confines of the reductive and essentialist models of etiology/pathology that have reigned in the past, especially in biological psychiatry. As Kendler, Zachar and Craver (2011) have argued, what is needed is a plurality of models, operating at multiple levels of analysis, which describe the mechanisms that produce and sustain disorders.

This raises an interesting question. When a philosopher such as Arthur Fine talks about the death of scientific realism, he is primarily writing about quantum physics. Upon realizing this, some readers may suspect that it is acceptable for physicists to assert that unobservables like charmed quarks are instruments for organizing and systematizing our observations, but diseases such as bipolar disorder are concrete processes. Shouldn't we expect that a good explanation of bipolar disorder would correspond to reality in the same way that a good explanation of tuberculosis does?

Schaffner's response would be that this argument about corresponding to reality misconstrues something important about explanatory projects, not only in psychiatry and psychology, but in biology as well. The kinds of mechanistic explanations we should be seeking would take the form of abstract models that allow us to integrate different levels of analysis—genetics, physiology, anatomy, cognition and emotion, behavior, interpersonal relationships, etc. For example, Bob Krueger's (Krueger and

Eaton, Chapter 10, this volume) behavioral genetic/structural model is an abstraction in this sense. As more levels of analysis are included in a model, it is going to become increasingly complex (and unwieldy). A model can get more detailed when it is examining connections between closely related levels of analysis, but as it spans more levels, it will be more coarse-grained. No single model can contain all the information and those that contain less may be easier to use for many purposes. Mechanistic models, therefore, are what philosophers such as Ronald Giere (1999) call partial representations. Such a view of models (and reality) opposes construing the goal of science as discovering a definite world structure that can be called the True Theory.

Schaffner says that the best way to think about this model-based perspective is along the lines of prototype models. The abstraction is the prototype. An example might be a causal model of major depression that describes the causal relationship between genetics, neuroanatomy and cognitive functions, but ignores the social environment and culture. The way prototype categories work is some cases match the prototype reasonably well, but others less well. A more successful explanatory psychiatry would contain families of related models, with different models emphasizing one level or process more than others. Which levels are considered relevant in a model would be influenced by our particular scientific and clinical goals.

Schaffner emphasizes that in medicine, the clinical reality of patent's panic attacks and phobias is a solid reality. If we can gain information about panic by looking at genetics and physiology then we should, but we should not believe that phenomenology is a fiction and the genetics are "really real." *Clinical validity* will use information from any level of analysis that contributes to its improvement. One of his implicit arguments here is that geneticists have given up trying to understand genetic products using reductionist "molecule only" models—such models are simply empirically inadequate. Given that the science of genetics is increasingly non-reductive, the reductive approach to psychopathology will be undermined whenever genetics are a target of the reductions. Another way to put it is this—if you set yourself the goal of reducing psychopathology to genetics, in order to be successful, you will have to abandon hardcore reductionism.

9.14 **Conclusion**

All of these philosophical cartwheels raise an important question—what practical advantages exist for psychiatry and clinical psychology in thinking about instrumentalism and scientific realism with respect to the validity of psychiatric classification? What has been suggested in this commentary is that one does not have to take a position on the instrumentalism versus scientific realism debate because scientific psychiatry can progress by means of the minimalist core position itself. Fine's Natural Ontological Attitude and Schaffner's Conditionalized Realism are designed to move us beyond this debate.

I also disagree, at least in one sense, with the goal of moving beyond instrumentalism and scientific realism. Studying and thinking about the philosophical issues involved in instrumentalism and scientific realism is still important. Why? Because in addition to foot stomping and desk thumping, there is quite a bit of essentialist chest pumping that occurs in psychiatry and clinical psychology, especially regarding talk about carving nature at the joints, exaggerated science versus pseudoscience rhetoric and, yes, construing big "V" validity as correspondence to external reality. The issue is not so much in setting up scientific realism as a regulative ideal, but in the hinting that some version of one's pet theory is just a few more studies away from carving nature at the joints. One of the things that studying the philosophy of science and the philosophy of psychiatry does is to show that things are not as tidy as they are made out to be, thus providing a little intellectual humility to the exploration of these vexing problems.

Acknowledgments

Thanks to Ken Schaffner, Michael First and Bob Krueger for helpful comments on an early version of this commentary.

Endnotes

1 Nor would he condone the notion that scientifically valid means "true representation of an objective external reality."

2 Fine considers instrumentalism to be a kind of anti-realism. He criticizes anti-realists for their own philosophical addition onto the core position in the form of new theories about the nature of truth or elaborate theories about what counts as observable. Fine's calls his own position non-realism.

3 It is important to note that Fine also accepts degrees of belief—so the evidence available to support assertions about bipolar disorder in psychiatry likely does not engender the same degree of beliefs/assent as the evidence supporting assertions about black holes in astronomy.

Comments References

Fine, A. (1986). *The shaky game: Einstein, realism, and the quantum theory*. Chicago, IL: University of Chicago Press, pp. xi, 186.

Giere, R. N. (1999). *Science without laws*. Chicago, IL: University of Chicago Press.

Kendell, R. and Jablensky, A. (2003). Distinguishing between the validity and utility of psychiatric diagnoses. *American Journal of Psychiatry*, **160**(1), 4.

Kendler, K. S. and Schaffner, K. F. (2011). The dopamine hypothesis of schizophrenia: An historical and philosophical analysis. *Philosophy, Psychiatry, & Psychology*, **18**(1), 41–63.

Kendler, K. S., Zachar, P. and Craver, C. (2011). What kinds of things are psychiatric disorders? *Psychological Medicine*, **41**, 1143–50.

Laudan, L. (1981). A confutation of convergent realism. *Philosophy of Science*, **48**(1), 19–49.

Meehl, P. E. (1972). Why I do not attend case conferences. In: Meehl, P. E. (ed.), *Psychodiagnosis: Selected papers*. Minneapolis, MO: University of Minnesota Press, pp. 225–302.

Meehl, P. E. (1978). Theoretical risks and tabular asterisks: Sir Karl, Sir Ronald, and the slow progress of soft psychology. *Journal of Consulting and Clinical Psychology*, **46**(4), 806–34.

Meehl, P. E. (1995). Bootstraps taxometrics: Solving the classification problem in psychopathology. *American Psychologist*, **50**(4), 266–75.

Skinner, B. F. (1953). *Science and Human Behavior*. Oxford: Macmillan.

Introduction

Kenneth S. Kendler

In this broad and informative chapter, Krueger and Eaton (K&E) provide a strong psychometric critique of the current psychiatric nosologic process. This paper well illustrates the tension seen elsewhere in this volume between the clinical-historical approach that psychiatry has typically adopted toward its diagnostic categories and the psychometric, measurement-oriented approach that has been cultivated for decades in the discipline of psychology.

After a brief review of the concept of reliability, the authors turn to their central concept of validity. The term "validity" is one of the most promiscuous in our field being used in many many ways. K&E begin by making an important distinction between external and structural validity. By external validity, I think they mean "looking out in the world and seeing whether by assigning a diagnosis to an individual, we also learn important other things about them such as their response to treatment, family history, and/or course of illness." They contrast this concept of validity with what they term "structural validity." While they do not provide us with a single definition, their meaning is relatively clear. Diagnostic criteria or the broader organization of disorders into categories is structurally valid to the degree to which it represents how symptoms and disorders occur in the real world.

As they note, much more of the DSM enterprise has focused on external validity than on the problems of structural validity, in part because structural validity and the measurement tradition that it represents has been much more the province of the field of psychology than psychiatry. They appropriately contrast what they call the "hypothetico-deductive spiral of reasoning" used in the development of a psychological test with the clinical-historical approach typically used in medicine and psychiatry.

The contrast here is a very interesting one that I cannot help trying to briefly illustrate. Psychologists typically start out with the concept of a trait they want to measure, for example, shyness. They then develop many self-report test items, some from the literature and perhaps some they write themselves. They then give these to several hundred college undergraduates (or, if they are more careful, as Dr Krueger often is, to a more representative sample of subjects). They analyze the results—reject the poor items, develop new ones and try again and again using a range of statistical methods to hone their scale. Typically a series of iterations are needed and tests in different populations before they can assure themselves that the items are performing well in assessing the underlying construct. Such a test would, if well developed, have a high degree of structural validity.

This is, of course, completely different from what happens in clinical medicine and psychiatry. Patients come for treatment. Doctors notice patterns. Some patients seem to present with similar symptoms. They then might go on to notice that patients with these similar symptoms have a similar course, or respond to treatment in the same way. They then propose this as a syndrome and write articles about it, trying to convince their colleagues of the validity of their proposal. If it is accepted, then medical scientists will try to study groups of patients with this syndrome seeking to uncover its pathophysiology and/or etiology.

K&E are rather critical of official psychiatric nosologies which they characterize as "self-perpetuating feedback loops." This is not the place to debate this issue in any depth. Surely some of their criticisms have merit. But, if this were entirely the case, why have other areas of medicine been so successful, using similar methods, at delineating true diseases (such as the distinction between juvenile and adult-onset diabetes)? Even in psychiatry, this clinical method produced the distinction between bipolar and unipolar affective illness and panic disorder and other anxiety disorders—both distinctions that have been validated from a number of perspectives. I might frame the question a bit differently from K&E. That is, how can we combine the best of the clinical and psychometric traditions to produce an optimally effective nosology?

In the latter parts of their essay, K&E point out the limitations of a nosology with inadequate structural validity and then begin to map out how such a situation might be ameliorated. They make the key point that any such effort will be driven by the data that is collected for such analyses.

K&E then review the seminal work, in which Krueger was a leader, looking at the structure of common psychopathology. The evidence is now quite substantial that much of the comorbidity observed in common psychiatric and substance use disorders can be explained by two broad dimensions of psychopathology named from terms borrowed from child psychiatry: internalizing and externalizing. K&E raise the issue of whether the assignment of disorders within DSM-5 should be altered to be consistent with this impressive body of evidence.

They also review psychometric approaches to studying individual criterion and how helpful psychometric methods can be in evaluating the performance of the criteria created by committees. Do the individual items measure what we want them to? Do they perform the same way in men versus women? How about in the young versus the old or in Americans versus Chinese?

I would like to conclude with what I hope might be a stimulating thought experiment. What would it be like to try to create an entire psychiatric nosology using the methods traditionally utilized by psychologists for constructing scales? The goal would be to maximize structural validity. The first question would be to define the population to be studied. Would it be the general population? Psychiatric out-patients? Psychiatric in-patients? What sort of samples would be needed to insure enough cases of rare syndromes like schizophrenia or anorexia nervosa or those requiring very sensitive questions such as the sexual paraphilias? What would come next? Would it be efforts to determine if the clinical phenomenon were truly categorical or dimensional and then how to optimally measure them? What would such an exercise produce and how closely, if at all, would it resemble our current nosology? If it was radically different, how easy would it be to change the behavior of psychiatrists, psychologists and insurance companies who were used to the older categories?

Chapter 10

Structural validity and the classification of mental disorders

Robert F. Krueger and Nicholas R. Eaton

In conceptualizing mental disorders, reliability and validity are fundamental concepts. Perhaps most frequently, the mental health field focuses on investigations of reliability, by one of several possible routes. Reliability studies often examine a particular assessment *instrument*—for instance, how similar are two scores on the Beck Depression Inventory when administered 1 hour apart? In addition to evaluating an assessment instrument's reliability, one can also examine the reliability of mental disorder *diagnoses*. For instance, investigators might have several trained clinicians interview each of a number of patients and then examine inter-rater agreement and reliability of their resulting diagnoses.

In general, the reliability of mental disorder diagnoses can be thought of as a fraction, with a numerator representing the signal of interest (true score) and a denominator representing the signal *plus* noise (observed score). As the noise associated with each diagnosis decreases, the numerator and denominator approach equivalence. Thus, when the noise is zero, the two quantities are the same, and the diagnosis (true score) can be made in an error free manner. In that case, the reliability would equal 1.00. As this illustration demonstrates, when one defines and classifies mental disorders based on reliability concerns, the primary goal is to reduce diagnostic noise, typically by reducing measurement error in assessment instruments.

Reliability is of greater than purely academic importance. Efforts to maximize diagnostic reliability have had a major impact on the way that mental disorders are classified, and thereby, on the way they are typically conceptualized in clinical settings. We need only look back to the precursors to the current nosology, DSM-IV-TR, to see this is the case. The early DSMs classified psychopathology into somewhat generalized disorders, often defined by a narrative paragraph designed to describe the "flavor" of the disorder in question. Later DSMs switched to providing a more specific list of diagnostic criteria, and diagnostic thresholds (e.g., five of nine diagnostic criteria must be present). Why was this change made? It was made primarily to enhance reliability. Narrative paragraphs produced unreliability in that they failed to maximize signal. The move to clearly delineated criterion sets helped to solve this problem, as it laid out specifically which signal(s) were of interest, which were not, and how much signal needed to be received before a diagnosis should be made.

10.1 **External validity and its limitations**

There is no denying that the changes to the DSMs over time—efforts to raise reliability by including sets of clearly delineated diagnostic criteria—were watershed events in the history of mental disorder nosology. The focus on reliability had a price, however, in that it shifted focus away from deeper questions of validity. In other words, the later DSMs, including DSM-IV-TR, strive to reduce noise. But are we focusing on the *correct* signals?

This question is deep but cannot be avoided. Indeed, there is a growing realization in the mental health field that most of the diagnoses enshrined in the DSMs are probably not true categorical entities in nature. Instead, many appear to index underlying dimensions of severity, and these dimensions seem to cut across current diagnostic constructs rather than following DSM-defined boundaries. Indeed, some have argued that the reification of diagnostic classifications as they stand is a major impediment to research that might eventuate in a valid nosology (Hyman 2010).

As with reliability, there are multiple types of validity that one can consider. The type of validity often invoked to evaluate mental disorder diagnoses is *external validity*. Researchers taking this approach might demonstrate that a disorder diagnosis is associated with poor functioning, such as undergoing divorce, being severed at the workplace, spending more days hospitalized, and so on. This perspective on validity is unquestionably important, and it highlights the marked impairments associated with mental disorder. However, these external validity approaches do not speak directly to the question of the optimal way to parse psychopathological phenomena. To provide a concrete example: it may be that major depression is associated with more days hospitalized, but it is likely that the presence of panic disorder, borderline personality disorder, schizophrenia, alcohol dependence and sleep disorders are similarly related to increases in hospitalization, when persons meeting criteria for these disorders are compared with persons who do not meet criteria. Contemporary DSM categories are associated with poorer functioning, but this does not mean that contemporary DSM categories represent the true nature of psychopathological variation.

To illustrate this point further, let us consider a particular disorder. DSM-IV-TR includes many culture-bound syndromes, such as *hwa-byung*, a Korean folk syndrome with symptoms of fatigue, fear of death, insomnia, panic, indigestion, anorexia, palpitations, aches and dysphoric affect. Thus, *hwa-byung* seems to cut across the DSM-IV-TR diagnostic categories: It appears to include aspects of mood disturbance as well as panic disorder, sleep disorder, hypochondriasis, and other disorders. Clearly, this disorder does not fit neatly into the categories Western psychiatric nosologies include, and academics in the United States or Europe probably would not argue that *hwa-byung* represents a fundamental diagnosis akin to major depression or schizophrenia. However, if one were to do an external validity study, it is almost assured that European or North American persons meeting criteria for *hwa-byung* would be more impaired than a comparison group; indeed, any one of the many diverse symptoms in the *hwa-byung* category would likely be associated with impairment. While this example might seem strange to some, it is no different from external validity studies used in "support" of the diagnostic validity of any disorder enshrined in the DSM-IV-TR.

10.2 **Structural validity**

If external validity is not a sufficient concept for carving psychopathology at its joints, what concept might be better suited to framing this task? The answer may be found in the work of Jane Loevinger, who explicated various conceptions of validity in a seminal 1957 monograph. Loevinger (1957) laid out the concept of *structural validity*, particularly in the context of psychological assessment. By structural validity, she was referring primarily to parallelism between psychological test item structure (the way test items tend to be correlated with each other) and the structure of extra-test behaviors (the way behaviors outside of the test, that should be correlated with the test, are correlated with each other). We believe that this notion of structural validity can be profitably applied to mental disorder classification and can help clarify how psychopathology might best be conceptualized.

Before we proceed further, an illustration of structural validity seems warranted. Consider the idea of a general and continuous dimension underlying intellectual (IQ) test performance—the so-called g factor. This g factor saturates the sub-tests of IQ batteries and leads to a positive manifold, wherein all subtests are positively correlated with one another. Indeed, it was the observation of this positive correlation matrix that first gave rise to the notion of a possible general factor of intelligence, g, in the first place. The existence of such a general factor is also inferred from evidence that essentially all reliable intellectual assessment instruments measure the same g (i.e., g estimates are very highly correlated between instruments), albeit to different extents (Johnson et al. 2004). If we apply the notion of structural validity here, we can state that extra-test behaviors should show much the same structure as the test itself. For example, persons who perform well in mathematics classes should tend to perform well in language classes. This would be a reasonable hypothesis given that people who do well on IQ test scales indexing mathematical ability also tend to do well on scales indexing verbal ability. Importantly, these patterns refer to the structure of individual differences, not the structure of abilities or qualities within specific people. Moreover, these patterns are probabilistic. Hence, it is possible to find specific persons who may be harder to fit within the model (e.g., a person with unusually strong mathematical ability but very weak verbal ability). However, to the extent that the model fits observed data and is structurally valid, such persons should be rare relative to persons where both mathematical and verbal talents are found (or are lacking) together.

10.3 **Alternative approaches to instrument and nosology design**

Loevinger's concept of structural validity had an important impact on psychological assessment and the study of individual differences because it focused thinking and research on the map connecting within-test behaviors with behaviors in the world outside of the test. By comparison, structural validity has had less influence on discussions of the validity of psychiatric classifications. This lack of explicit focus on structural validity likely arose because psychological assessment instruments and psychiatric nosologies arise from different frameworks. Psychological tests are often the result of a hypothetico-deductive spiral of reasoning. In this sort of reasoning, hypotheses are posited, data are collected, hypotheses are adjusted given the data, new data reflecting the modified hypotheses are collected, and so on. This is an iterative process by which the test instrument, and the hypotheses (the theoretical model), are refined over successive rounds of data collection and analysis. An example of such an approach can be seen in Tellegen's development of the Multidimensional Personality Questionnaire (MPQ; Tellegen and Waller in press). Originally planning to develop a measurement instrument to capture trait absorption (theorized to be predictive of hypnotizability), Tellegen created a list of hypothetically relevant items. Upon analysis of the structure of these items, he found that other latent factors had influence over the covariance within the item pool. He included additional items to flesh out these factors, which revealed the presence of additional latent factors. Eventually, his intended measure of absorption had expanded, through the hypothetico-deductive spiral, to be an omnibus measure of personality, of which absorption was only a single component.

Official mental disorder classification system development does not typically follow this hypothetico-deductive spiral. Nosologies are developed in a more of a self-reifying feedback loop. Notions about what constitutes a cogent set of psychopathological signs and symptoms, composing a mental disorder, are derived initially from clinical observation. Publications, both case studies and more formal empirical studies, emerge in the literature, and the disorder may eventually gain enough professional traction to warrant being included in the diagnostic manual. In the case of modern classification systems, the decision of what disorders to include is left up to a committee of experts, who consider clinical experiences and the scholarly literature in their deliberations. Clinical practice and the scientific research agenda then change to accept and apply these diagnoses, and a literature develops around the corresponding disorders. Assessment instruments are developed, interventions are tested, patient advocacy groups are formed, and managed care entities negotiate reimbursements for treatment. In the end, subsequent editions of the diagnostic manual tend to retain the diagnosis (sometimes in modified form, sometimes not) on the basis of this literature—which was spurred from the inclusion of the disorder in the manual in the first place.

The self-reifying disorders included in manuals are assumed to be valid by fiat and are therefore treated as "real" entities by clinicians, researchers and the public at large. What they actually are, however, is the result of an interaction of clinical and political forces that, by design, almost certainly do not represent the actual nature of psychopathology in terms of structural validity. Nevertheless, the necessary focus on reliability and validity quickly switches from the disorders themselves to their operationalizations in assessment instruments. To the extent that a specific operationalization of a mental disorder in an assessment tool fails to perform as expected in an empirical context, the presumption is usually that something is wrong with the assessment tool; a concern that the mental disorder the tool was designed to assess might be flawed at the conceptual level is raised more rarely. One can imagine that, if diagnoses made using a newly developed interview for a panoply of mood and anxiety disorders produced highly intercorrelated diagnoses across domains, many researchers might suggest that the new interview was suboptimal, because it did not properly discriminate between numerous distinct forms of mood and anxiety psychopathology. An alternative explanation—compatible with the exact same observation—would be that the interview reliably assessed the invalid mental disorders of the classification system. In structural validity terms in this scenario, the hypothesized within-test structure (distinctions between mood and anxiety disorder diagnoses) did not mirror the structure of behaviors outside of the test (co-occurrence of mood and anxiety symptomatology that, in nature, does not conform to notions derived primarily from clinical observation).

In sum, traditional official nosologies are self-perpetuating feedback loops. They begin from the "top-down," with expert definitions. If data do not conform to expert opinion, the expert opinion is rarely questioned, and the expert opinion continues to perpetuate a fixed set of constructs. By contrast, a focus on structural validity is a focus on working from the "bottom up." More basic data units (e.g., specific clinical phenomena, such as "delusions of reference" or "manipulativeness") are the core elements, and statistical methods can be used to assemble these units into empirically derived mental disorder constructs.

10.4 Other limitations of the current approach to classification

Contemporary nosologies are further compromised by assumptions that are placed on psychopathology conceptualizations a priori. For example, mental disorders are defined by fiat as dichotomous entities in nature, which are either present or absent in a given individual. An implication of this assumption is that the empirical distribution of mental disorder symptoms should be essentially bimodal. However, studies of many mental disorders have found that they are better captured as dimensional, rather than categorical entities. For instance, in the case of the personality disorders, accumulating research has demonstrated that these disorders are likely dimensional (Clark 2007).

Another result of the categorical classification of the myriad mental disorders in DSM-IV-TR is the implication that putatively distinct mental disorders are unrelated to one another. For instance, mood and anxiety psychopathology is parsed into numerous categorical disorders, and these disorders are listed in separate chapters of the diagnostic manual. Certainly, this organization into multiple disorders, separated by chapter, suggests meaningful boundaries between these disorders—otherwise, why not classify them together? This is a question of structural validity. How frequently do mood and anxiety disorders co-occur? Based on the DSM-IV-TR framework, one might expect that these disorders should be unrelated; as such, they would co-occur at rates based on their individual prevalence rates. Departures from this rate of expected co-occurrence would suggest that the current, multiply parsed classification fails to capture, in a structurally valid way, the interrelations among the diagnoses as they actually occur.

Studies of the issue of co-occurrence between mood and anxiety disorders have demonstrated that comorbidity between mood and anxiety disorders is the rule rather than the exception (Watson 2009), indicating that the perceived boundaries between these disorders are at least somewhat artificial. As illustrated using prevalence rate data from the Midlife Development in the United States (MIDUS) study, one would expect, based on these disorders being unrelated, four individuals out of 1000 to have comorbid major depression and generalized anxiety disorder (Eaton et al. 2010). The observed values, however, are 17 out of 1000—a rate of more than 400% of what is expected based on the disorders being independent. This highlights the close interrelations among these putatively independent disorders. Examples like this clearly illustrate that the "within-test structure" of the classification system (e.g., distinct mood and anxiety disorders, separated by chapter) does not mirror the structure of these constructs "outside of the test." Clearly, the DSM system is lacking in structural validity.

10.5 **Consequences of structural invalidity**

Departures from structural validity contribute error to the enterprise of understanding, assessing, and ameliorating psychopathology. When researchers examine the causal links between disorder X and an important outcome, say, suicide, the true relations are obscured to the extent that disorder X as classified does not represent how Disorder X is structured in nature. Imagine a hypothetical construct in nature, which we will call "emotionally labile disinhibition" and imagine, just for the sake of argument, that this construct captures a major and coherent axis of biological variation in humans. This construct might relate strongly to suicidality. If this construct were improperly parsed in the diagnostic manual into mental disorders Y (emotionally labile component) and Z (disinhibition), each of which were a categorical diagnosis, we can see that the relations between emotionally labile disinhibition and suicide could be unclear. Structural validity in a nosology is critical if one wishes to capture accurately the relations among mental disorders and also the associations of mental disorders with outcomes of importance.

Another consequence of using a structurally invalid system is the expense associated with pursing mental disorders of questionable accuracy. The costs—in time, grant funding, resources and so on—that have been put toward examining disorders that are non-optimal operationalizations of deleterious forms of psychopathology are very real. How much of clinicians', and patients', valuable time has been spent in differential diagnosis between two or more disorders that may or may not have accurate boundaries between them in the first place?

Structurally invalid classification systems can also mislead the scientific research enterprise or diminish its ability to accumulate an accurate body of literature. As noted earlier, research on mental disorders can have a self-reifying quality about it, which prevents movement toward uncovering the true structure of psychopathology. We can imagine that, if major depression and generalized anxiety disorder are actually closely related as suggested above, studies of one disorder that have exclusion criteria for the other for participants are biasing their samples. Further, it is possible that, when fine-grained analysis, such as genome-wide association studies (GWAS) is required, structurally invalid classifications thwart progress. For instance, Dick and colleagues (2008) suggested that one possible reason that the molecular genetic underpinnings of psychopathology have yet to be uncovered is that we may be focusing on improperly parsed constructs; rather, focusing on latent liabilities to broad types of psychopathology might prove more profitable, as they are presumably closer to the biological substrates of mental disorders.

Finally, let us consider the cost to the patients themselves, who frequently receive one or more diagnoses from a flawed classification system. These individuals often internalize their diagnoses and come to associate with them. They may start support groups or advocacy organizations for their disorder. And, unfortunately, many of them become saddled by two, three, or more diagnoses—a truly stigmatizing, disempowering situation that portrays the patient as afflicted by a multiplicity of different mental disorders. We may well be doing our patients a great disservice by categorizing them into multiple, fine-grained diagnoses if those diagnoses do not accurately represent the structure of psychopathology in nature. Putting aside that treatment decisions, managed care reimbursement plans, and so on are frequently based on particular diagnoses, this issue of "over-pathologizing" the patient warrants close consideration in discussions of the structural validity of our systems of mental disorder classification.

10.6 Developing a structurally valid nosology

Thinking through the examples given earlier leads us to the conclusion that structural validity may be a concept with great utility at this juncture in the development of psychiatric nosologies. Standard categorical mental disorder concepts developed by fiat are known to result in a variety of conceptual conundrums when they encounter data. As we now turn our attention to the development of a mental disorder classification system that is structurally valid, we must recognize the importance of data (Krueger and Eaton 2010). The problems with the current nosology likely emerged from placing less emphasis on data, particularly in earlier phases of construct development, relative to implicit clinical theories (e.g., that mental disorders are categories and that clinical observation and expert discussion can identify those categories). By bringing data into the construct development process earlier, we can better ensure that the structure of the diagnostic system maps onto the empirical structure of psychopathological signs and symptoms.

Theory will always precede data somewhat, because hypotheses about relevant variables will impact data collection. However, as we have noted earlier, this process does not tether the emergent classification system wholly to the original hypotheses, especially when a hypothetico-deductive approach is taken. It seems probable that many, if not most, of the signs and symptoms of psychopathology have been documented over the past century. Clearly, some mental disorder involves depressed mood; it is less clear that depressed mood is best conceptualized as its own, distinct construct. If we include assessments of depressed mood in our data collection, along with other indicators of psychopathology, we can analytically tease apart its relations with other symptoms or "core criteria," such as "refusal to maintain body weight," "use of illicit substances," and "excessive worry." In this way, we can "bootstrap" from an imperfect system, to a better system, which can inform further data collection, and so on.

There are several approaches one could take toward developing a structurally valid, data-driven classification system. One of the more common ways to achieve this goal is through latent variable modeling, including exploratory and confirmatory factor analysis, latent class analysis, and so on. These approaches clarify latent structures, usually either underlying liability dimensions or liability classes, which underlie the relations between constructs of interest. Another important approach, not discussed here, is to use biological markers and putative endophenotypes, such as brain activation in fMRI (functional magnetic resonance imaging) scans, to classify mental disorders. This approach has recently gained a great deal of traction with the National Institutes of Mental Health Research Domain Criteria (RDoC) program (see Insell and Cuthbert 2009). Although this chapter will focus on latent variable modeling of directly observable signs and symptoms, converging evidence from approaches like the RDoC will be critical to articulating a structurally valid nosology.

Starting with observable signs and symptoms (as opposed to more intermediate neurobiological phenotypes), there are at least two main initial units of observation: diagnoses and symptoms. The majority of the work that has been done toward uncovering a structurally valid understanding of the latent constructs underlying observed psychopathology has examined diagnoses, mostly because the data are available in epidemiologic samples; large samples are typically required for this type of structural modeling. In addition, diagnostic data are typically computationally tractable, as the information contained in a multitude of criteria has been condensed down into a single binary variable (0 = disorder absent, 1 = disorder present). Also, modeling diagnoses in a multivariate context helps to understand diagnostic comorbidity patterns, rather than symptom comorbidity patterns, which may be of substantive interest to the researcher (e.g., in determining the source of prevalence rate differences between women and men; Eaton et al. in press). This being said, it should be clear to the reader that there are also limitations associated with statistically modeling diagnoses, including their reliance on potentially arbitrary diagnostic thresholds.

Another approach, closely related to the analysis of mental disorder *diagnoses*, is to model mental disorders in a non-categorical way. This approach is sometimes taken to avoid the problems of questionable diagnostic thresholds and, historically, the somewhat complex nature of categorical observed variables in latent variable analysis. Researchers pursuing this avenue of analysis typically use a dimensional "criterion count" variable, as opposed to a dichotomous diagnosis, where the criteria endorsed are summed to a single number. While this method removes any effect of arbitrary diagnostic thresholds, it still parses psychopathology into the constructs defined by the classification system—for example, major depression criterion count variable still assumes that each of the criteria included in (and excluded from) the major depression diagnostic criteria represents a structurally valid inference. Thus, this approach relies on the current nosology's organization of symptoms/criteria into disorders and influences how they sum. Further, criterion counting assumes, as does DSM-IV-TR, that each criterion is associated with the same "amount" of the disorder as any other, but this too may be somewhat inaccurate. Item response theory (IRT) modeling of criteria within disorders indicates that endorsement of each criterion is associated with a different level of the latent construct. By summing criteria with unit weight (e.g., each criterion counts as a value of 1), we are assuming that, for major depression, a change in appetite/weight shows the same relation to major depression as does recurrent thoughts of death/suicidality. Based on IRT studies, this is likely not a structurally valid assumption (Aggen et al. 2005).

A third approach, which researchers have only recently begun applying in earnest, is symptom-level analysis. Latent variable modeling of symptoms is computationally complex and complicated further by frequent use of "skip-out" rules in epidemiologic interviews. However, in instances when these issues can be overcome, symptom-level analysis is a powerful analytic tool for building empirically derived, structurally valid nosologies. Unlike the examination of diagnoses, the use of symptoms (and signs, if such data exist) allows for a truly bottom-up explication of the relations between symptoms, which can then be used to infer the structure of disorder constructs. While researchers must be careful to ensure that the universe of content is adequate when doing these sorts of analyses, they are an excellent means of building a structurally valid nosology from the ground up.

Building off the earlier discussion, much can be learned via IRT modeling of existing mental disorder constructs (see Reise and Waller 2009). Researchers could apply IRT methods to the symptoms/criteria of each currently defined disorder and thereby develop an understanding of how each criterion relates (or fails to relate) to the construct of interest. In doing so, the problem of unit weight criterion counting toward a diagnostic threshold is mitigated, because IRT provides a direct estimation of "how much" of a disorder construct is associated with endorsing each criterion. For example, if criterion X tends to indicate a z-score depression trait level of 2.5 (i.e., 2.5 standard deviations above the population mean value of zero), and criterion Y is associated with a depression trait level of 0.5, we can see that endorsing criterion X indicates a much greater level of depression than does endorsing criterion Y; in a unit weight criterion counting approach, an individual who endorsed criterion X or criterion Y is assumed to have the same level of depression. Further, IRT allows for investigation of how criteria relate to the construct of interest in different groups, a phenomenon called differential item functioning (DIF). One study of endorsement patterns of seven personality disorders in younger and older adults found that 29% of diagnostic criteria contained age bias (e.g., endorsement of the schizoid personality disorder criterion of little interest in sex was associated with a schizoid trait z-score of 1.12 in younger adults but of -0.08 in older adults; Balsis et al. 2007). Approaches such as these can help refine the symptoms/criteria of an already defined disorder construct. These methods might be desired as a transitional step between nosologies, or as a means of preserving particular constructs for clinical or political reasons. While it is unlikely that the results of this approach would be truly structurally valid, it would likely yield a more valid conceptualization of each disorder than the more basic, unit weight criterion counting approach employed in the current classification manual.

10.7 What is the state of structural knowledge?

Given the previous discussion, it seems reasonable to summarize briefly the current state of structural knowledge about mental disorders. Interested readers are referred to recent reviews of this topic for a more in-depth account (see, e.g., Eaton et al. 2010; Krueger and Markon 2006). As such, we will focus briefly on the major themes of structural psychopathology research, which is currently a rapidly evolving and active area.

Seminal work by Achenbach and Edelbrock (1978, 1984) examined the structure of child psychopathology and, through factor analysis, determined that a wide variety of problem behaviors and symptoms tended to group into two groups of internalizing and externalizing problems. Subsequent research, primarily with adults (e.g., Kendler et al. 2003; Krueger 1999; Krueger et al. 1998; Slade and Watson 2006; Vollebergh et al. 2001), has replicated this finding.

Comorbidity within each group of mental disorders appears to be due to a stable (Eaton et al. in press; Fergusson et al. 2006; Krueger et al. 1998; Vollebergh et al. 2001) latent liability to experience disorders in each group. Both internalizing and externalizing have been shown to emerge in large part from underlying genetic effects acting coherently and in concert (Kendler et al. 2003, 2011) and to serve as the primary causal pathway for the continuity of psychopathology and lifetime comorbidity of disorders (Kessler et al. 2011).

Let us consider the externalizing spectrum in greater detail, with an eye toward explicating its basic nature. Externalizing is the shared (common) liability to experience a variety of mental disorders, including antisocial personality disorder, alcohol dependence, nicotine dependence, and dependence on illegal substances such as heroin, cocaine, marijuana, and so on. The structure of the externalizing liability itself has been investigated in several studies, and it appears that this liability has a dimensional nature, as opposed to being composed of latent liability classes or a mixture of dimensions and classes (Markon and Krueger 2005; Walton et al. 2011). In addition, the externalizing liability is closely related to the normal personality trait of disinhibition/impulsivity (Krueger et al. 2002).

In contrast, internalizing is the shared (common) liability to experience mental disorders such as major depression, dysthymia, generalized anxiety disorder, panic disorder, specific phobia, social phobia, hypochondriasis, obsessive–compulsive disorder, post-traumatic stress disorder, eating disorders and so on. Thus, internalizing captures a wide variety of psychopathology—primarily mood and anxiety disorders, but it is associated with other types of disorders as well. Like externalizing, the internalizing liability also shows relations to normal personality traits; internalizing correlates essentially perfectly ($r=0.98$) with trait neuroticism (Griffith et al. 2010).

Unlike externalizing, the precise structure of internalizing has not been fully resolved. Typical studies of internalizing liability model the construct as dimensional, but the precise number of dimensions necessary to capture internalizing disorders' comorbidity is somewhat unclear. Many studies model the comorbidity between these disorders as a single liability dimension (Eaton et al. in press; Fergusson et al. 2006; Krueger et al. 1998). Other studies have found, both through exploratory and confirmatory factor analyses, that the internalizing liability is best represented as a set of two correlated subfactors, distress and fear (Eaton et al., in press; Krueger 1999; Slade and Watson 2006; Vollebergh et al. 2001). In such studies, a higher-order general internalizing liability is typically parameterized as the correlation between these two subfactors. Distress primarily represents the liability to major depression, dysthymia and generalized anxiety disorder; fear primarily represents the liability to social phobia, specific phobia and panic disorder. Few investigations have directly compared these two competing models of internalizing liability, and thus its structure remains somewhat unresolved.

One interesting point about this research is that not all disorders have been found to load optimally on internalizing *or* externalizing. Rather, some disorders show meaningful cross-loadings on both. For instance, borderline personality disorder is primarily an internalizing disorder, but it shows notable relations with latent externalizing as well (Eaton et al. 2011). This highlights the heterogeneity of mental disorders as they are currently defined. If we accept that latent internalizing and externalizing liabilities are fundamental building blocks of psychopathology, then the borderline personality disorder diagnosis is a rather complex combination of two such components rather than a discrete and singular diagnosis.

Internalizing–externalizing's implications for nosology

The replication of these internalizing and externalizing structures have led some to call for a reshuffling of the classification manual such that the "meta-structure"—the broad organizational framework—of the upcoming DSM-5 would reflect this knowledge about how disorders group together (Andrews et al. 2009; Regier et al. 2011). Rather than theoretically derived chapters such as "mood disorders" and "anxiety disorders," a more empirically based nosology would likely have sections for internalizing and externalizing disorders, and perhaps subheadings within the former to characterize rubrics such as distress and fear. As more research accumulates on this topic, it may well become clear that the current parsing of these common mental disorders may be in need of serious reclassification to reflect internalizing and externalizing liabilities more accurately. This would represent a notable step toward a structurally valid classification system. As it stands now, it is clear that the current organization does not represent the state of mental disorders in nature and, is thus, not structurally valid.

10.8 **Future directions**

Internalizing and externalizing capture only some of the myriad manifestations of psychopathology that individuals experience. This is largely a function of the nature of the data available. Epidemiologic studies frequently do not assess less common mental disorders. In addition, endorsement rates of these disorders are so low that they are not easily amenable to statistical modeling. This will likely be an important area for future structural psychopathology research. For example, Kotov et al. (2011) examined the structure of diverse mental disorders in a clinical sample and found evidence for internalizing and externalizing spectrums, but also evidence for additional antagonistic (indicated by e.g., narcissistic personality disorder), somatoform (e.g., hypochondriasis), and thought disorder (e.g., schizotypal personality disorder) spectrums.

An additional symptom-level study in a general population sample found that hallucinations and delusions, paranoia, eccentricity, and schizoid symptom clusters defined a latent factor the author called thought disorder (Markon 2010). The thought disorder factor correlated with internalizing ($r=0.72$) and externalizing ($r=0.58$) liabilities, but it was best modeled as a separate factor. Diverse personality disorders (beyond antisocial personality disorder) are also rarely examined in the context of underlying structure. Recent research, however, supports the notion that these disorders fit well into the internalizing-externalizing structure of psychopathology (Kendler et al. 2011).

In sum, by elaborating these models, and building them from approaches that utilize both mental disorders and symptoms, it seems likely that a structurally valid nosology is within reach. This is an exciting proposition, because such an endeavor could revolutionize the mental health field as we know it. Although there would be considerable difficulties associated with this kind of endeavor—such as political pushback, redefining managed care payments, linking the extant literature on old constructs with new constructs—these issues are not insurmountable if approached in a systematic way. Ultimately, the goals of mental health efforts are to understand and ameliorate suffering due to psychopathology, and these goals will be furthered by ensuring that our working definitions of psychopathology closely mirror the way it actually occurs. A focus on structural validity aims to ensure this congruence between the nosology and phenomena the nosology is designed to parse.

Chapter References

Achenbach, T. M. and Edelbrock, C. S. (1978). The classification of child psychopathology: A review and analysis of empirical efforts. *Psychological Bulletin, 85*(6), 1275–301.

Achenbach, T. M. and Edelbrock, C. S. (1984). Psychopathology of childhood. *Annual Review of Psychology, 35*, 227–56.

Aggen, S. H., Neale, M. C. and Kendler, K. S. (2005). DSM criteria for major depression: Evaluating symptom patterns using latent-trait item response models. *Psychological Medicine, 35*, 475–87.

Andrews, G., Goldberg, D. P., Krueger, R. F., Carpenter, W. T., Jr., Hyman, S. E., Sachdev, P., et al. (2009). Exploring the feasibility of a meta-structure for DSM-V and ICD-11: Could it improve utility and validity? *Psychological Medicine, 39*, 1993–2000.

Balsis, S., Gleason, M. E. J., Woods, C. M. and Oltmanns, T. F. (2007). An item response theory analysis of DSM-IV personality disorder criteria across younger and older age groups. *Psychology and Aging, 22*, 171–85.

Clark, L. A. (2007). Assessment and diagnosis of personality disorder: Perennial issues and an emerging reconceptualization. *Annual Review of Psychology, 58*, 227–57.

Dick, D. M., Aliev, F., Wang, J. C., Grucza, R. A., Schuckit, M., Kuperman, S., et al. (2008). Using dimensional models of externalizing psychopathology to aid in gene identification. *Archives of General Psychiatry, 65*, 310–18.

Eaton, N. R., Keyes, K. M., Krueger, R. F., Balsis, S., Skodol, A. E., Markon, K. E., et al. (2011). An invariant dimensional liability model of gender differences in mental disorder prevalence: Evidence from a national sample. *Journal of Abnormal Psychology.* August 15, Advance online publication. doi: 10.1037/a0024780.

Eaton, N. R., Krueger, R. F. and Oltmanns, T. F. (2011). Aging and the structure and long-term stability of the internalizing spectrum of personality and psychopathology. *Psychology and Aging, 26*(4), 987–93.

Eaton, N., Krueger, R. F., Keyes, K. M., Skodol, A. E., Markon, K. E., Grant, B. F., *et al.* (2011). Borderline personality disorder co-morbidity: Relationship to the internalizing-externalizing structure of common mental disorders. *Psychological Medicine*, **41**(5), 1041–50.

Eaton, N., South, S. and Krueger, R. F. (2010). The meaning of comorbidity among common mental disorders. In T. Millon, R. Krueger and E. Simonsen (eds.), *Contemporary Directions in Psychopathology: Scientific Foundations of the DSM-V and ICD-11*. New York: Guilford Press, pp. 223–41.

Fergusson, D. M., Horwood, L. J. and Boden, J. M. (2006). Structure of internalizing symptoms in early adulthood. *British Journal of Psychiatry*, **189**, 540–6.

Griffith, J. W., Zinbarg, R. E., Craske, M. G., Mineka, S., Rose, R. D., Waters, A. M., *et al.* (2010). Neuroticism as a common dimension in the internalizing disorders. *Psychological Medicine*, **40**, 1125–36.

Hyman, S. E. (2010). The diagnosis of mental disorders: The problem of reification. *Annual Review of Clinical Psychology*, **6**, 155–79.

Insel, T. R. and Cuthbert, B. N. (2009). Endophenotypes: Bridging genomic complexity and disorder heterogeneity. *Biological Psychiatry*, **66**(11), 988–9.

Johnson, W., Bouchard, T. J., Jr., Krueger, R. F., McGue, M. and Gottesman, I. I. (2004). Just one g: Consistent results from three test batteries. *Intelligence*, **32**, 95–107.

Kendler, K. S., Aggen, S. H., Knudsen, G. P., Røysamb, E., Neale, M. C., and Reichborn-Kjennerud, T. (2011). The structure of genetic and environmental risk factors for syndromal and subsyndromal common DSM-IV axis I and all axis II disorders. *American Journal of Psychiatry*, **168**, 29–39.

Kendler, K. S., Prescott, C. A., Myers, J. and Neale, M. C. (2003). The structure of genetic and environmental risk factors for common psychiatric and substance use disorders in men and women. *Archives of General Psychiatry*, **60**, 929–37.

Kessler, R. C., Ormel, J., Petukhova, M., McLaughlin, K. A., Green, J. G., Russo, L. J., *et al.* (2011). Development of lifetime comorbidity in the World Health Organization World Mental Health Surveys. *Archives of General Psychiatry*, **68**, 90–100.

Kotov, R., Ruggero, C. J., Krueger, R. F., Watson, D., Yuan, Q., and Zimmerman, M. (2011). New dimensions in the quantitative classification of mental illness. *Archives of General Psychiatry*, **68**(10), 1003–11.

Krueger, R. F. (1999). The structure of common mental disorders. *Archives of General Psychiatry*, **56**, 921–6.

Krueger, R. F., Caspi, A., Moffitt, T. E. and Silva, P. A. (1998). The structure and stability of common mental disorders (DSM-III-R): A longitudinal-epidemiological study. *Journal of Abnormal Psychology*, **107**(2), 216–27.

Krueger, R. F. and Eaton, N. R. (2010). Personality traits and the classification of mental disorders: Toward a more complete integration in DSM-5 and an empirical model of psychopathology. *Personality Disorders: Theory, Research, and Treatment*, **1**, 97–118.

Krueger, R. F., Hicks, B. M., Patrick, C. J., Carlson, S. R., Iacono, W. G. and McGue, M. (2002) Etiologic connections among substance dependence, antisocial behavior, and personality: Modeling the externalizing spectrum. *Journal of Abnormal Psychology*, **3**, 411–24.

Krueger, R. F. and Markon, K. E. (2006). Reinterpreting comorbidity: A model-based approach to understanding and classifying psychopathology. *Annual Review of Clinical Psychology*, **2**, 111–33.

Loevinger, J. (1957). Objective tests as instruments of psychological theory. *Psychological Reports*, **3**, 635–94.

Markon, K. E. (2010). Modeling psychopathology structure: A symptom-level analysis of Axis I and II disorders. *Psychological Medicine, 40*, 273–88.

Markon, K. E. and Krueger, R. F. (2005). Categorical and continuous models of liability to externalizing disorders: A direct comparison in NESARC. *Archives of General Psychiatry, 62*, 1352–9.

Regier, D. A., Narrow, W. E., Kuhl, E. A., and Kupfer, D. J. (eds.). (2011*). The conceptual evolution of DSM-5*. Arlington, VA: American Psychiatric Publishing, Inc.

Reise, S. P. and Waller, N. G. (2009). Item response theory and clinical measurement. *Annual Review of Clinical Psychology, 5*, 27–48.

Slade, T. and Watson, D. (2006). The structure of common DSM-IV and ICD-10 mental disorders in the Australian general population. *Psychological Medicine, 36*, 1593–600.

Tellegen, A. and Waller, N. G. (2008). Exploring personality through test construction: Development of the Multidimensional Personality Questionnaire. In G. J. Boyle, G. Matthews, and D. H. Saklofske (eds.), *The SAGE Handbook of personality theory and assessment: Personality measurement and testing* (Vol. 2). London: Sage.

Vollebergh, W. A. M., Iedema, J., Bijl, R. V., de Graaf, R., Smit, F. and Ormel, J. (2001). The structure and stability of common mental disorders: The NEMESIS study. *Archives of General Psychiatry, 58*, 597–603.

Walton, K. E., Ormel, J., and Krueger, R. F. (2011). The dimensional nature of externalizing behaviors in adolescence: Evidence from a direct comparison of categorical, dimensional, and hybrid models. *Journal of Abnormal Child Psychology, 39*(4), 553–61.

Watson, D. (2009). Differentiating the mood and anxiety disorders: A quadripartite model. *Annual Review of Clinical Psychology, 5*, 221–47.

Chapter 10: Comments

Seeing sense in psychiatric diagnoses

Paul R. McHugh

This essay splendidly depicts and elucidates the current problems that DSM-driven psychiatry faces—namely how to refine its classificatory and diagnostic task while remaining committed to the appearance-based identification method that these authors acknowledge has "enshrined" diagnoses false to nature in the discipline. Amongst the benefits a reader garners from Krueger and Eaton—not surprising perhaps given the great traditions of psychological methodology found at their University of Minnesota—one must include the helpful distinctions they draw between the concepts of reliability and validity that emerged from the science of psychological testing and the way these concepts were employed in DSM-III/IV (where, as they say, officially endorsed diagnoses tend to be "self-reifying" and "assumed to be valid by fiat" with all that implies in social and political terms.) These authors are not timid in identifying how these built-in misconceptions of purpose hinder the psychiatric enterprises of explaining and relieving psychopathology and speak compellingly about the costs of such misconceptions in terms of time, money, and effort.

As they turn to propose a "structurally valid nosology" they emphasize the impor-tance of it being "data-driven" and acknowledge that data are never "theory free" especially in our field. With this sort of goal in mind they conscientiously review the several methods of working with diagnostic symptoms and concepts in ways that take into account the defining weight of different items in discerning and distinguishing conditions. Here they anticipate progress through a growing understanding of dimen-sional features tied to diagnostic "entities." Their views on these matters are illuminating.

They especially emphasize how current psychiatric diagnoses have underplayed—even neglected—the interesting distinctions drawn by Achenbach and Edelbrock (1978, 1984) between the "internalizing" and "externalizing" problems reflected in human psychological symptoms of disorder and distress. The "externalizing" liability reflected in such disorders as alcohol dependence is clearly of a dimensional nature in the population. The "internalizing" liability expressed in such disorders as major depression and social phobia may best be represented by the subfactors of dis-tress and fear. Further work here is needed, they believe, as some disorders such as borderline personality have loadings of both externalizing and internalizing factors.

Although these authors acknowledge that other bodies of concept and data may add to the formation of a structure for validity, the internalizing-externalizing distinction holds the greatest promise for them.

What I find most welcome in this essay is how it identifies the disciplinary burden brought about by the contemporary diagnostic methods and how the resolution of this burden calls for psychiatrists to commit to "bottom-up" approaches in evaluating and treating their patients. As a further take on this essay I want to emphasize that classifications in biological sciences and medicine have two purposes best working in tandem namely: (1) for identification and (2) for separating natural groups. That is simply to say that developed classifications should satisfy both the denotative and connotative functions tied to naming.

It is ever a vulnerability for biologists and physicians to fall under what amounts to an hypnotic spell for developing classificatory names sanctioned by usage and based on easily observed appearances of entities as in this way they find consistent identification simple to apply and teach. From this commitment to the denotative function emerges the naturalist's field guide with all its confidence building for consistency in terminology and identification. And DSM-III/IV is a field guide.

All biologists and physicians know that they must fight the temptation to stop with the field guide (denotative) version of their classifications. Essential to scientific and clinical progress are efforts developing a classificatory nomenclature that derives from the rules of generation of entities and conditions and that provides the connotative sense to a terminology. This after all characterized the Darwinian advance on the Linnaean classificatory system in biology that had suited biological scientists for a century.

The connotative rules of generation though demand to be understood, exemplified and practiced in order for them to become applied with consistency in medicine. And, they become refined over time by their successes and failures in provoking better understandings of natural groups and better practices with them.

It is for this reason that I've taken to emphasizing the path of "intelligibility first, explanation second" to replace the mantra of "reliability first, validity second" that underpins faith in DSM-III/IV. Whether these authors' emphasis on internalizing as against externalizing factors will do what I and they want remains something of an empirical and practical question open to the tests of time. Something of the connotative kind though that speaks to generation and distinctions of nature are certainly needed now in psychological medicine.

Our emphasis at Johns Hopkins on what we have called the Perspectives of Psychiatry (McHugh and Slavney 1998) through which we differentiate mental disorders according to the most obvious aspects of their generative natures has been spelled out in my chapter in this text and it has exactly the same aim and purpose as these authors. It's ever encouraging as here to encounter colleagues who see the same problems in one's discipline and who offer solutions. Would that those responsible for the next iteration of the DSM listen carefully to both the serious concerns with its approach we have found identified here and some of the solutions suggested.

Comments References

Achenbach, T. M. and Edelbrock, C. S. (1978). The classification of child psychopathology: A review and analysis of empirical efforts. *Psychological Bulletin*, **85**, 1275–301.

Achenbach T. M. and Edelbrock, C. S. (1984). Psychopathology of childhood. *Annual Review of Psychology*, **35**, 227–56.

McHugh P. R. and Slavney P. R. (1998). *The Perspectives of Psychiatry* (2nd ed.). Baltimore MD: Johns Hopkins University Press.

Part IV

Application to major depression and schizophrenia

Chapter 11

Introduction

Josef Parnas

This chapter tries to address one of the central issues in the contemporary nosological puzzle, namely what is a clinically significant depression?

The nosological difficulties encountered in the domain of schizophrenia spectrum disorders pale in comparison to those encountered in affective disorders, and that is for obvious reasons. We all experience fluctuations in our mood, energy level, performance and well-being. It is also not uncommon to develop sadness in response to a loss of a close figure or to a life change having a similar emotional significance. Humans are often unhappy, irritable, angry, but only a fraction of that malaise is considered as a clinically significant condition, deserving some form of psychiatric attention and treatment. Obviously, a non-arbitrary selection of this fraction is not only a headache for the clinicians but is also a crucial issue for the pathogenetic research. Maj outlines, and briefly evaluates, pros and cons of three possible approaches to delimit a clinically significant depression:

1. Following Wakefield, to exclude from clinical depression the cases of normal sadness, the latter being considered as a normal reaction to a relevant adverse life event. Maj is skeptical with respect to this solution.

2. To deepen our knowledge of phenomenology of depression in order to be able to distinguish the "true depressive states" (marked by a qualitatively distinct feel) from a ragbag of heterogeneous cases of normal sadness and varieties of discomfort. It can be added that the DSM-IV section of mood disorders contains 10 disorders, each with various specifiers. One can doubt whether we can reliably perform these distinctions without having a better grasp of what constitutes a clinically significant depression. The psychiatric sources, including easily available textbooks and the manuals of DSM-IV and ICD-10, are rather vague on the question of "what it is like to be depressed" (apart from references to sadness and irritability). To explore this phenomenological approach, says Maj, we need more empirical research data. It is difficult, but not impossible, to envisage how such a qualitative phenomenological research could be translated into a more operational format.

3. The third approach, based on the assumption of a certain dimensionality of the number of depressive features in the transitions between normality, sadness and clinical depression, advocates an increase in the number of features required by the DSM-IV for the diagnosis of a "major depression" (or elevating a corresponding score on the HDSD-10). This is a pragmatic approach with certain empirical support.

The question addressed by Maj has some urgency and tremendous social significance, given the astronomic worldwide prevalence figures of "major depression" and the commercial interests of pharmaceutical industry to medicalize "the human condition." It is not uncommon today to see general practitioners using simplified Hamilton Depression Scale for *diagnosis* and treatment indication. Some colleagues support the wide-spread use of selective serotonin reuptake inhibitor drugs on the ground that the operational improvement of our diagnostic means now correctly picks up a specific "brain disease." They suggest that the previously untreated cases only now have an access to relevant treatment.

Chapter 11

When does depression become a mental disorder?

Mario Maj

Major depressive disorder is reported to be the most common mental disorder, with a lifetime prevalence in the community ranging from 10 to 25% in women and from 5 to 12% in men (American Psychiatric Association 1994). According to the World Health Organization, it will, by the year 2020, be the second leading cause of worldwide disability (Murrey and Lopez 1996), an estimate based on the above-mentioned data on its prevalence in the community and on a severity score according to which major depression is placed in the second most severe category of illness, the same category as paraplegia and blindness.

These figures are frequently quoted in the psychiatric literature, but are viewed by many, both outside and within the psychiatric field, with a substantial degree of skepticism.

From outside the psychiatric field, it has been pointed out that "determining when relatively common experiences such as. . . sadness. . . should be considered evidence of some disorder requires the setting of boundaries that are largely arbitrary, not scientific, unlike setting the boundaries for what constitutes cancer or pneumonia" (Kutchins and Kirk 1997). From within the psychiatric field, it has been stated that "based on the high prevalence rates identified in both the ECA and the NCS, it is reasonable to hypothesize that some syndromes in the community represent transient homeostatic responses to internal or external stimuli that do not represent true psychopathologic disorders" (Regier et al. 1998).

According to Horwitz and Wakefield (2007), "the DSM definition of major depressive disorder. . . fails to exclude from the disorder category intense sadness. . . that arises from the way human beings naturally respond to major losses." As a consequence of this, normal sadness is sometimes treated as if it were depressive disorder, which "may undermine normal recovery. . . by disrupting normal coping processes and use of informal support networks."

This argument is likely to be increasingly endorsed by the public opinion in the years to come, and it is therefore crucial for our profession to articulate a convincing response to the question "When does depression become a mental disorder?" In this paper, I will summarize three approaches to this issue, pointing out their weaknesses and the lessons we may take from each of them.

The first approach I will consider is the one proposed by Jerome Wakefield, emphasizing the context in which depressive symptoms occur. According to Wakefield

(1997), the diagnosis of depression should be "excluded if the sadness response is caused by a real loss that is proportional in magnitude to the intensity and duration of the response." It is useful to notice that this criterion of "proportionality" already appears in some other DSM-IV diagnostic categories (for instance, in the narrative description of generalized anxiety disorder, where it is stated that "the intensity, duration or frequency of the anxiety and worry is far out of proportion to the actual likelihood or impact of the feared event").

Wakefield's approach is certainly appealing to many clinicians and lay people, but has some important weaknesses.

First, it is well known that the presence itself of a depressive state may affect the individual's accuracy in reporting life events. It has been documented that the experimental induction of depressed mood can lead to a significant increase in reports of recent stressful events (Cohen and Winokur 1988). Actually, many depressed patients try to find a meaning in their depressive state, by attributing a significance to events which are in themselves neutral. Not surprisingly, Wakefield himself, in his Archives study based on a community sample, found that as many as 95% of depressive episodes were reported by the respondents to have been triggered by a life event (Wakefield et al. 2007).

Second, the presence of a depressive state may expose a person to adverse life events. In fact, the relationship between depression and so-called "dependent" events, i.e., events which can be interpreted as a consequence of the depressive state, such as being fired from a job or being left by a fiancé, is much stronger than the relationship between depression and other events (Williamson et al. 1995).

Third, whether an adverse life event has been really decisive in triggering a depressive state may be difficult to establish in several cases, and in any case will require a subjective judgment by the clinician, with a high risk for a low reliability. This is well known since the 1930s, when Sir Aubrey Lewis, testing a set of criteria aimed to distinguish between "contextual" and "endogenous" depression, concluded that most depressive cases were "examples of the interaction of organism and environment," so that "it was impossible to say which of the factors was decidedly preponderant" (Lewis 1934).

Fourth, the few studies which have compared definitely situational with definitely non-situational major depressive disorder, defined according to Research Diagnostic Criteria, reported that the two conditions were not different with respect to several demographic, clinical and psychosocial variables (Hirschfeld et al. 1985). Similarly, in a study comparing five groups of depressed patients differing by the level of psychosocial adversity experienced prior to the depressive episode, Kendler et al. (2010) found that the groups did not differ significantly on several clinical, historical and demographic variables.

Finally, the clinical utility of the distinction proposed by Wakefield in terms of prediction of treatment response appears very uncertain. Actually, currently available research evidence suggests that response to antidepressant medication in major depressive disorder is not related to whether or not the depressive state was preceded by a major life event (Andreson et al. 2000).

Further research is clearly needed to explore the applicability and reliability of the contextual exclusion criterion proposed by Wakefield, and its clinical utility for the prediction of treatment response and clinical outcome. However, at the present state of knowledge, it would be unwise to disallow the diagnosis of major depression, in a person meeting the current severity, duration and impairment criteria for that diagnosis, just because the depressive state occurs in the context of a significant life event (Maj 2008).

The second approach to our question "When does depression become a mental disorder?" is the one endorsed by several European psychopathologists, according to whom there is always a qualitative difference between true depression and normal sadness, a difference which has been lost in the recent process of oversimplification of psychopathology. The oversimplification, according to this approach, has occurred at two levels: at the level of individual phenomena, where the need for specific professional expertise to discriminate psychopathological manifestations from other expressions of impaired mental well-being has been de-emphasized, and at the level of syndromal description, where the fact that there is a *gestalt* of the depressive syndrome, beyond the sum of depressive symptoms, has been ignored (Helmchen and Linden 2000; van Praag 1998).

Within this approach, it has been maintained that "normal forms of negative mood, such as despair or sadness, must not be mistaken as depressed mood, characterized by a lack of holothymia and being an emotional feeling only known to depressed persons" (Helmchen and Linden 2000).

Indeed, the notion that depressed mood, at least in endogenous depression, is perceived by the patient as being qualitatively different from the feeling he/she would have following the death of a loved one, has a long tradition (e.g., Kiloh and Garside 1963). However, in which way the perception of depressed mood is actually different from the experience of ordinary sadness has not been clarified in the literature.

This issue has been addressed in some studies. A good example is a qualitative study by Healy (1993). In the first part of the study, a sample of depressed patients were asked to describe in their own words their current mood. "The commonest primary description was of the experience of lethargy and inability to do things, whether because of tiredness, a specific inability to summon up effort, a feeling of being inhibited or an inability to envisage the future." "The next most common description was of a sense of detachment from the environment." "The next most common descriptor was of physical changes that were described in terms of feeling that the subject was coming down with a viral illness, either influenza or glandular fever, along with descriptions of aches and pains and, in particular, headaches or numbness of the head or tight bands around the head." In the second part of the study, the patients were asked to select, from a list of adjectives, those best describing their current mood. The words from the list that were endorsed most frequently were as follows: dispirited, sluggish, wretched, empty, washed out, awful, dull, bothered, listless, tightened up, exhausted, gloomy, burdened. The author emphasizes that both the descriptions and the selected adjectives are different from those that people who are simply miserable or unhappy would be likely to offer spontaneously.

Along the same line, some studies carried out in patients with severe or chronic physical illness have described the differential features between true depression and "demoralization." According to Clarke and Kissane (2002), a depressed person has lost the ability to experience pleasure generally, whereas a demoralized person is able to experience pleasure when he/she is distracted from thoughts concerning the demoralizing event. The demoralized person feels inhibited in action by not knowing what to do, feeling helpless and incompetent; the depressed person has lost motivation and drive, and is unable to act even when an appropriate direction of action is known.

The fact is, however, that taxonic research on depression, based on Meehl's taxometric methods and latent class analysis (e.g., Ruscio and Ruscio 2000), has failed to support the idea that a latent qualitative difference exists between diagnosable depression and milder mood states, arguing instead in favor of a continuum of depressive states, but with the possible existence of a subtype, grossly corresponding to DSM-IV major depression with melancholia, which may be qualitatively different (Grove et al. 1987). It is possible, therefore, that the qualitative differences suggested by the earlier-mentioned studies apply to a subtype of depression rather than to major depressive disorder as a whole.

Further research is clearly needed to explore the nature of the subjective experience of depressed persons, and its differences with respect to the perception of ordinary sadness. A more precise characterization of the individual depressive symptoms is needed, as well as an exploration of the predictive value of each of them, and of clusters of them. Further studies on the validity and the clinical utility of the construct of melancholia are also warranted. For the time being, however, it would be hard to maintain that the difference between depression and ordinary sadness is always a qualitative one.

The third approach to our question ("When does depression become a mental disorder?") is the one championed by Kendell and Jablensky (2003), according to which, since "the variation between extensive, handicapping symptoms or pathology and an almost total absence of symptoms or pathology appears to be continuous... the boundary between normality and disorder has to be decided arbitrarily on pragmatic grounds." This is what the DSM-IV actually tries to achieve, regarding depression as a "disorder" when it reaches a given threshold in terms of severity, duration and degree of suffering or functional impairment, thus deserving clinical attention.

The problem is, however, that the threshold fixed by the DSM-IV for the diagnosis of major depression is not only arbitrary, but also not based on reasonably solid pragmatic grounds. In particular, the number of depressive symptoms required by the DSM-IV criteria does not have at the moment an acceptable empirical support. An increasing number of DSM-IV depressive symptoms has indeed been found to predict in a monotonic fashion a greater risk for future depressive episodes, a greater functional impairment, a higher physical comorbidity, and a more frequent parental history of mental disorders (Kessler et al. 1997) but, when a point of rarity was reported, it usually corresponded to a threshold higher than that fixed by the DSM-IV. For instance, Kendler and Gardner (1998) found that the risk for future depressive episodes was substantially greater in subjects with seven or more symptoms (odds ratio (OR)=6.50 and 13.26, respectively) than in those with 6 symptoms (OR=3.17), and

Klein (1990) reported that the risk for mood disorder and for hospitalized mood disorder was significantly higher in relatives of patients with six or more depressive symptoms than in both those with four or five symptoms and those with non-affective disorder.

The notion that the threshold fixed by the DSM-IV and its precursors may be too low is also supported by some research concerning prediction of response to pharmacological treatment.

Paykel et al. (1988) found that the superiority of amitriptyline over placebo was more substantial when the initial score on the 17-item Hamilton Rating Scale for Depression (HRSD-17) was 16–24, less substantial when it was 13–15, and non-significant when it was 6–12. The authors reported that 13% of patients with RDC major depression were among those with an HRSD-17 score 6–12, while 34% had a score of 13–15. So, almost one half of the patients with a diagnosis of major depression were in the groups showing a non-significant or "less substantial" response. Similarly, Elkin et al. (1989) found that, among patients with an RDC diagnosis of major depressive disorder, those with an initial score of less than 20 on the HRSD-17 (who were more than 60% of the sample) did not recover more frequently with imipramine than with placebo plus clinical management, whereas patients with an initial score of 20 or more did significantly better.

On the other hand, it has been repeatedly reported that the psychosocial impairment associated with the presence of two to four depressive symptoms is comparable to that associated with the presence of five or more symptoms (e.g., Broadhead et al. 1990). Furthermore, Thase (2003) reported a point of rarity between depressed patients seeking outpatient care and age-matched healthy controls corresponding to an HRSD-17 score of 7–10 (which is likely to be lower than that the threshold fixed by the DSM-IV). A score of 7 was at least three standard deviation units below the mean, which conveyed a probability of more than 99% not to be depressed.

These findings clearly require replication, but seem to suggest that more than one threshold may be needed in the characterization of depressive states, in order to maximize clinical utility. These thresholds may need to be based on the overall severity of depressive symptoms rather than, or in addition to, their number. This may, however, generate a tension between the need to use a validated rating scale and the feasibility of its use in ordinary clinical practice.

Overall, there are lessons to be taken from each of these approaches.

The lesson we can take from Wakefield's approach is that the contextualization of a depressive state is important, if not in the diagnosis of depression, at least in the subsequent stage of clinical characterization of the individual case, which is the one that guides the choice of treatment. In particular, the decision whether to implement a psychotherapy and the choice of the type of psychotherapy should be based on this contextualization of the depressive state rather than on the clinician's theoretical orientation.

The lesson which can be taken from the second approach is that we need a more in-depth exploration of the subjective experience of depressed persons and of its differences with respect to the perception of ordinary sadness. We may need a more precise description of individual depressive symptoms (the glossary of terms which appears as an appendix in the DSM-IV appears insufficient in this respect). The individual depressive symptoms, and clusters of them, should be weighed with respect to their predictive value, especially concerning clinical outcome and treatment response. In addition, the validity and clinical utility of the construct of melancholia should be further explored. Even if melancholia is not a distinct disease entity but just an expression of the most severe degree of depression, it may be associated with the recruitment of further cerebral structures or circuits in addition to those involved in non-melancholic depression. The issue of whether the presence of melancholia has a predictive value in terms of treatment response remains controversial and requires further investigation in larger samples.

The lesson we can take from the third approach is that our clinical practice and our research on depression should be informed by the currently predominant evidence of the existence of a continuum of depressive states. Depression should not be conceptualized and presented as an all-or-none disease, and biological research based on that assumption is probably bound to fail. The threshold for a depressive state requiring clinical attention may be lower than that fixed by the DSM-IV, but the threshold for a depressive state requiring pharmacological treatment is likely to be higher. This explains, along with the increasing difficulty in recruiting severely depressed patients for clinical trials, why the efficacy gap between antidepressants and placebo is found today to be much narrower than some decades ago.

In conclusion, of the three approaches to the issue "When does depression become a mental disorder?" considered in this paper, the first two, which are probably more appealing and easier to explain to patients, families, students, residents, journalists and the general public, are not supported by currently available research evidence, whereas the third, which is certainly more difficult to explain to lay people, has at the moment some empirical support. In interacting with lay people, we may use the analogy between depression and some common physical diseases such as hypertension and diabetes, which also occur on a continuum, with the possibility to identify two thresholds: one for a condition deserving clinical attention and one for a state requiring pharmacological treatment. The counterargument will be that in the case of those diseases the continuum is delineated on the basis of objective measurements, while in the case of depression it is mostly based on subjective judgments. What is much worse, however, is that we have to acknowledge that the only threshold along the continuum fixed by our most influential diagnostic system does not have a solid empirical basis. This is a very sensitive issue, which has to be addressed urgently. The more the question of the distinction between depression and ordinary sadness appears to be loaded with philosophical, ethical, social and political—in addition to clinical and scientific—implications, the more it requires a truly convincing and unequivocal research evidence.

Chapter References

American Psychiatric Association (1994). *Diagnostic and Statistical Manual of Mental Disorders* (4th ed.). Washington, DC: American Psychiatric Association.

Anderson, I. M., Nutt, D. J., Deakin, J. F. W., on behalf of the Consensus Meeting and endorsed by the British Association for Psychopharmacology (2000). Evidence-based guidelines for treating depressive disorders with antidepressants: a revision of the 1993 British Association for Psychopharmacology guidelines. *Journal of Psychopharmacology*, **14**, 3–20.

Broadhead, W. E., Blazer, D. G., George, L. K. andTse, C. K. (1990). Depression, disability days, and days lost from work in a prospective epidemiologic survey. *Journal of the American Medical Association*, **264**, 2524–8.

Clarke, D.M. and Kissane, D.W. (2002). Demoralization: its phenomenology and importance. *Australian and New Zealand Journal of Psychiatry*, **36**, 733–42.

Cohen, M.R. and Winokur, G. (1988). The clinical classification of depressive disorders. In: J. J. Mann (ed), *Phenomenology of Depressive Illness*. New York: Human Sciences Press, pp. 75–96.

Elkin, I., Shea, T., Watkins, J. T., Imber, S. D., Sotsky, S. M., Collins, J. F., *et al.* (1989). National Institute of Mental Health Treatment of Depression Collaborative Research Program. General effectiveness of treatments. *Archives of General Psychiatry*, **46**, 971–82.

Grove, W.M., Andreasen, N.C., Young, M. Endicott, J., Keller, M. B., Hirschfeld, R. M., *et al.* (1987). Isolation and characterization of a nuclear depressive syndrome. *Psychological Medicine*, **17**, 471–84.

Healy, D. (1993). Dysphoria. In C. G. Costello (ed). *Symptoms of Depression*. New York: Wiley, 23–42.

Helmchen, H. and Linden, M. (2000). Subthreshold disorders in psychiatry: clinical reality, methodological artifact, and the double-threshold problem. *Comprehensive Psychiatry*, **41**(Suppl. 1), 1–7.

Hirschfeld, R. M. A., Klerman, G. L., Andreasen, N. C., Clayton, P. J., and Keller, M. B. (1985) Situational major depressive disorder. *Archives of General Psychiatry*, **42**, 1109–14.

Horwitz, A. V. and Wakefield, J. C. (2007). *The Loss of Sadness. How Psychiatry Transformed Normal Sorrow into Depressive Disorder*. Oxford: Oxford University Press.

Kendell, R. and Jablensky, A. (2003). Distinguishing between the validity and utility of psychiatric diagnoses. *American Journal of Psychiatry*, **160**, 4–12.

Kendler, K.S. and Gardner, C.O., Jr. (1998). Boundaries of major depression: an evaluation of DSM-IV criteria. *American Journal of Psychiatry*, **155**, 172–7.

Kendler, K. S., Myers, J. and Halberstadt, L. J. (2010). Should the diagnosis of major depression be made independent of or dependent upon the psychosocial context? *Psychological Medicine*, **40**, 771–80.

Kessler, R. C., Zhao, S., Blazer, D. G. and Swartz, M. (1997). Prevalence, correlates, and course of minor depression and major depression in the National Comorbidity Survey. *Journal of Affective Disorders*, **45**, 19–30.

Kiloh, L. G. and Garside, R. F. (1963). The independence of neurotic depression and endogenous depression. *British Journal of Psychiatry*, **109**, 451–63.

Klein, D. N. (1990) Symptom criteria and family history in major depression. *American Journal of Psychiatry*, **147**, 850–854.

Kutchins, H. and Kirk, S. A. (1997). *Making Us Crazy. DSM: the Psychiatric Bible and the Creation of Mental Disorders*. New York: Free Press.

Lewis, A. (1934). Melancholia: a clinical survey of depressive states. *Journal of Mental Sciences*, **80**, 277–378.

Maj, M. (2008). Depression, bereavement, and "understandable" intense sadness: should the DSM-IV approach be revised? *American Journal of Psychiatry*, **165**, 1373–5.

Murray, C. J. and Lopez, A. D. (1996). *The Global Burden of Disease*. Geneva: World Health Organization, Harvard School of Public Health, World Bank.

Paykel, E. S., Hollyman, J. A., Freeling, P. and Sedwick, P. (1988). Predictors of therapeutic benefit from amitriptyline in mild depression: a general practice placebo-controlled trial. *Journal of Affective Disorders*, **14**, 83–95.

Regier, D. A., Kaelber, C. T., Rae, D. S., Farmer, M. E., Knauper, B., Kessler, R. C., *et al.* (1998). Limitations of diagnostic criteria and assessment instruments for mental disorders: implications for research and policy. *Archives of General Psychiatry*, **55**, 109–115.

Ruscio, J. and Ruscio, A. M. (2000). Informing the continuity controversy: a taxometric analysis of depression. *Journal of Abnormal Psychology*, **109**, 473–87.

Thase, M. E. (2003). Evaluating antidepressant therapies: remission as the optical outcome. *Journal of Clinical Psychiatry*, **64**(Suppl. 13), 18–25.

van Praag, H. M. (1998). The diagnosis of depression in disorder. *Australian and New Zealand Journal of Psychiatry*, **32**, 767–72.

Wakefield, J. C. (1997). Diagnosing DSM-IV. 1. DSM-IV and the concept of disorder. *Behavioral Research Therapy*, **35**, 633–49.

Wakefield, J. C., Schmitz, M. F., First, M. B., and Horwitz, A. V. (2007). Extending the bereavement exclusion for major depression to other losses: evidence from the National Comorbidity Survey. *Archives of General Psychiatry*, **64**, 433–40.

Williamson, D. E., Birmaher, B., Anderson, B. P., Al-Shabbout, M. and Ryan, N. D. (1995) Stressful life events in depressed adolescents: the role of dependent events during the depressive episode. *Journal of the Academy of Child and Adolescent Psychiatry*, **34**, 591–8.

A sea of distress

Josef Parnas

Depression is declared by the WHO as the most burdensome mental disorder. Maj's chapter touches therefore upon the issue of immense societal importance. In this commentary, I will focus on: (1) the borders of depression, i.e., primarily, on a dividing line, if such exists, between affective and bipolar disorders on the one hand, and the schizophrenic spectrum disorders, on the other, and (2) the issue of heterogeneity of depression versus the "true" depression. This second section will touch upon the question of melancholic depression as a paradigmatic true depression.

11.1 **Affective disorders and the schizophrenia spectrum**

In the Introduction to Regier, Kenneth Kendler (Chapter 14, this volume) recalls his first encounter with the structured interviewing with the aid of SADS-L (Schedule for Affective Disorders and Schizophrenia-Lifetime). SADS-L was also my first exposure to structured interviewing, as a member of a small group of research assistants who, after completing residency, were being trained for the US-DK adoption- and High-Risk-studies. We were surprised by the finding that many patients with fairly typical schizophrenia apparently also suffered from a "major depressive" episode and, following the SADS-L/Research Diagnostic Criteria (RDC) diagnostic algorithm were "schizoaffective" (the SADS-L's opening section contains a list of depressive symptoms). Years later, I participated in an international workshop, scheduled to discuss which psychiatric interview to use in epidemiological and genetic research. We were shown two different, video-taped structured interviews with the same patient, a middle-aged lady with a monotonously vigilant attitude, wearing dark glasses, and spontaneously complaining of a distressing cognitive predicament: each time she was thinking a thought in the "right side of the brain," a "counter-thought" arose "in the left side," preventing her from concluding the train of thoughts, let alone take any decision. During the diagnostic and technical discussion (schizophrenia or affective illness?) nobody mentioned (or dared to mention; personally, I did not want to appear old-fashioned) ambivalence, experiential concreteness and the disorders of rapport. Anyhow, there was no place to score these features in either interview schedule.

We have known for some time that depressive symptoms and syndromes are very frequent in schizophrenia (Conrad 1958; Häffner et al. 2005; Jäger et al. 2008) and that excluding diagnosis of schizophrenia on the basis of a history of a prior depressive episode is not warranted by empirical data.

Moreover, for some years now we have witnessed a vigorous revival of "Unitary Psychosis." This idea is typically supported by "dimensionality" in symptomatic transitions, findings of shared genetic markers and some similarities in the neurocognitive profiles. Yet, as Lawrie et al. (2010) notes, this unitary proposal is quite vaguely articulated. One can add that the psychopathological distinction between schizophrenia and affective illness (including bipolar) should be ideally linked to the considerations on the "whatness" of these disorders (see Parnas, Chapter 12, this volume), which include a bottom-up reconstruction of the illness history (see McHugh, Chapter 13, this volume), rather than relying predominantly on checklist scores on affective, positive and negative symptoms. Consider these two contrastively constructed cases:

A. Bipolar disorder. 40 years old, married man, owner of a successful business, energetic, efficient, sociable, outgoing, history of two severe manic episodes, one necessitating involuntary admission. Prophylactic lithium treatment.

B. Schizophrenia spectrum. 40 years old, single and living alone, unemployed man, who always had a sense of confinement to the interiority of his mind, a diminished sense of bodily self-presence, feeling profoundly different from other people, unable to reach out to others and become immersed, isolated, spending his time visiting para-psychological websites. Three past hospitalizations with a paranoid-hallucinatory condition. On continuous antipsychotic medication.

Does it make sense to claim that these two patients suffer from *the same* disorder because there is some genetic vulnerability overlap? No, I think, rather, that this scenario emphasizes the fact that the ontology of the psychiatric object (i.e., the patient's experience and existence) plays a foundational role in any sensical psychiatric classification (see Bolton, Chapter 1, this volume).

11.2 **Heterogeneity and searching for the true depression**

The vast majority of psychiatric patients are not happy and that applies also to a substantial proportion of general population, familiar with antidepressant medication. The prevalence and heterogeneity problems in depression research and treatment are reflected in the findings of temporal instability of depression across relapses (Mann 2010; see also other comments in this issue of the journal). Such instability was, e.g., found across prospective, temporally fixed follow-ups, utilizing Hamilton Depression Scale scores, mathematically derived factors, and scores on the individual scale items (Oquendo et al. 2004).

One important quandary of the entire research field stems from the very polysemic nature of the word "depression." This is a lay and medical expression, signifying, by and large, some sort of distress and ill-being, not limited to negative affect or mood. Unfortunately, the question of "what it is like to be depressed" is insufficiently answered in the contemporary textbooks and diagnostic manuals. It is no longer studied and existing sources are gone into oblivion.[1] The problem can be illustrated very simply. When a patient says "I feel depressed, sad, or down," such a statement may signify, if further explored, a bewildering variety and range of experiences (apart from depressed mood): feelings of emptiness, loss of meaning, poverty of ideation, varieties of fatigue and inactivity, ambivalence, painful ruminations (of different kinds), irritation, anger, hyper-reflectivity, thought pressure, anhedonia, apathy, devitalization, constant psychic anxiety, varieties of depersonalization, etc. The list is almost infinite. It requires some interviewing effort to enucleate the salient profile of the presented distress. It is therefore unlikely that a checklist of depressive features has an adequate potential to clarify the matter. *There is no other way than to talk to the patient* and illuminate his experience in its context of other experiences, expressions, behaviors and developmental historical aspects. As McHugh advocates, such interview should include: "(1) an extensive personal background history from birth to presentation, (2) a thorough description of the onset and progress of the presenting illness or disorder, (3) a complete mental status examination as the patient first appeared to the psychiatrist, and, whenever possible, (4) inquiry with 'external informants' who knew the patient and could provide contexts and continuities enriching what the distressed patient could report" (McHugh, Chapter 13, this volume).

Unless we are prepared to call the entire sea of unhappiness, a "depression" (mood disorder), we still need, what was once called a differential diagnosis, perhaps in addition to more specific diagnostic criteria.

Here, it is appropriate to address briefly what the concept of mood signifies. We are always in a mood, a pervasive, pre-reflective and passively lived dimension of our being in the world. In other words, mood is not only an "inner mental state" but is an affective tonality that colors both the world and the experiencing subject, e.g., the world as a stage of possibilities or, on the contrary, as something blocked and inaccessible (the DSM-IV emphasizes the pervasiveness of mood and its specific coloring of perception). This existential significance of mood is sometimes called with terms "situatedness" or "attunement" (in German, Befindlichkeit and Stimmung). Mood is intimately linked to our self-temporalization. Mood is not an *isolated mental object*, easily dissociated from its experiential context and identified in an act of introspection (i.e., converted to a reportable symptom). It is, so to say, a pre-given and pre-reflective manner of our experiencing (Gallagher and Zahavi, 2008; Tallon, 1997).[2] We *are* mood rather than we *have* mood. This pre-reflective pervasive nature of mood is, of course, one source of diagnostic difficulties. We cannot completely dissociate a pure mood from cognitions, feelings, and behaviors. Therefore, the effort to grasp the patient's mood includes an assessment of his world experience, feelings, cognitive processes, their contents, and, not least the temporal aspects of the experience (e.g., inhibition and psychomotor retardation are not identical concepts). In a typical, melancholic depression, the dominating, pervasive painful experience is that of "not being able to. . ." (von Gebsattel 1938; Tellenbach, 1980). As a central complaint there is a sense of *despair* rather than of *hopelessness* (however, the latter is listed in the diagnostic manuals). Hopelessness is a painful conviction that there is no hope left. Despair is an active, ongoing *struggle*: the faults should be corrected but there is no possible way to cope or escape. The sometimes present "omega-sign" (like the Greek letter Ω), a characteristic fold in the forehead just above the root of the nose, expresses this ongoing struggle of despair. I will abstain from further description, but only add that a "typical" or "true" depression exhibits a certain phenomenological *coherence*. You do not, for example, encounter a patient, reproaching himself for stealing at the age of 8, $5 from his father (and claiming that this theft has irreparable, though unclear, consequences) but, who, at the same time, is manipulative and blaming others. This notion of coherence also points to the inherent limitations of a checklist-based diagnostic approach.

Maj's very wise proposal of more descriptive research in depression is nonetheless difficult to reconcile with the prevailing epistemological position. The structured interviews are gold standard, data collections are performed by multiple checklists targeting multiple domains, and the insight into the investigated matter is solely expected to emerge from the statistical analyses of the checklist data. When Max Hamilton created his severity of depression scale (HDS), he emphasized its primary goal, which was *a detection of change* in the quantitative scale score under treatment of a patient, who, in advance (already), was *clinically diagnosed with depression*. Today, we have diagnostic criteria nearly isomorphic with HDS items and diagnostic practices where the HDS items are used for a quick diagnosis. Perhaps, the epistemological problems have a major share in the apparent heterogeneity and confusion which beset the issue of major depression.

It is also worrisome, because likely, that a further, reliability-driven simplification of psychopathology (diminished number and complexity of symptoms and signs *legalized to exist* by, and in, the diagnostic systems) will inevitably contribute to blurring the borders between the categories, compromise empirical research, and, in the long run, lead to eliminativist psychiatry, i.e., a psychiatry without psyche.

Endnotes

1 There is an obvious possibility of historic-cultural influences at the level of the *content*, e.g., the contemporary Western culture is certainly less guilt-ridden than its closest predecessors.
2 Tallon's (1997) book is an excellent, terminologically clear, and easily readable introduction to the phenomenology of emotion, feeling, and mood. It provides very helpful and important conceptual distinctions.

Chapter References

Conrad, K. (1958). *Die beginnende Schizophrenie. Versuch einer Gestaltanalyse des Wahns.* Stuttgart: Thieme.

Gallagher, S. and Zahavi, D. (2008). *The Phenomenological Mind: Introduction to Phenomenology and Cognitive Science.* New York: Routledge.

Häfner, H., Maurer, K., Trendler, G., Schmidt, M. and Konnecke, R. (2005). Schizophrenia and depression: challenging the paradigm of two separate diseases a controlled study of schizophrenia, depression and healthy controls. *Schizophrenia Research*, **77**, 11–24.

Jäger, M., Riedel, M., Schmauss, M., Pfeiffer, H., Laux, G., Naber, D., *et al.* (2008). Depression during an acute episode of schizophrenia or schizophreniform disorder and its impact on treatment response. *Psychiatry Research*, **158**, 297–305.

Lawrie, M. S., Hall, J., McIntosh, A. M., and Owens, D. G. C. (2010). The "continuum of psychosis": scientifically unproven and clinically impractical. *British Journal of Psychiatry*, **197**, 423–5.

Mann, J. J. (2010). Clinical pleomorphism of major depression as a challenge to study of its pathophysiology. *World Psychiatry*, **9**(3), 167–8.

Oquendo, M. A., Barrera, A., Stevens, P. E., Li, S., Burke, A. K., Grunebaum, M., *et al.* (2004). Instability of symptoms in recurrent major depression: A prospective study. *American Journal of Psychiatry*, **161**, 255–61.

Tallon, A. (1997). *Head and Heart. Affection, Cognition, Volition as Triune Consciousness.* New York: Fordham University Press.

Tellenbach, H. (1980). *Melancholy.* Pittsburgh, PA: Duquesne University Press.

von Gebsattel, V. E. (1939). Die Störungen des Werdens und des Zeiterlebens im Rahmen psychiatrischer Erkrankungen. In Roggenbau C. (ed.), *Gegenwartsprobleme der psychiatrisch-neurologischen Forschung, Ferdinand Enke.* Stuttgart: Verlag, pp. 54–71.

Chapter 12

Introduction

Assen Jablensky

This chapter grasps the reader's attention from its first page. It is a rich, scholarly discourse on the nature of schizophrenia, anchored in the tradition and conceptual apparatus of psychiatric phenomenology, now sorely missing in "mainstream" classifications, teaching and clinical practice. The phenomenological school of thought, broadly exemplified in the contributions of Jaspers, Gruhle, Berze, Minkowski and many others, regarded schizophrenia as a prototypical disorder of the structure of conscious experience that could only be understood as a *gestalt*, a fundamental whole which is only partly revealed in its individual symptoms and signs. In his article "Patterns of mental disorders" (*Die Erscheinungsformen des Irreseins*), Kraepelin (1920/1974) acknowledged that "the affective and schizophrenic forms of mental disorder do not represent the expression of particular pathological processes, but rather indicate the areas of our personality in which these processes unfold. . . it is conceivable that these two illnesses may. . . at times spread beyond the framework of their usual syndromes." Similarly, Bleuler based his construct of "the schizophrenias" on profound and complex disturbances of thought, affect and will, resulting in autistic dereism. Finally, Parnas points out that this perspective on the "whatness" (*quiddity*) of schizophrenia was retained in the ICD-8 Glossary of Mental Disorders (1974) which referred to a "disturbance involving the most basic functions that give the normal person a feeling of individuality, uniqueness, and self-direction" (text originally drafted, on behalf of the World Health Organization (WHO), by Sir Aubrey Lewis). This perspective has faded away in subsequent revisions of ICD, and has never penetrated DSM.

A good deal of the chapter focuses on Schneider's first-rank symptoms (FRS) which have been given particular (and possibly undue) prominence in the DSM-IV diagnostic criteria and the ICD-10 diagnostic guidelines (Jablensky 2010). Parnas's main point is that the FRS have been taken out of their original context, presented in an abridged format, and misinterpreted. While Schneider referred to the *experience* of thought insertion, or *experience* of replacement of will as *primary* and irreducible psychopathological phenomena, these symptoms are presented in DSM-IV as interpretative *delusions* of thought insertion or passivity—i.e., as errors of judgment.

In contrast, Parnas highlights the importance of primary delusions, subjective thought disorder (audible thoughts, thought broadcast, insertion and echo) and passivity experiences as pointers to the same fundamental, qualitative alteration of the structure of experiencing that was regarded as the hallmark of schizophrenia in

European psychiatry. Other important points in his discussion concern (1) the "comorbidity" issue in DSM-IV, which results from the inherent "atomization" of psychopathology and affects the placement of depressive, obsessive–compulsive, and anxiety symptoms in the diagnostic category of schizophrenia; and (2) the simplistic split of symptomatology into "positive," "negative" and "disorganized" symptoms. The bottom line of all this is that the "first-person" perspective on the core phenomena of schizophrenia is being lost, replaced by a "third-person" stance where core symptoms are regarded as "things" out there, or attributes unrelated to the unity of the person's wholeness which is retained even in schizophrenia as a deviant (and painful) "mode of being" in a shared world. While the "third person" perspective may work well in somatic medicine, psychiatry needs to assert its legitimate concern with the private worlds of patients. This should not be interpreted as opening the way to idiosyncratic, subjective interpretations based on uncontrolled "empathy" but rather as being anchored in the general rules of the phenomenological method, lucidly outlined in Jaspers's magisterial opus.

Parnas appeals for a reinstatement of the gestalt approach to the clinical evaluation and the scientific study of schizophrenia, "because the fundamental phenotypes of schizophrenia—the starting point of all research—are seriously distorted." But research today is heavily dependent on our ability to operationalize and quantify the units of analysis. The limited success, so far, of genome-wide association studies, suggests that a fallible phenotype may be largely responsible. How exactly can the gestalt understanding of schizophrenia, based on a phenomenological exploration of the patients' inner worlds, be adequately operationalized to yield quantifiable, real-world phenotypes? This question remains unanswered, but in the wake of the forthcoming revisions of DSM and ICD it attains some urgency.

Everything being said, Parnas's chapter, offering as he states an "anachronistic and anarchic" point of view on the current conceptualization of schizophrenia, merits deep thought and attention.

Introduction References

Jablensky, A. (2010). The diagnostic concept of schizophrenia: its history, evolution, and future prospects. *Dialogues Clin Neurosci*, **12**, 271–87.

Kraepelin, E. (1920/1974). Die Erscheinungsformen des Irreseins. *Zeitschrift für die gesammte Neurologie und Psychiatrie*, **62**, 1–29. English translation by H. Marshall (1974). Patterns of mental disorder. In S. R. Hirsch and M. Shepherd (eds.), *Themes and Variations in European Psychiatry*. Bristol: John Wright & Sons, pp. 7–30.

Chapter 12

DSM-IV and the founding prototype of schizophrenia: are we regressing to a pre-Kraepelinian nosology?

Josef Parnas

12.1 **Introduction**

This contribution will be both anachronistic and anarchic. Anachronistic, because it will seriously take up Bolton's (Chapter 1, this volume) emphasis on the constitutive dimension of distress for psychiatric classification, and the equally fundamental remark of Berrios (Chapter 6, this volume), that the conceptualization of the "psychiatric object" (symptoms and signs) remains today the most challenging task confronting psychiatric nosology. The anachronistic element will be visible through an appeal to a phenomenological perspective as the most adequate for addressing the concerns of Bolton, Berrios and others. It is a perspective where a psychiatrist, through a conversation with her patient, explores, conceptualizes and grasps the patient's experience ("inner life"), not only in its content but its structure as well (Parnas and Zahavi 2002). This (mainly) European perspective is now almost forgotten in the Anglophone world (if it had ever been voiced), and if occasionally remembered, then either as a superfluous or no longer necessary detour on psychiatry's path to scientific fulfillment. It is also an anarchic essay, not only because of its unorthodox appeal to phenomenology, but also due to a rather skeptical view of a widespread, mainstream representation of a formidable progress of psychiatric nosology over the last 30 years, and equally critical of the mainstream epistemology.

This essay compares the concept of schizophrenia described in the DSM-IV-TR (APA 2000) with the continental European concept from 1974—described in the glossary of ICD-8 (which later served as a template for the DSM-III) (WHO 1974). This prototype may be seen as a zenith achievement of psychopathologic research in Europe, providing the basis for the first major scientific achievements in the study of schizophrenia, e.g., the foundational Scandinavian epidemiological studies, the US-DK Adoption studies, the US-DK High-Risk studies, and the WHO's International Pilot Studies of Schizophrenia (Bøjholm and Strömgren 1989; Jablensky and Sartorius 2008; Kety 1988; Mednick et al. 1987).

The transition to DSM-IV entailed important modifications. First, it reduced its utility for diagnosing non-paranoid schizophrenia (hebephrenia). Second, in the process of operational transformation, the very gestalt or *prototype* of *what schizophre-nia is*, has vanished, suffering from a progressive oblivion.

We will first deal with the question of DSM-IV's affinity to the Schneiderian concept of schizophrenia. This issue will be examined in some detail, especially the phenomenological features which are *omitted* in the DSM. This will be followed by presenting the phenomenology of the core gestalt of schizophrenia, as it was conceived of in the European prototype, and its prime embodiment in the form of hebephrenia (non-paranoid schizophrenia). I will end by briefly addressing the epistemological/metaphysical underpinning of the "operational revolution," an aspect which is necessary to illuminate in order to assess the potential nosological gains brought forth by the contemporary diagnostic systems. These crucial clinical and conceptual issues are unaddressed in the recent reviews (Tandon et al. 2009; Van Os 2010).[1]

12.2 **The DSM-IV-TR criteria of schizophrenia**

The formation of DSM-III and its subsequent editions (-R, -IV,-IV-TR; APA 1980–2000) have been mainly inspired by the concerns of reliability (First, Chapter 7; Pincus, Chapter 8, this volume). This process did not only affect the criteria *retained* as diagnostic, but, importantly, the features that were *omitted* from the diagnostic concept, and ultimately forgotten. The DSM is not only a diagnostic manual. In fact, the diagnostic criteria and their epistemological assumptions have monopolized the entire descriptive and conceptual universe of psychopathology, including its language and institutions.[2] Symptoms outside the diagnostic boxes went into oblivion, with dramatic consequences for the general level of psychopathological competence and scholarship. A prominent, original advocate of operationalism and biological reductionism, describes in the hindsight these consequences:

> Because DSM is often used as a primary textbook or the major diagnostic resource in many clinical and research settings, students typically do not know about other potentially important or interesting signs and symptoms that are not included in DSM. Second, DSM has had a dehumanizing impact on the practice of psychiatry. History taking – the central evaluation tool in psychiatry – has frequently been reduced to the use of DSM checklists. DSM discourages clinicians from getting to know the patient as an individual person (. . .). Third, validity has been sacrificed to achieve reliability. DSM diagnoses have given researchers a common nomenclature – but probably *the wrong one* (Andreasen 2007).

The wording of DSM-IV, including its 'Glossary of Technical Terms', is very carefully crafted, with an impressive paucity of descriptive content, probably motivated by a desire to present a medical, "scientific" air, while simultaneously reducing potential exposure to criticism (there is not much to criticize). It is consistently written in a lay language, making it readable to non-specialists.

The DSM-IV-TR (APA 2000) defines schizophrenia in the following way in: "The essential features of schizophrenia are a mixture of characteristic (. . .) positive and negative [symptoms] that have been present for a significant portion of time (. . .), associated with marked social and occupational dysfunction. The disturbance is *not better accounted for by*. . .(exclusion criteria; italics added)." Thus, the DSM does not offer any general account of *what schizophrenia is* but rather what it is not (non-organic, non-affective etc.) (Maj 1998; Maj, Chapter 8, this volume, commentary on Pincus). The issue taken up by Maj is that of "whatness" (quiddity). It refers to the properties that a particular category (e.g., a person) shares with others of its kind. Posing such a question, however, does not presuppose any commitment to realism about natural kinds. "What (quid) is it?" simply asks for a general description by way of commonality. Questioning *what schizophrenia is*, implies that schizophrenia displays a characteristic gestalt, a certain *typicality* or proto-typicality, which we need to be familiar with when performing a (differential and early) diagnosis or in studying schizophrenia's extra-clinical associations.

It seems that the DSM-IV criteria favor a *chronic* paranoid schizophrenia marked by prominent delusions or hallucinations, with a pathognomonic status of certain Schneiderian first-rank symptoms. This emphasis on Schneiderian symptoms is usually understood as reflecting a turn from Bleuler–Kraepelin to Schneider. Schneider himself is frequently portrayed as a forerunner of a reliable diagnosis, a sort of a pioneer operationalist (Nordgaard et al. 2008). We will therefore examine this issue more closely.

12.3 **Kurt Schneider on schizophrenia**

Schneider was a phenomenologically oriented professor of psychiatry in Heidelberg.[3] He had regular exchanges with psychiatrist (and later, an acclaimed philosopher) Karl Jaspers. The majority of Jaspers's (1963) distinctions are incorporated in Schneider's (1950/1959) *Clinical Psychopathology*, one of two major texts of Schneider available in English translation. The first draft of this text, describing the (later) so-called "first-rank" symptoms, was published in a journal for medical practitioners in 1939. Schneider described here certain characteristic *symptoms of schizophrenia*, which he claimed were easier for the clinicians to identify than the more difficult and ephemeral Bleulerian "fundamental" symptoms. It should be noted that these "Schneiderian" symptoms were all familiar to the student of psychiatry from the second half of the 19th century. We find their descriptions in Kraepelin, Bleuler and countless other authors. However, their explicit listing for the diagnostic purposes was new. Schneider claimed that these symptoms were pathognomonic of schizophrenia. Yet, it is important to realize that Schneider would never have accepted something remotely resembling contemporary methodological behaviorism in psychiatry (e.g., with structured interviews done by non-clinicians). Like the majority of German psychiatrists, he advocated phenomenology, "the methods of clinical interview . . . [that] were established decades ago by Karl Jaspers" as a descriptive and conceptual tool in psychiatry, "possible for an ordinary clinician."

Schneider was not a reductionist but held a phenomenological view of a certain gestalt of interrelated elements that was characteristic of schizophrenia:

> Schizophrenia always involves an *overall change*... individual phenomena have only a limited diagnostic claim. . . . A psychotic symptom is not like a defective stone in an otherwise perfect mosaic. *Psychotic individuals are as much closed microcosms as normal persons* (Schneider 1950/1959, p. 95).

The specificity of certain of the first-rank symptoms (FRS) was to be sought in the structural changes of self-consciousness (to which we will return later):

> Among the basic characteristics of experience, certain disturbances of self-experience show the *greatest degree of schizophrenic specificity*. Here we refer to those disturbances of *first-personal-givenness* (Ich-heit) or *mineness* (Meinhaftigkeit) which consist of one's own acts and states not being experienced as one's own … (Schneider 1950/1959, p. 58)

Ichheit and Meinhaftigkeit have roots in the philosophical phenomenology. "Mineness" (or "for-me-ness") is not something that one instigates; it is simply an automatically given *structural aspect of all experience*. All experience is given to me as mine, as an experience "for me" (in the first person perspective). Schneider and other seminal psychiatrists (Berze 1914; Blankenburg 1971; Gruhle 1929; Kronfeld 1922; Minkowski 1926, 1927), considered instability of the sense of "mineness" of experience as a severe abnormality in the structure of self-awareness, essential and diagnostic of schizophrenia.

In the European concept of schizophrenia (e.g., ICD-8), the FRS were considered as one possible, *non-pathognomonic*, psychotic manifestation of the disorder, as being *complementary* rather than *alternative* to the relational and expressive disorders, originally emphasized by Bleuler and Kraepelin ("fundamental" symptoms).

12.4 First-rank symptoms: Schneider and DSM-IV-TR

The number of features enumerated by Schneider as being of first rank is larger than in the DSM-IV (Table 12.1) and they are differently described. It is important to note that Schneider considered all FRS as being of a diagnostic first rank, *only on the condition* of a preservation of clear or *lucid* consciousness (Besonnenheit; composure), i.e., excluding patients with impaired consciousness due to organic causes or acute, severely agitated conditions with pronounced *affective turbulence*, anger, agitation, panic or

Table 12.1 Schneider's list of first-rank symptoms and their counterparts in the DSM-IV-TR

Primary delusions, especially but not only, in the mode of perception	
Audible thoughts (echo phenomena)	
Loss of the sense of privacy: thought diffusion	
Experience of thought block, thought insertion, thought deprivation	*Delusion* of thought insertion
	Delusion of thought deprivation
Other passivity *experiences*	*Delusion* of external control
in the domain of thought, body, movement, feeling, impulse, volition	
Voices conversing	Voices conversing
Voices as commentary to ongoing activity	Voices as commentary to ongoing activity

with markedly elevated, ecstatic mood (Sigmund and Mundt 1999). In the DSM and ICD-10, there is no reference to Besonnenheit or considerations on the status of FRS in acutely disturbed consciousness. This lacuna is perhaps partly responsible for the disputes about the specificity of FRS for schizophrenia (see Nordgaard et al. 2008).

Primary delusions

Primary delusion is a characteristic mode of experience—in which the content of any experience, e.g., an occurrent perception, thought, imagination or recollection— articulates or unfolds a delusional significance in a direct, un-mediated way. "Immediately" is the word used in the English translation of Jaspers (1963), but the original adjective in German is "unmittelbar," i.e., not only temporally instantaneous, but entailing a *modal sense* as well, i.e., in *a direct way, non-mediated by reflection or inference.* The delusional meaning, e.g., in a percept, articulates itself in the perceptual content like a revelation, formally similar to a strong esthetic experience (Blankenburg 1965).

> A patient walking up the staircase to his psychiatrist's office, noticed through a window, a canvas with intense blue color, among some furniture stabled in the yard. Seeing the painting with its blue color, the patient became aware of being insane [an example of empirically true delusion] (Blankenburg 1965).

This characteristic, *primary*, articulation of delusional meaning is not empathically understandable, because it is not mediated by inferential reflection that the psychiatrist can simulate in his own mind. Primary delusion is thus not an inferential or empirical error, a mistaken view of reality. It is *primary* in the developmental or pathogenetic, rather than a temporal sense. It reflects a fundamental shattering of experience that does not involve formation of inferential, *secondary* delusions (Jaspers 1963; Schneider 1949). Jaspers wrote: "To say simply that a delusion is a mistaken idea which is firmly held by the patient and which cannot be corrected gives only a superficial and incorrect answer to the problem. . ." A true delusion is a pathological *primary experience,* implying a transformation of the patient's total awareness of reality. What is changed is not an *opinion* about reality but the very structure of the global perspective on reality: the patient's existential framework. True delusion should not be considered as a *knowledge statement about empirical matters* (i.e., beliefs) but rather as a metaphor (Blondel 1914; Parnas 2004; Spitzer 1990) for the changes *in the structure of experience*, affecting the very sense of presence to the world and self-presence, i.e., the existential feelings (Ratclifffe 2008). These changes are related to the structural disorders of self-awareness to which Schneider alluded in a quote presented earlier. For the patient, his delusional "evidence" and conviction stem primarily from an unreflected (non-conceptual) *felt* experience, the latter being a touchstone of a private, unique and absolute sense of conviction (Müller-Suur 1950, 1954, 1962). "The significance is of a special kind; it always carries a great import, is urgent and personal, *a sign or message from another world*" (Schneider 1959, p. 104). The sense of conviction, even if *thematically* vague in the nascent stages of delusional experience is nonetheless overwhelming from the very start (Müller-Suur 1950). Delusional disorder patients (paranoia) believe in their basic experience only with relative, more or less compelling certainty, and their certainty increases through reflections over time. By contrast, the patients with schizophrenia experience *absolute certainty*, even if the contents of their delusions are nascent or plainly absurd. The schizophrenic certainty is a "suffered" certainty (*erlittene Gewissheit*), i.e., it emerges passively, like a sensation, whereas the "paranoiac" delusional certainty is "achieved" (*errungene Gewissheit*), i.e., it is hard-earned, through observation and reflection. Primary delusion cannot be challenged by some more fundamental dataset. The patients typically do not seek social validation, are indifferent to empirical proofs and only rarely act upon their delusions (Parnas 2004). The sense of certainty often persists, even after the patient is said to have remitted from a frankly delusional condition.

The DSM-IV (and ICD-10) category of *bizarre* delusion is a *hybrid* of (1) the concept of delusion as a *false belief due to incorrect inference* (which Jaspers categorized as secondary delusions, and which were considered by Schneider as being of a second diagnostic rank, (not specific to schizophrenia), and (2) a particular delusional *content* that is considered "bizarre," and defined as "physically impossible," "totally implausible," "un-understandable," etc., and epitomized by the FRS passivity phenomena. The new category of "bizarre" delusion was justified by a cursory reference to Kraepelin's remark that schizophrenic delusions often were "nonsensical" and to Jaspers, according to whom they were "un-understandable" (Spitzer et al. 1993).[4] Since the delusions based on passivity experiences (e.g., thought insertion, deprivation) are of an explanatory kind, they all fall into the category of Japers–Schneider's secondary delusions. For a detailed analysis of the notion of "bizarreness" and "incomprehensibility," see Parnas and Sass (2008) and Cermolacce et al. (2010).

Audible thoughts (Gedankenlautwerden, l'écho de pensée)

Gedankenlautwerden is *a group of phenomena* in which thinking loses its normal phenomenal quality and acquires acoustic and audible character (Durand 1909). The patient is said to hear his own thoughts aloud, spoken with his own voice (Leuret 1834, 2007; "la pensée parlée"), a symptom that often precedes auditory-verbal hallucinations.

Certain phenomenological aspects of cognition need to be understood in describing and grasping of this feature. Normally, thinking is phenomenally transparent ("non-iconic"), i.e., it has no definite or distinct phenomenal embodiment, but rather consists of a stream of thoughts, articulated as a chain of semantic meanings or senses (see Leuret 1834, p. 125). Thinking may also happen through the medium of "inner speech," a distinct modality of consciousness. Here, thinking may have a linguistic sign format, which is perhaps comparable to short stenographic notes (i.e., we do not think in fully formed sentences, but rather through the flashes of single word meanings). The *inner speech has no spatial characteristics*, and hence no sound. Normal inner speech has an "expressive" function which means that the signifier or the *vehicle* of thought (the inner speech) and the *meaning* (sense) of thought *are but one* (Husserl 1900/1970). Thus the meaning/sense emerges as the very substance of my thought. If I "say to myself" (in my inner speech): "now, I will take a break," the particular meaning of the thought ("to take a break") and the sense of the "I" or of "me," who does the thinking, are inseparable, they form a single unified whole. In other words, I do not *inspect* my thinking or *listen* to my inner speech *in order to know* what I am thinking. It borders on incoherence to say that "*I know what I am thinking*" (there is no knowledge relation here, just thinking). Thinking is always *mine* because it happens in the first person perspective (*vide supra*: the concepts of Meinhaftigkeit and Ichheit). The subject of thinking is in the midst of the thought itself. It is on the basis of such certainty that Descartes claimed "I think therefore I am" (Jaspers claimed that this certitude was characteristically shattered in schizophrenia). This unity of signifier (sign), signified (meaning, sense), and the sense of self, breaks apart (or lacks) in the schizophrenia spectrum conditions. The self no longer permeates the thinking as its first-person perspective. There emerges a distance or gulf between the self and the thinking. The patient starts to *inspect his thoughts*, which become reified, spatialized, akin to physical objects. Eventually, the inner speech may acquire a quasi-perceptual, acoustic character. The patient now *listens* to his thoughts. The *expressive* function of inner speech [Husserl 1900/1970; vide supra] is replaced by the *indicative* function, i.e., the spoken words [signifiers] *refer to* an independent layer of thought meaning [signified]. A fading of first person perspective in thinking was described in the following way by one of our patients:

> A female patient distinguished between *being thoughts* and *having thoughts*. She explained that "'being' thoughts is equal to filling them up as 'me,' saturating them." By contrast, in the "having" mode, "the thoughts are *delimited*; you can hear or see them, but they are not spread out in the body; they are incomplete, they are not real."

Some patients are able to contrast Gedankenlautwerden, usually intensified in solitary reflection, from a normal mode of "inconspicuous thinking," which prevails when they are world-engaged. Related phenomena comprise "reading and writing echo" ("l'écho de la lecture" and "l'écho de l'ecriture"), where writing and reading is accompanied by loud thinking. Thinking may also be doubled as a sort of soundless echo, and finally, the patient may experience his thinking as sentences "seen" in his inner space, as if on a screen; finally the reading process may be accompanied by a feeling that the text had just been read (déjà lu).

None of these phenomena are mentioned in the DSM-IV-TR and they are increasingly unfamiliar to clinicians. In the ICD-10, Gedankenlautwerden is listed as a FRS if associated with thought-diffusion (transmission, broadcasting). The patient must express or enact a worry that others are able to participate in (often, but not necessarily, hear) his thinking, before the symptom can be rated as present.

Thought diffusion (transmission, broadcasting, Gedankenaussbreitung)

This symptom is not listed under the DSM-IV-TR diagnostic criteria (pp. 298–312), but appears in the glossary of technical terms as a subtype of delusion (p. 822): "The delusion that one's thoughts are being broadcast out loud so that they can be perceived by others." For Schneider, thought diffusion was an aspect of the fundamental change in the structure of consciousness, i.e., a fading first person perspective and inability to distinguish between the inner and the outer (loss of the sense of *privacy of the first person perspective*; "loss of ego-boundaries"). *It is primarily a change of experience.* Thus the patient may complain of feeling permanently "open," "naked," "thin-skinned," "transparent"—complaints that may express an unpleasant experience of being excessively accessible for others. It is a qualitatively different experience from a common impression that others *do* indeed have access to the contents of one's mental states via our expressivity (mainly affectivity). In thought diffusion, the patient *feels* that the privacy (or intimacy) of his first person perspective (his "inner world") is *uncertain* or compromised but such experience is not yet interpreted through explanatory delusions. Thought diffusion is closely linked to self-reference and, sometimes, to a sense of resonance between one's thoughts and external events or a sense of a strange synchrony between one's own and others' movements (Grivois 1992). Thought diffusion and audible thoughts often go together (Durand 1909). A phenomenon, associated with the disorders of self-awareness in schizophrenia (Parnas and Handest 2003), and always considered of particular importance (but omitted from the current DSM and ICD descriptions) is the so-called "mirror-phenomenon" ("signe du miroir," "Spiegelphänomen"). "Mirror phenomenon" is the behavior enacting the patient's insecure sense of selfhood. The patient may inspect his face excessively, especially the eyes, e.g., trying to grasp his own gaze (which is an impossible task), searching for potential morphological changes, to verify his existence, to check upon and adjust his expression, or to identify a visible basis of his felt porosity and accessibility to others, etc.

Passivity phenomena

This group of phenomena comprises different alienations in nearly all modalities of experience (thought, feelings-emotions-impulses, bodily and motor phenomena). Common to them all is that the subjectivity of experience is lost, and may be replaced by some kind of feeling of external manipulation. These phenomena were regularly described since the beginning of modern French, German and British psychiatry. Schneider considered them to be of a prime diagnostic specificity to schizophrenia, because—as pointed out earlier—they reflected a structural change of consciousness, a diminished or shattered first person perspective or "mineness." It was this anomalous configuration of experience that was diagnostically specific, rather than the secondary delusional elaborations, explaining the experience (primarily to the patient himself and to others).

Clear example of the diagnostic emphasis on the *experiential nature* of the anomalies, prior to their delusional elaborations, are explicitly described by Schneider (1950/1959). *Thought block* is described in the following way: "A schizophrenic woman said: when I want to hang on my thoughts, they break off" (p. 100). In other words, a characteristic experience of sudden block or break in the stream of thoughts already counts as FRS rather than its delusional articulation in terms of externally instigated thought deprivation. Another female patient described her bodily feelings as "a sort of intercourse, as if a man was really there. *He was not there of course*, nobody was there. I was quite alone but it was *as if* a man was with me, as though we were having intercourse" (p. 97).

It is clear that the delusional explanations, in which "interferences are (. . .) attributed to various devices, rays, suggestions, hypnotic influences" (p. 97), strengthen the reliability of schizophrenia diagnosis. Thus, a pure experience of thought block may be difficult or impossible to distinguish from normal feelings of absent-mindedness— especially if the patient's subjective life is not assessed adequately (or not at all).

The original focus on passivity *experience* (loss of mineness) became transformed in the DSM-IV into an emphasis on explanatory delusions with propositional contents related to passivity experiences (insertion, deprivation, other type of manipulation from without).

12.5 **FRS and DSM: a conclusion**

The diagnosis of schizophrenia in the DSM-IV (and the ICD-10) cannot claim a faithful epistemological-conceptual or phenomenological continuity with Schneider. There is in the DSM no trace of Schneider's observations on the underlying structure of the FRS in particular, or on the nature of schizophrenia in general. On the concrete, practical level, the number of FRS became restricted and those retained, underwent important modification. Original emphasis on *anomalies of experience* was replaced by the requirements of fully-formed *explanatory delusions*.

It is likely that the changes in the number and nature of the FRS have had a negative impact on the overall sensitivity of the DSM-IV schizophrenia, if compared to the original Schneiderian concept. Such claim is consistent with a recent review of poly-diagnostic studies (studies applying different diagnostic criteria in the same patient group) (Jansson and Parnas 2007). The use of the FRS (as singly diagnostically sufficient) results in approximately twice as many schizophrenia cases than it is the case with the DSM-proximate definitions. Moreover, the emphasis on the well-articulated explanatory delusions automatically makes the schizophrenia concept more chronic, independently of the duration criterion. Indeed, the duration of illness must be sufficiently long as to allow for the elaboration of thematically complex delusions.

12.6 **Mood and affectivity**

In the Bleulerian prototype, mood, emotion and affect changes are considered as frequent: depression, (silly) elation, excitement, indifference, dysphoria, irritability, etc. This change is often the first sign of the disease noticed by the patient's relatives. It was once a common knowledge that the onset of schizophrenia was often preceded by the "initial depression" (Conrad 1949).[5] Affective changes were described as being qualitatively different from depressive *state*-features of a true affective illness, e.g., *trait*-anhedonia, sense of emptiness, loss of meaning, and loss of basic motivation, oppressing solitude (Kepinski 1974). Yet, even in the typical cases of melancholia, a presence of enduring schizophrenia features (e.g., formal thought disorder, primary delusions) justified a schizophrenia diagnosis (Kraepelin 1919).

Anxiety is not mentioned in the context of DSM-IV schizophrenia concept (with the exception of one sentence on associated features). Yet anxiety, qualitatively quite distinct, is a significant aspect of schizophrenia, especially in the early stages of the disorder (see Parnas et al. (2005b) for a phenomenological description and Saks (2007), for first-person account).

The issue of a "third psychosis" was in Europe regularly invoked since Wernicke (1900) and, more recently by Leonhardt (1999). These acute "cycloid" psychoses (sometimes designated as "schizoaffective") were characterized by severe emotional turbulence manifest in several psychopathological dimensions (anxiety-happiness, akinesis-hyperkinesis, schizophasia), often leading to a *compromised lucidity (composure)* of consciousness (Sigmund and Mundt 1999). The creation of the contemporary schizoaffective diagnosis in the DSM-ICD took, however, another route. Affective features became simply evacuated from schizophrenia, and an independent schizoaffective diagnosis emerged from a symptomatic mixture of schizophrenic and affective symptoms.

12.7 **The negative and disorganized symptoms**

The division of schizophrenic symptoms into negative, positive and disorganized has a long history (Schneider 1930). Mathematically, it was for the first time demonstrated on a large patient sample by (Wittman and Sheldon 1948) but in a slightly different terminology (negative=schizoid, positive=paranoid, and disorganized=heboid). In the DSM tradition, the negative symptoms are conceived of as quantitative *deficits*, *fall-outs* of normal functions i ("too little") signaled by the deprivative α: a-logia, a-volition, an-ergia, and an-hedonia. This *deficit* concept has a very limited relation to the original gestalt of schizophrenia (see later) (Parnas and Bovet 1994). Since these features, considered as simple deficits are ubiquitous and non-specific (McGory et al. 1995), the DSM-IV goes into great lengths in emphasizing the high severity level that is required for crossing the diagnostic threshold. In the case of affective flattening, we are reminded of that it is "useful to observe the person's interacting with peers to determine if affective flattening is sufficiently persistent" (p. 301), whereas in the case of alogia, "observation over time and in a variety of situations," is recommended. The concept of disorganized speech is in the DSM-IV described in a lay language and does not contain any trace of the previously developed distinctions of formally disordered discourse and thought (Andreasen 1986; Johnston and Holzman 1979). Rather, the severity is emphasized: "[disorganized speech] must be sufficiently severe to *substantially* impair communication."

One consequence of such a severity level is an increasing inability of psychiatrists to identify, grasp and describe in detail clinically significant formal thought disorder, disorders of discourse as well as varieties of disintegrated expressivity.

Thus, the DSM-IV-TR negative and disorganized symptoms function as diagnostic of schizophrenia on the condition of being so severe that *they are mainly useful for a diagnosis of chronic schizophrenia*. Most cases of today's hebephrenic cases fall below this severity threshold. Similar problems are encountered by the ICD-10.

12.8 **Gestalt and prototype**

It is now necessary to take a detour to the notions of gestalt and prototype in order to understand how these notions are relevant in the domain of nosology and diagnosis (excellently described by Schwarz and Wiggins (1987a, 1987b); see also Parnas and Bovet (1995)). *Gestalt elements are always present* in the clinical process, and the quality of a typification process is not independent of the accumulated experience and skill of the clinician.

A prototype is a *central example of a category in question*; a sparrow is a more typical bird than is a penguin or an ostrich. A prototypical gestalt is a salient *unity* or organization of phenomenal aspects which articulates itself in an epistemic relation (e.g., in a diagnostic interview). This unity emerges from the relations between component features (part-whole relations) but cannot be reduced to their simple aggregate ("whole is more than the sum of its parts"). A gestalt notion transcends the dichotomies of "inner and outer," "form and content," "universal and particular" (Merleau-Ponty 1942). The salience of, e.g., interpersonal encounter does not normally emerge in piecemeal disconnected allusions to the patient's inner life on the one hand, in addition to independently salient fragments of his visible expressions, on the other hand. Rather, the person articulates himself through certain wholes, *jointly constituted* by his experience, belief, and expression ("inner and outer"). "*What*" he says (content) is always molded by the "*how*" (form) of his way of thinking and experiencing. A gestalt instantiates a certain *generality of type* (e.g., this patient is typical of a category X), but this typicality is always modified, because it is necessarily embodied by a particular, concrete individual, thus deforming the ideal clarity of type ("universal and particular").

The gestalt's *aspects* are inter-dependent in a mutually constitutive and implicative manner (Sass and Parnas 2007)[6] and the whole of gestalt co-determines the nature *and specificity* of its particular aspects, while, at the same time, the whole receives from the single aspects its concrete clinical rootedness. It means that a symptom only articulates itself as a delimited entity through the relations to other features, context, and a more encompassing whole.

Imagine a case of "social phobia," motivated by fear of physical/tactile contact with other people, a proximity experienced as engulfing, fusing, and annihilating. You would probably not consider such "phobia" as an isolated behavioral dysfunction but rather as being indicative of insecure identity and porous self-demarcation, with avoidant coping behavior ensuing by implication. We can also consider an example of "mumbling speech." In itself it is perhaps characteristic of 5% of a random sample of people. Yet, in a psychiatric context, e.g., associated with stereotypies and inappropriate affect, it acquires a diagnosis-relevant status.

More detailed conceptual determinations of the gestalt proceed through the steps of psychiatric typifications, excellently described by Schwartz and Wiggins (1987a, 1987b) in two seminal papers. *The clinical task is to allow the gestalt to manifest itself in more detail*; to let its latent or unexpected profiles become apparent and to conceptualize and flesh out these originally only dimly apprehended or non-apprehended aspects. Some typifications happen automatically and pre-reflectively, whereas others imply a more explicit attention and reflection. All typifications should be subjected to ongoing critical reflection, and therefore necessitate training, teaching of concepts, and acquisition of skills and expertise. They are open to intersubjective judgment, may be shared by other psychiatrists (Parnas and Zahavi 2002; Schwartz and Wiggins 1987). In summary, they may be assessed with respect to inter-rater reliability. Moreover, a psychopathological emphasis on gestaltic nature of "mental object" does not preclude that the final, formal diagnosis follows a list of prespecified (e.g., polythetic) criteria, because nothing a priori prevents constructing a list of criteria with strong affinities to the gestalt features.

12.9 **The core gestalt of schizophrenia in European psychopathology**

All European psychopathologists agree about something phenomenologically distinctive, characteristic and typical about schizophrenia, a "something," "whatness," alluded to in the introduction but absent in the DSM-IV (Maj 1998). The "whatness" of schizophrenia is a prototypical *core*, whose properties are not contingent surface symptoms (state phenomena), but rather reflect a phenomenological *depth* or a generative structure of the disorder. It is important to emphasize that the core is not just a theoretical construct but has a phenomenological reality; it is perceivable and accessible to observation.

European psychiatry proposed many designations for this core, some of which are listed in Table 12.2. The differences between these individual positions are more nominal than substantial.

There was a reasonable consensus that the specificity of schizophrenia was not to be found in the fleeting positive psychotic symptoms. Rather, what seems to be at stake is a more pervasive change, pointing to a *profoundly changed mental life*. It is the basic congruence between the modes and contents of consciousness, its self-coherence, its basic subject-world directedness, and its contextual adequacy, that strikes one as being fundamentally disturbed. When, paraphrasing Jaspers and others, we say "un-understandable," impenetrable, or "bizarre" (Cermolacce et al. 2010) we refer to our sense of confronting a *trait condition*, not only marked by circumscribed abnormal contents, but by *a structural change of subjectivity* (consciousness). The enigmatic character of this trait condition stems from the impossibility to anchor it into a particular, isolated feature or symptom. The disorder is manifest across a manifold of symptoms in the patient's self-relation (self-disorders), relation to the world (ambivalence, lack of meaning, lack of attunement), and sociality (isolation/poor interpersonal relations/

Table 12.2 Designations of the core of schizophrenia

Le syndrome de discordance (Chaslin 1912)
Disunity of consciousness (Kraepelin 1919)
Intrapsychic ataxia (Stransky 1904)
Autism/Spaltung (Eugen Bleuler 1911/1950; Manfred Bleuler 1983)
Autisme/Perte du contact vital (Minkowski 1926, 1927)
Anthropological disproportion/Breakdown of natural experience (Binswanger 1956)
Crisis of "common sense"/lack of natural self-evidence (Blankenburg 1971)
Schizophrene Grundstimmung: Ich-Störung (Gruhle 1929; Berze 1914)
Changed modality of being [Eine Daseinsweise] (Wyrsch 1946)

eccentricity) (Parnas and Handest 2003; Parnas and Sass 2008; Parnas et al. 2002). The core disorder (Minkowski 1926, 1997) has a fundamental or generative status because it subordinates psychotic state features, often conferring on these symptoms a certain fractal-quality.[7] Thus the single symptoms may appear colored by the overall gestalt of the illness (e.g., see the descriptions of Schneiderian symptoms earlier as examples of such coloring; see also earlier: part-whole relations of gestalt).

No wonder that Bleuler (1911/1950) needed 31 pages to describe the "complex fundamental symptoms," most importantly *schizophrenic autism*, a description that came to include interrelated *expressive, behavioral, subjective (cognitive, affective)*, and *existential* aspects (see Parnas and Bovet 1991, for a detailed analysis, and Parnas et al. 2002, for a more general discussion). Other "fundamental" symptoms (formal thought disorder, peculiar affectivity, *lack of rapport reciprocity* and ambivalence) pop up in the autism section as well. Such panoply is clearly beyond what *the notion of a symptom* can contain. Aware of the problem (but not of the solution), Bleuler qualified autism as a "*complex*" symptom. Phenomenological notions of gestalt and prototype[8] offer conceptually better and more adequate resources: the schizophrenic autism is not an atomic symptom but a disordered structure of subjectivity, manifest through manifold phenomenological and existential changes.

Thus the ICD-8 Glossary[9] defines the core feature of schizophrenia as a change in the patient's structure (or framework) of subjectivity: it is "the fundamental disturbance of personality [self], [which] involves its most basic functions, those that give the normal person his *feeling of individuality, uniqueness, and self-direction*" (p. 27).

Recently, we have indeed *rediscovered* the disorders of self-awareness in schizophrenia spectrum conditions[10] (self-disorders) (Parnas and Handest 2003; Parnas et al. 1998, 2005a, 2005b, 2011; Raballo and Parnas 2011; Raballo et al. 2011; Sass and Parnas 2003). These are *disorders of self-experience* and *not* delusions or hallucinations. They comprise a pervasively diminished sense of existing as an embodied subject, various distortions of first-person perspective, feelings of disembodiment, anonymization of the field of awareness with deficient "mineness" ("my thoughts have no respect for me"), inadequate ego-demarcation, and, very importantly, a lack of attunement to, and immersion in the world ("I only live in my head").

12.10 **Hebephrenia and non-paranoid schizophrenia**

In relation to the "whatness" of schizophrenia, hebephrenia, or more broadly, non-paranoid schizophrenia, occupy a privileged position. It was always considered as a *paradigmatic subtype* of schizophrenia, instantiating *in a nutshell* its fundamental gestalt. It was emblematic or *educational of what schizophrenia was about*. There has been a decrease of flamboyant, "silly hebephrenia," parallel to that of catatonia over 1920–1960, probably due to cultural and iatrogenic influences[11] (Morrisson 1974).

Most of hebephrenic features are "the core features" described previously, *trait-like features*, often also present to a subtle degree among vulnerable people, prodromally, and in remitted schizophrenia. The so-called simple schizophrenia (with absent hallucinations and delusions, and usually, but not always, with paucity of ideation) is often assimilated into the non-paranoid continuum. Kahlbaum (1890) and Hecker

(1871), who founded the notion of hebephrenia, believed that the latter formed a "hebetic" spectrum of disorders with variable severity—a notion very similar to, and overlapping, Kety's construct of the schizophrenic spectrum of disorders. The cases of "schizoidia," "latent," or "borderline" schizophrenia (Kety 1988) became eventually formalized as schizotypal disorders in the ICD-10 (Axis I) and the DSM-III (Axis II) (for a detailed phenomenological description, see Parnas et al. (2005c)).

Hebephrenia is marked by a gestalt of *disintegration* or *discordance*, both *between* and *within* modalities of consciousness: expression, affect, thought, speech, mood, willing and behavior and a severely defective emotional rapport.

Henri Ey (1977) summarized the manifestations of "discordance" in four general dimensions (p. 53):

> 1) *Ambivalence*: a division of all states or operations of the mind into contradictory tendencies: desire/fear-repulsion; willing/not willing; affirmation/negation. 2) *Bizarreness*: impression of a strangeness that seems to reflect a disconcerting intention of the paradoxical or the illogical. 3) *Impenetrability*: all schizophrenic symptoms appear to be imbued by an enigmatic tonality; there is always some opacity in the relations of understanding between the patient and the other. 4) *Detachment*: loss of vital contact with reality (Minkowski 1927) [lack of attunement, loss of the world's natural self-evidence, inability of immersion in the world, solipsism].[12]

To these four dimensions we can add a *disorder of consciousness* (not in the sense of clarity) but as a change in the structure of experiencing (self-disorders; vide supra), which Ey considered as intrinsic to schizophrenia (with the term "destructuration of consciousness"; Ey 1977, 1978).

Feelings, thoughts and affects are incongruous, expression may vary in different parts of the face, the temporal contour of affect is often unpredictable, and there is a tendency to subtle parakinetic or stereotypic movements, especially in the oral or paraocular muscles. There may be a mannerist expression and rich varieties of formal thought disorder, interpersonal and social dysfunctions (sometimes with indifference, withdrawal, poor motivation, hostility or fleeting, inconsequential, fragmentary engagements, "crazy projects"). Mood is shallow and monotonous, or dysphoric and chaotic, sometimes inappropriately elated. The inner life is severely disorganized with an unstable sense of subjecthood, and other disorders of self-experience (e.g., diminished sense of self, ambivalence, perplexity, thought pressure-, interference-, block or emptiness).[13] The patient is severely dislocated from shared values and social frameworks, living an apathetic, detached, "alternative" or bizarre existence, or acting inappropriately, out of proportion. Some of these actions deserve to be called psychotic because of their plain irrationality (Parnas et al. 2010). Minkowski talked here of "psychosis through action" (délire en acte) and Conrad of "crazy actions" (Unsinnige Handlung). This "non-propositional" irrationality manifests itself through affectivity, expressivity, or action (e.g., with certain less flamboyant catatonic features, odd behavioral style [e.g., a Danish patient, sitting in a yoga position on the floor of the hospital's waiting room, would, most likely, turn out upon closer examination, to be psychotic]— e.g., like sudden aimless trips ("voyage pathologique"), unprovoked homicide etc). The post-hoc explanations are typically evasive, vague or illogical—and they can be barely (and only with some difficulty and distortion) translated into a clear proposi-tional delusional "belief-format." Many of these patients, the label "non-paranoid" notwithstanding, suffer from a variety of fleeting psychotic symptoms seen in para-noid patients: e.g., phenomena of somatic depersonalization with bizarre hypochon-driac explanations, audible thoughts, inappropriate-strange, disorganized behaviors, and varying degrees of hallucinations and delusions (including passivity phenomena). Yet, the general initial clinical presentation is typically of non-paranoid nature, with the following, overlapping, "surface presentations": apathy, depression, "neurasthenic"-hypochondriac complaints, or puerile or impulsive behavior (including self-mutila-tion). Many patients are pushed into psychiatry because of their poor school/work performance, drifting around or transgressive behavior.

12.11 Non-paranoid schizophrenia/hebephrenia in the DSM-IV and ICD-10

The criteria of DSM-IV and ICD-10 do not allow for a substantial number of hebe-phrenic and other non-paranoid patients to be so diagnosed.[14] First, the negative- and disorganized- symptom criteria, through which the patient may enter the schizophre-nia diagnosis, are, as already mentioned, stipulated at such a high severity level that, in today's Europe, is mainly seen during exacerbations and in *chronic* and neglected course. Second, and more importantly, clinicians are today typically *not taught* and therefore not aware of the characteristic gestalt of schizophrenia, about its "whatness." This prototype, so salient in hebephrenia, eludes the psychopathological radar of con-temporary psychiatrists, no longer trained in an in-depth psychopathological evalua-tion of their patients (Andreasen 2007). An impression, a suspicion of this gestalt commands a comprehensive and detailed psychopathological assessment, an assess-ment that simply does not take place when the gestalt is unsighted. Instead, the patient is diagnosed on the basis of a contingently presenting prominent feature. Typically, he is diagnosed as suffering from a variety of non-schizophrenia spectrum diagnoses: borderline personality disorder, social phobia, anxiety disorders, obsessive–compul-sive disorder and, quite frequently, affective disorder. To phrase it provocatively: we seem to be in a full regression to a pre-Kraepelinian predicament of multiple unrelated disorders, inviting endless comorbidity research.

We know from the Danish ICD-10 hospital statistics that the frequency of border-line disorder has increased immensely. The percentage of hebephrenia among first hospitalized schizophrenia patients is now down to around 1%, i.e., in practical terms, almost non-existent. There is no reason to believe that this situation is dramatically dissimilar for the DSM-IV.

12.12 Epistemological considerations

Andreasen's (2007) assessment of decline in psychopathology fails to consider the pos-sibility that the "unintended consequences" of the DSM-project which she describes, may not be independent of its *intended* epistemology and metaphysics. The DSM project—a response to reliability crisis and a reaction to psychoanalysis—embraced two basic assumptions: explicit behaviorism and more implicit physicalism.

The main idea in the DSM is that the psychiatric "symptoms and signs" should be ideally considered as third person data, namely as reified (thing-like), mutually independent (atomic) entities, *devoid of meaning*, suitable for context-independent definitions. Preference is given to "external behavior," with skeptical, if not aversive, attitude towards the subjective experience. The latter is not accessible to a third-person observation and description and may require reflection (inference). A physicalist (neo-Kraepelinian) research program amplified this tendency of reification and atomization of psychopathological phenomena, in the hope of their ultimate reduction to modular defects in the neural substrate, "carving nature at its joints." It is as if the symptom/sign and its causal substrate were assumed to exhibit the same descriptive nature: both are spatio-temporally delimited objects, i.e., things. In this paradigm—adequate and fruitful in *medicine*, from which it originates—the symptoms and signs have *no* intrinsic *sense or meaning*. They are almost entirely *referring*, pointing to the underlying abnormalities of anatomo-physiological substrate. This background scheme of "symptoms=causal-referents" is automatically activated in the mind of every physician confronting a medical-somatic illness. Yet the psychiatrist, who confronts a "psychiatric object," finds himself in a situation *without analogue in the somatic medicine* (Jaspers 1963; Spitzer 1988). The psychiatrist confronts a *person*, and not a leg, an abdomen, or a skin surface, *not a thing*, but broadly speaking, another embodied consciousness in all its dimensions. What the patient manifests is not isolated *symptoms with referring function* but rather certain wholes of mutually implicative, interpenetrating experiences, feelings, beliefs, expressions, and actions, all permeated by biographical detail. The psychiatric typifications and reflections start from these meaning-wholes. *The latter are not constituted by a referential symptom function but by their meaning.* We do not (with few exceptions) know potential causal referents in any pragmatically useful sense. Our approach is a second-person approach guided by phenomenological distinctions, a process through which we extract, represent and individuate from the flow of the patient's subjective life certain repeatable constellations of experience, certain meaningful wholes. A psychiatric symptom or sign only emerges as an *individuated entity* (as *this* or *that* symptom) in a *context* of other, simultaneous, preceding and succeeding, experiences.

An important epistemological point to note is that clinicians *always* perceive their patients in a gestaltic manner, not in defiance of current epistemic dogma but because the prototypical lens is built into the human cognition (Schwartz and Wiggins, 1987a, 1987b). A psychiatric teaching or training that omits or discourages the prototypes from its curriculum is *a non-starter*. Such training produces an unarmed clinician who finds himself in a position of confronting a chaotic myriad of unconnected data, where each individual signal is a priori worth of attention, acting as a fulcrum for a potential diagnostic class. When prototypes are not taught systematically, the clinicians inevitably acquire *their own private* prototypes, but in a way that is not subjected to disciplined, critical and peer-shared reflection. Such "private" prototypes cannot resist becoming anchored in the single, contingently protuberant clinical features that happen to hit a matching aspect of a contingent diagnostic category. Here, a decisive role may be even played by the very first verbalizations of the complaint. Someone, who says: "I feel depressed" will be very likely diagnosed with "depression"; someone who says: "I have a habit of cutting myself" will be diagnosed as "borderline." If a 30-year-old habitually dysfunctional bachelor says that he was diagnosed with obsessive–compulsive disorder at the age of 17, the likelihood of a thorough assessment of his inner life is small (e.g., what does the word "obsession" mean to him, is it given as a thought, fantasy, urge, image or even picture? Is there automatic resistance? Etc.).

Thus, we need a methodological approach that is faithful to reality rather than the approach that models the reality in order to make it fit to its own prejudice. To faithfully assess another person's anomalies of experience, belief, expression, and behavior (*the second person perspective*), adds certain specific demands to our clinical skills and analytic-conceptual knowledge, constituting psychiatry also as an *academic and scholarly endeavors*,[15] while at the same time providing solid foundations for achieving empirical objectivity. It seems to me that the nosological progress cannot happen unless these basic epistemological issues haunting psychopathology are addressed, discussed, and re-dressed. Should it indeed happen, it will entail a dramatic and massive re-learning of what psychiatry is about and how it should be exercised.

12.13 **The consequences summarized**

Seymour Kety—a very distinguished scientist and a major figure behind the foundational adoption studies in schizophrenia—was worried by the Schneiderian criteria of schizophrenia proposed for the DSM-III. He suggested that this new definition should also have a new name because it failed to correspond to the essential Kraepelinian–Bleulerian prototype. Unfortunately, these worries have not been unfounded.

The concept of schizophrenia became narrowed into a predominantly *chronic delusional-hallucinatory* syndrome. All links to the constitutive ideas on the psychopathological nature of schizophrenia by Kraepelin, Eugene and Manfred Bleuler, Minkowski, Jaspers, Schneider, Blankenburg and many other prominent European psychopathologists have vanished (Figure 12.1).

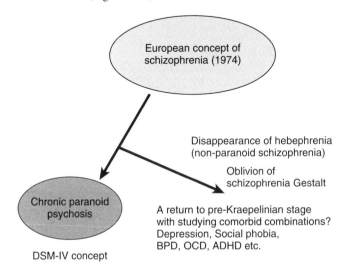

Figure 12.1 Regression to a "pre-Kraepelinian" nosology.

This has a profound impact on daily clinical practice. This impact is especially pronounced at the illness onset, efforts of early detection and early treatment. We may safely assume that it has also research consequences, especially in the domain of etiology and pathogenesis, because the fundamental phenotypes of schizophrenia—the starting point of all research—are seriously distorted.

Endnotes

1 In a recent editorial, Taylor et al. (2010), disenchanted with the current DSM-definition of schizophrenia (because of lack of visible etiological and pathogenetic progress) advocate its replacement with hebephrenia. Unfortunately, the latter is conceived of as a "natural kind"—well-delimited disease.

2 It changed from nomenclature to "Nomenklatura". The term "Nomenklatura," very much used in the French debate, stems from the Soviet era. It denotes people and institutions in power, who carve out a permissible semantic universe that prefigures ideologically/politically correct questions and answers.

3 His reputation in the Anglophone world greatly overshot that in Germany.

4 There is a long European discussion of the questions of typicality of content of delusions in schizophrenia (see Schmidt 1940; Jaspers 1963; Bovet and Parnas 1995), but there is no indication that this literature was consulted in connection in the process of creation of DSM concept of "bizarre delusions."

5 In the DSM-IV affective symptoms are mentioned as associated features (APA 2000, p. 304) but mood symptoms are said not to meet the full severity of a mood-episode (p. 310).

6 This is, of course, of paramount epistemological importance and makes the operationalist project of counting number of symptoms for a diagnostic purpose highly problematic

7 "Fractal" is a geometric shape that can be iteratively split into increasingly smaller parts, each of which is a reduced-size copy of the original whole (a property called "self-similarity").

8 Prototype or gestalt has affinities to Wittgenstein's concept of "family resemblance" (Wittgenstein 1953). Here the typicality resides in the recognition of "crisscrossing network of analogous relations." All these concepts are far from ephemeral and may be expressed in polythetic criteria for empirical research.

9 It is retained, in a diluted version, in the ICD-10.

10 Self-disorders are described by many European authors: Kraepelin (1919), E. Bleuler (1911/1950), Berze (1914), Schneider (1950/1959), Blankenburg (1971, 1988), Ey (1978), Gruhle (1929), Kronfeld (1922); see also Spitzer, (1988).

11 Several authors believe that schizophrenia has generally become a "milder" disease over the post-World War II period.

12 My translation and my additions in square brackets.

13 There is a disunity of consciousness (Kraepelin). A prerequisite for unity and coherence of consciousness is an intact first person perspective. Different, variable, simultaneous and successive mental contents are unified into the same stream or one field of consciousness because they are experienced by, or given to, the same subject (Parnas and Sass 2011; Zahavi 2005).

14 This problem is more pronounced for ICD-10 than for DSM-IV; however it is better manageable in the ICD-10 due to hierarchy rules. Here the schizotypal disorder diagnosis

is located on Axis I, following schizophrenia, and therefore useful in picking up the below-threshold cases (Handest and Parnas 2005; Parnas et al. 2011).

15 Because of its lack of own conceptual resources, psychopathology is today being invaded by phenomenologically undigested constructs from cognitive science, e.g., "mentalizing," "monitoring," "metarepresentation" etc.

Chapter References

American Psychiatric Association (1980). *Diagnostic and Statistical Manual of Mental Disorders* (3rd ed.). Washington DC: American Psychiatric Association.

American Psychiatric Association (1987). *Diagnostic and Statistical Manual of Mental Disorders* (3rd ed., revised (DSM-III-R)). Washington, DC: American Psychiatric Association.

American Psychiatric Association (2000). *Diagnostic and Statistical Manual of Mental Disorders* (4th ed., Text Revision). Washington DC: American Psychiatric Association.

Andreasen, N.C. (1986). Scale for the Assessment of Thought, Language, and Communication (TLC). *Schizophrenia Bulletin*, **12**, 473–82.

Andreasen, N. C. (2007). DSM and the death of phenomenology in America: An example of unintended consequences. *Schizophrenia Bulletin*, **33**(1), 108–12.

Berze, J. (1914). *Die primäre Insuffizienz der psychischen Aktivität: Ihr Wesen, ihre Erscheinungen und ihre Bedeutung als Grundstörungen der Dementia Praecox und der hypophrenen überhaupt*. Leipzig: Frank Deuticke.

Binswanger, L. (1956). *Drei Formen Misglückten Daseins: Verstiegenheit, Verschrobenheit, Manieriertheit*. Tübingen: Niemeyer.

Blankenburg, W. (1965). Zur Differentialphänomenologie der Wahrnehmung. Eine Studie über abnormes Bedeutungserleben. *Nervenarzt*, **36**, 285–298.

Blankenburg, W. (1971). *Der Verlust der natürlichen Selbstverständlichkeit. Ein Beitrag zur Psychopathologie symptomarmer Schizophrenien*. Stuttgart: Enke.

Blankenburg, W. (1988). *Zur Psychopathologie des Ich-Erlebens Schizophrener*. In: M. Spitzer, F. A. Uehlein, and G. Oepen (eds.), *Psychopathology and Philosophy*. Berlin: Springer, pp. 184–197.

Bleuler, E. (1911/1950). Dementia Praecox oder Gruppe der Schizophrenien. In: G. Aschaffenburg (ed.). *Handbuch der Psychiatrie*. Spezieller Teil, 4. Abteilung, 1. Hšlfte. Leipzig: Deuticke. Zinkin J. and Lewis, N. D. C. (trans.) (1950). *Dementia Praecox or the Group of Schizophrenias*. New York: International University Press.

Bleuler, M. (1983). *Lehrbuch der Psychiatrie. 15 Aufgabe*. Heidelberg: Springer Verlag.

Blondel, C. (1914). *La Conscience Morbide. Essai de Psychopathologie Générale*. Paris: Alcan.

Bøjholm, S. and Strömgren, E. (1989). Prevalence of schizophrenia on the island of Bornholm in 1935 and in 1983. *Acta Psychiatrica Scandinavica*, Suppl. **348**, 157–66.

Bovet, P. and Parnas, J. (1995). Schizophrenic delusions: A phenomenological approach. *Schizophrenia Bulletin 1993*, **1**, 579–97.

Cermolacce, M., Sass, L.A. and Parnas, J. (2010). What is bizarre in bizarre delusions? A critical review. *Schizophrenia Bulletin*, **34**(6), 667–79.

Chaslin, P. (1912). *Éléments de Sémiologie et de Clinique Mentale*. Paris: Asselin et Houzea.

Conrad, K. (1958). *Die beginnende Schizophrenie. Versuch einer Gestaltanalyse des Wahns*. Stuttgart: Thieme.

Cutting, J. and Shepherd, M. (1987). *The Clinical Roots of the Schizophrenia Concept*. Cambridge: Cambridge University Press.

Durand, C. (1909). *L'écho de la pensée*. Paris: Doin & Cie.

Ey, H. (1977). *La notion de schizophrénie. Séminaire de Thuir, Février-Juin 1975*. Paris: Descler de Brouwer.

Ey, H. (1978) *Consciousness. A Phenomenological Study of Being Conscious and Becoming Conscious*. (Flodstrom J. H. (trans.) (1963). *La conscience*. Paris: PUF). Bloomington, IN: Indiana University Press.

Ey, H. (1996). *Schizophrénie. Collection des études cliniques et psychopathologiques*. Les Plessis-Robinson: Synthelabo.

Grivois, H. (1992) *Naître à la folie*. Paris: Les Émpêcheurs de penser en rond.

Gruhle, H. (1929). *Schizophrene Grundstimmung (Ich-Störrung). In J*. Berze and H. Gruhle (eds.), *Psychologie der Schizophrenie*. Berlin: Springer Verlag, pp. 86–94.

Hecker, E. (1871) Die Hebephrenie. Ein Beitrag zur klinischen Psychiatrie. *Archiv für patologische Anatomie und Physiologie und für Klinische Medizin*, **25**, 394–429.

Husserl, E. (1900/1970). *Logische Untersuchungen*. Halle: Niemeyer. Findlay, J.N. (trans.) (1970). *Logical Investigations*. London: Routledge & Kegan Paul.

Jablensky, A. and Sartorius, N. (2008). What did the WHO studies really find? *Schizophrenia Bulletin*, **34**(2), 253–5.

Jansson, L. B. and Parnas, J. (2007). Competing definitions of schizophrenia: what can be learned from polydiagnostic studies? *Schizophrenia Bulletin*, **33**(5), 1178–200.

Jaspers, K. (1959/1963). *Allgemeine Psychopathologie* (7th ed.). Berlin: Springer. Hoenig, J., and Hamilton, M. W. (trans.) (1963). *General Psychopathology*. Chicago, IL: University of Chicago Press.

Johnston, M. H. and Holzman, P. S. (1979). *Assessing Schizophrenic Thinking*. San Francisco, CA: Jossey-Bass.

Kahlbaum, K. (1890). Über Heboïdophrenie. *Allgemeine Zeitschrift für Psychiatrie*, **46**, 461–74.

Kepinski, A. (1974). *Schizofrenia*. Warsaw: Panstwowy Zaklad Wydawnictw Lekarskich.

Kety, S. S. (1988). Schizophrenic illness in the families of schizophrenic adoptees: findings from the Danish national sample. *Schizophrenia Bulletin*, **14**(2), 217–22.

Kraepelin, E. (1919). *Dementia Praecox und Paraphrenie*. Leipzig: Barth. R.M. Barclay and G.M. Robertson (trans.) (1919). *Dementia Praecox and Paraphrenia*. Edinburgh: Livingstone, reprinted 1971.

Kronfeld, A. (1922). Über schizophrene Veränderungen des Bewustsseins der Aktivität. *Zeitschrift für die gesamte Neurologie und Psychiatrie*, **74**, 15–68.

Leonhard, K. (1999). *Classification of Endogenous Psychoses and their Differentiated Etiology* (2nd ed.) (ed. H. Beckmann ed.). New York: Springer Verlag.

Leuret, F. (1834/2007). *Fragments psychologiques de la folie*. Paris: Éditions Frison-Roche.

Maj, M. (1998). *The critique of DSM-IV operational criteria for schizophrenia*. **172**, 458–60.

McGorry, P. D., McFarlane, C., Patton, G. C., Bell, R., Hibbert, M. E., Jackson, H. J., *et al.* (1995). The prevalence of prodromal features of schizophrenia in adolescence: A preliminary study. *Acta Psychiatrica Scandinavica*, **92**, 241–249.

Mednick, S. A., Parnas, J. and Schulsinger, F. (1987). The Copenhagen High-Risk Project. 1962–1986. *Schizophrenia Bulletin*, **13**, 485–95.

Merleau-Ponty, M. (1942). *La structure du comportement*. Paris : Presses Universitaires de France.

Minkowski, E. (1926). *La notion de perte de contact vital avec la réalité et ses applications en psychopathologie*. Paris: Jouve & Cie.

Minkowski, E. (1927). *La schizophrénie. Psychopathologie des schizoïdes et des schizophrenes.* Paris: Payot.

Minkowski, E. (1928/1997). *"Du symptome au trouble gènèrateur" (originally in Archives suisses de neurologie et de psychiatrie, 22). In Au-delà du rationalisme morbide.* Paris: Éditions L'Harmattan, pp. 93–124.

Møller, P. and Husby, R. (2000). The initial prodrome in schizophrenia: searching for naturalistic core dimensions of experience and behavior. *Schizophrenia Bulletin,* **26**, 217–32.

Morrison, J. R. (1974). Changes in subtype diagnosis of schizophrenia: 1920–1966. *American Journal of Psychiatry,* **131**, 674–7.

Müller-Suur, H. (1950). Das Gewi§heitsbewu§tsein beim schizophrenen und beim paranoischen Wahnerleben. *Fortschritte der Neurologie Psychiatrie und ihrer Grenzgebiete,* **18**, 44–51.

Müller-Suur, H. (1954). Die Wirksamkeit allgemeiner Sinnhorizonte im schizophrenen Wahnerleben. *Fortschritte der Neurologie Psychiatrie und ihrer Grenzgebiete,* **22**, 38–44.

Müller-Suur, H. (1962). *Das Schizophrene als Ereignis.* In H. Kranz (ed.), *Psychopathologie Heute.* Stuttgart: Thieme, pp. 81–93.

Nordgaard, J., Arnfred, S. M., Handest, P. and Parnas, J. (2008). The diagnostic status of first-rank symptoms. *Schizophrenia Bulletin,* **34**(1), 137–54.

Parnas, J. (2004). Belief and pathology of self-awareness: A phenomenological contribution to the classification of delusions. *Journal of Consciousness Studies,* **10–11**, 148–61.

Parnas, J., and Bovet, P. (1991). Autism in schizophrenia revisited. *Comprehensive Psychiatry,* **32**, 7–21.

Parnas, J. and Bovet, P. (1994). Negative/positive symptoms of schizophrenia: Clinical and conceptual issues. *Nordic Journal of Psychiatry (suppl. 31),* **48**, 5–14.

Parnas, J. and Bovet, P. (1995). Research in psychopathology: Epistemological issues. *Comprehensive Psychiatry,* **36**, 167–81.

Parnas, J., Bovet, P. and Licht, D. (2005c). Cluster A personality disorders: A review (followed by peer commentaries). In M. Maj, H. Aksiskal, J. E. Mezzich, and A. Okasha (eds.), *Personality Disorders* (World Psychiatric Association series in Evidence and Experience in Psychiatry). Chichester: John Wiley & Sons, pp. 1–74.

Parnas, J., Bovet, P. and Zahavi, D. (2002). Schizophrenic autism: Clinical phenomenology and pathogenetic implications. *World Psychiatry,* **1/3**, 131–5.

Parnas, J., and Handest, P. (2003). Phenomenology of anomalous self-experience in early schizophrenia, *Comprehensive Psychiatry,* **44**, 121–34.

Parnas, J., Handest, P., Jansson, L. and Sæbye, D. (2005a). Anomalous subjective experience among first admitted schizophrenia spectrum patients: Empirical investigation, *Psychopathology,* **38**, 259–67.

Parnas, J., Handest, P., Sæbye, D. and Jansson, L. (2003). Anomalies of subjective experience in schizophrenia and psychotic bipolar illness. *Acta Psychiatrica Scandinavica,* **108**, 126–33.

Parnas, J., Jansson, L., Sass, L. A. and Handest, P. (1998). Self-experience in the prodromal phases of schizophrenia: A pilot study of first admissions. *Neurology, Psychiatry and Brain Research,* **6**, 107–16.

Parnas, J., Moller, P., Kircher, T., Thalbitzer, J., Jansson, L., Handest, P., *et al.* (2005b). EASE: Examination of Anomalous Self-Experience. *Psychopathology,* **38**, 236–58.

Parnas, J., Nordgaard, J. and Varga, S. (2010). The concept of psychosis: A clinical and theoretical analysis. *Clinical Neuropsychiatry*, **7**, 32–7.

Parnas, J., Raballo, A., Handest, P., Vollmer-Larsen, A. and Sæbye, D. (2011). Self-experience in the early phases of schizophrenia: 5 years follow-up of the Copenhagen Prodromal Study. *World Psychiatry*, **10**(3), 200–4.

Parnas, J. and Sass, L. A. (2008). Varieties of "phenomenology": On description, understanding, and explanation in psychiatry. *In* K. Kendler and J. Parnas (eds.), *Philosophical Issues in Psychiatry: Explanation, Phenomenology, and Nosology.* Baltimore, MD: Johns Hopkins University Press, pp. 239–77.

Parnas, J. and Sass, L.A. (2011). *The structure of self-consciousness in schizophrenia.* In S. Gallagher (ed.), *The Oxford Encyclopedia of the Self.* Oxford: Oxford University Press, pp. 521–46.

Parnas, J. and Zahavi, D. (2002). The role of phenomenology in psychiatric classification and diagnosis. In M. Maj, W. Gaebel, J. J. Lopez- Ibor, and N. Sartorius (eds), *Psychiatric Diagnosis and Classification* (World Psychiatric Association series in Evidence and Experience in Psychiatry). Chichester: John Wiley & Sons Ltd., pp. 137–62.

Raballo, A. and Parnas, J. (2011). The silent side of the spectrum: Schizotypy and the schizotaxic self. *Schizophrenia Bulletin,* **37**(5), 1017–26.

Raballo, A., Saebye, D., and Parnas, J. (2011). Looking at the schizophrenia spectrum through the prism of self-disorders: An empirical study. *Schizophrenia Bulle*tin, **37**(2), 344–51.

Ratclifffe, M. (2008). *Feelings of being: Phenomenology, psychiatry and the sense og reality.* Oxford: Oxford University Press.

Rümke, H. C. (1951). *Significance of phenomenology for the clinical study of sufferers of delusion.* *In* F. Morel (ed.), *Psychopathologie des Délires* (Congrès International de Psychiatrie, Paris 1950). Paris: Herman & Cie, pp. 174–205.

Saks, E. (2007). *The Center Can Not Hold: Memoirs of My Schizophrenia.* London: Vargo.

Sass, L. A., and Parnas, J. (2003). Schizophrenia, consciousness, and the self. *Schizophrenia Bulletin*, **29**, 427–44.

Sass, L. A., and Parnas, J., (2007). Explaining schizophrenia: The relevance of phenomenology. In M. C. Chung, K. W. M. Fulford and G. Graham (eds.), *Reconceiving Schizophrenia.* Oxford: Oxford University Press, pp. 63–95.

Schmidt, G. (1940). Der Wahn im deutschschprachigen Schrifttum der letzten 25 Jahre (1914–1939). *Zentralblatt für die gesamte Neurologie und Psychiatrie*, **97**, 113–43.

Schneider, C. (1930). *Die Psychologie der Schizophrenen.* Leipzig: Georg Thieme Verlag.

Schneider, K. (1949). Zum Begriff des Wahns. *Fortschritte der Neurologie Psychiatrie und ihrer Grenzgebiete*, **17**, 26–31.

Schneider, K. (1950/1959). *Klinische Psychopathologie* (3. vermehrte Auflage der Beiträge zur Psychiatrie ed.) *Stuttgart: Thieme.* Hamilton, M. W. and Anderson, E. W. (trans.) (1959). *Clinical Psychopathology.* New York: Grune and Stratton.

Schwartz, M. A. and Wiggins, O. P. (1987a). Diagnosis and ideal types: A contribution to psychiatric classification. *Comprehensive Psychiatry*, **28**, 277–291.

Schwartz, M. A. and Wiggins, O. P. (1987b). Typifications: The first step for clinical diagnosis in psychiatry. *J Nerv Ment Dis*, **175**(2), 65–77.

Sigmund, D. and Mundt, C. (1999). The cycloid type and its differentiation from core schizophrenia: A phenomenological approach. *Comprehensive Psychiatry*, **40**, 4–18.

Spitzer, M. (1988a). Psychiatry, philosophy; The problem of description. In M. Spitzer, F. A. Uehlein and G. Oepen (eds.), *Psychopathology and Philosophy*. Berlin: Springer, pp. 3–18.

Spitzer, M. (1988b). Ichstšrungen: In search of a theory. In M. Spitzer, F. A. Uehlein and G. Oepen (eds.), *Psychopathology and Philosophy*. Berlin: Springer, pp. 167–183.

Spitzer, M. (1990). On defining delusions. *Comprehensive Psychiatry*, **31**, 377–397.

Spitzer, R.L., First, M.B., Kendler, K.S. and Stein, D.J. (1993). The reliability of three definitions of bizarre delusions. *American Journal of Psychiatry*, **150**(6), 880–4.

Stransky, E. (1904). Zur Auffassung gewisser Symptome der Dementia praecox. *Neurologisches Zentralblatt*. **23**, 1137–43.

Tandon, R., Nasrallah, H.A. and Keshavan, M.S. (2009). Schizophrenia, "just the facts" 4. Clinical features and conceptualization. *Schizophrenia Research*, **110**, 1–23.

Tatossian, A. (1979). *Phénoménologie des psychoses*. Paris: Masson.

Taylor, M.A., Shorter, E., Vaidya, N.A. and Fink, M (2010). The failure of the schizophrenia concept and the argument for its replacement by hebephrenia: applying the medical model for disease recognition. *Acta Psychiatrica Scandinavica, ***122**, 173–83.

Van Os, J. (2010). Are psychiatric diagnoses of psychosis scientific and useful? The case of schizophrenia. *Journal of Mental Health*, **19**(4), 305–17.

Vollmer-Larsen, A., Handest, P., and Parnas, J. (2007). Reliability of measuring anomalous experience: The Bonn Scale for the assessment of basic symptoms. *Psychopathology, ***40**(5), 345–8.

Wernicke, C. (1900) *Grundriss der Psychiatrie in klinischen Vorlesungen*. Leipzig: Thieme.

Wittgenstein, L. (1953). *Philosophical Investigation (tr. G.E.M. Anscombe)*. Oxford: Blackwell.

Wittman, P. and Sheldon, W. (1948). A proposed classification of psychotic behavior reactions. *American Journal of Psychiatry*, **105**, 124–8.

World Health Organization (1974). Glossary of terms. In *International Classification of Diseases* (8th ed.). Geneva: WHO.

World Health Organization (1974). *International Classification of Diseases* (8th ed.). Geneva: WHO.

World Health Organization (1992). *The ICD-10 Classification of Mental and Behavioural Disorders. Clinical descriptions and diagnostic guidelines*. Geneva: WHO.

Wyrsch, J. (1946). Über die Intuition bei der Erkennung der Schizophrenen. *Schweizerische Med. Wochenschrift*, **46**, 1173–6.

Zahavi, D. (2005). *Subjectivity and Selfhood: Investigating the First-Person Perspective*. Cambridge, MA: MIT Press.

Phenomenology, nosology and prototypes

Kenneth S. Kendler

There is much to be enthusiastic about in this chapter. It is beautifully written and, although not its primary intent, it in fact constitutes an excellent summary of a range of key psychopathological concepts in schizophrenia. I will refer trainees to this chapter for just that purpose. It also raises a range of conceptual, diagnostic and philosophical points only a subset of which can feasibly be dealt with here. However, I would be so bold as to speculate that its primary purpose was to provide a tough critique of what American psychiatry, in general, and the DSM process, more specifically, has done with the concept of schizophrenia. As an American-born and trained psychiatrist, and one who worked on DSM-III-R and DSM-IV, one who was, for DSM-IV, a member of the Psychotic Disorder Work-Group that produced the criteria for schizophrenia, and who is centrally involved in a number of debates about DSM-5, I am in a good position to respond to his critique.

To the main thrust of Dr Parnas's comments, my response can be succinctly summarized as a: "*Yes, but. . .*" Let's start with the "Yes" part. I fully share Dr Parnas's concern with, what I would call, the "cheapening of descriptive psychopathology" in American psychiatry, generally, and the DSM process, more specifically. American Psychiatry in the last 30 years, in part through DSM-III, has emerged as a dominant paradigm in the world. Also, for better and for worse, for a range of historical and cultural reasons, the tradition of descriptive psychopathology which was so influential in European psychiatry never took strong hold in the US. I cannot hope to give a thorough analysis of the reasons here, nor am I really qualified to do so. But here are my guesses of the key factors. First, we Americans see ourselves as a pragmatic people. We do not share the cultural fascination with intellectuals with a philosophical bent that has been especially common in France and Germany in the 20th century. Compare, for a moment, the figures of John Dewey, William James and (much more recently) John Searle, with the likes of Hegel, Husserl, Sartre, Heidegger and Merleau-Ponty. Quite a contrast! As John Searle popularly says, "Watch out for those damn German philosophers whose names starts with H!" Second, modern science, in general, and American psychiatry, in particular, suffers from a bad case of "Presentism." One is looked askance at referencing something 5 years old, let alone 50 or 100!

Third, it is difficult to underestimate the impact of the linguistic barrier. In what is surely a sad state of affairs, very few of the current leaders in American psychiatry born after 1940 are fluent in any language but English. While more and more high-quality descriptive psychopathology has become available in translation in the last 20 years (with one key contributor being the journal *History of Psychiatry*, edited by G. Berrios), very little of this is read by leading psychiatrists. Fourth, in America, more than in almost any country in Europe, psychoanalysis achieved widespread dominance in academic psychiatry from the 1930s through the 1960s. Famously, with a few exceptions, psychoanalysis was uninterested in diagnosis as they viewed symptoms and signs as merely "surface phenomenon." In the 1970s, we saw a rapid cultural-historical switch from psychoanalysis to biological psychiatry as the dominant paradigm. The latter was hardly more interested in the phenomenology of psychiatric illness than the former. They certainly accepted operationalized diagnostic criteria, but the interest largely ended there. The model would be the senior biological psychiatrist handing any one of a variety of structured interviews to his senior resident and telling him to, "Go get me 20 cases of RDC (Research Diagnostic Criteria (Spitzer et al. 1975)) schizophrenia."

Fifth, the key leaders in American psychiatric nosology—Eli Robins, Sam Guze, Bob Spitzer, Allen Frances and David Kupfer—were not chosen because of the level of knowledge or sophistication in Continental descriptive psychiatry, and certainly not of phenomenology. Rather, their focus was typically imminently practical—they wanted facts, simple diagnostic criteria, and clear empirical rules for deciding what diagnostic criteria to value.

So, do I share Dr Parnas's view that American psychiatry would be better off if its leaders and trainees were better versed in the history and practice of psychopathology in the European tradition? Absolutely! I also practice what I preach, as I do my best given my shameful linguistic limitations, to read widely and teach in this literature.

Now, let us come to the: "but." This has several parts. First, I am strongly influenced by Robins and Guze, Spitzer, and Anglo-American analytic philosophy and proud of some of the advances they made. I see problems with reliability to be very important to the scientific foundation of psychiatry. We cannot practically expect all psychiatrists, research interviewers or family doctors to be expert in phenomenology. For both routine clinical care and research, we need diagnostic tools that are as straightforward as possible and, critically, that can be reliably rated. I had a discussion with Bob Spitzer about why he selected some of Schneider's first-rank symptoms to be included in the RDC (Spitzer et al. 1975) and not others. His response was that he picked thought broadcasting, insertion and withdrawal because they could be easily explained to interviewers and elicited on structured interview. However, he singled out another of the first-rank symptoms, delusional percept (or as Parnas calls it, a "primary delusion"), as an example of a criterion he would want not to choose. He notes that he had a very hard time explaining to people what it meant and that, after reading Schneider and a few other German psychiatrists—several times—he wasn't exactly sure what they meant either! I have some sympathy with this position and to be fair, Dr Parnas agrees that DSM criteria have succeeded in at least this one aim: producing a reliable diagnosis of schizophrenia. (As a side note, at no point was it ever intended that all of Schneider's first-rank symptoms would or should be incorporated into the RDC or DSM systems, or that the DSM should, in Parnas's words, "claim a faithful epistemological-conceptual or phenomenological continuity with Schneider.")

My point can perhaps be best illustrated by a research project with which I was involved some years ago on definitions of bizarre delusions (Spitzer et al. 1993). Could we improve on the DSM-III-R (and DSM-IV) definition, which Dr Parnas criticizes, that runs basically like this: a phenomenon that the person's culture would regard as totally implausible? We examined two candidates, the first of which simply assessed the physical impossibility of the delusional belief. The second one, for which I advocated, was based on the Jasperian concept of "un-understandable" (Jaspers 1963). We recorded 180 independent delusions from patient charts and had a series of expert reviewers (including me). In preparing for the study, we had to prepare what we hoped would be a short sheet of explanations for our raters. We found that we could define the cultural implausibility and physical impossibility criteria with examples, each one short page in length. However, to explain and illustrate Jaspers's more subtle concept so that it would be clearly understood by these expert raters took more than two pages. My hope that Jaspers's concept—which I found more conceptually appealing—would perform better was not to be. Kappa reliability coefficients were moderate and nearly identical for the DSM cultural implausibility and the physical impossibility criteria: +0.64 and +0.65, respectively. Both were substantially higher than we observed for Jaspers's un-understandability criterion (+0.45). For me, this project starkly highlighted the conflict between the conceptual appeal of rich psychopathological concepts and the practical problems of implementing them in research settings. The ideas might be great, but getting them to be reliably rated can be problematic. That said, if we had interviewed our patients directly and tried to obtain a more in-depth picture of their delusional beliefs and experiences (which we did not in this study), the results might have been different.

So, I view Dr Parnas's concerns from the perspective of someone who has run large-scale field studies where our goals were to interview thousands of subjects. While I appreciate the subtle information that can be obtained by a detailed interview with a skilled and learned clinician, that is just not always feasible in such situations. Scientific advances require some sacrifice in terms of subtlety to be able to scale up to the numbers needed, for example, to clarify the action of genetic risk factors.

Dr Parnas's response might well be that we are sacrificing validity on the altar of reliability. My response to him would be simple: "Prove it." By the traditional validators that we use to evaluate our diagnostic categories (Kendler 1980; Robins and Guze 1970), the DSM diagnosis of schizophrenia does pretty well. It is good at predicting outcome and familial aggregation. Diagnostic stability is substantial and it is validated by a number of anatomic changes in the brain and neuropsychological correlates. If we adopted his diagnostic approach to schizophrenia, how much better would it perform on these tried and true measures? Would it be equally reliable in the hands of less skilled clinicians? Remember, if the evaluation takes three times as long and results in only a modest improvement in validity, for some large-scale studies that might not be a good tradeoff.

I am not entirely convinced about his interpretation of the fate of hebephrenia. In the Roscommon Family study, where we used blind best estimate diagnosis based on both high-quality interviews and hospital records, we diagnosed hebephrenia in 17.5% of the schizophrenia probands (Kendler et al. 1994). Admittedly, this was with DSM-III-R, which had somewhat broader criteria for the disorganized subtype than DSM-IV. Also, this study was done in the 1980s so I cannot address his claim of a more recent decline in prevalence of hebephrenic schizophrenia. However, we saw a number of meaningful differences in terms of age of onset and course, between the disorganized and paranoid subtypes. So the diagnoses carried some predictive validity.

Another point that deserves mention is that all the important features of a disorder need not be included in diagnostic criteria. Diagnostic criteria have important pragmatic aims—to classify accurately with maximal efficiency. Subtle phenomenological features of the experience of individuals with schizophrenia are important to help us understand important features of the disorder and can help us clinically in individual cases. But that does not mean that they have to be part of the diagnostic criteria if (a big if admittedly) their assessment is not required to identify accurately affected people. If possible, it is better to select diagnostic criteria that are easily and reliably assessed.

Finally, let me comment briefly on the rich topic of "gestalt and prototype." Again, the Atlantic is a potent divide. I cannot recall at any point in the dozens and dozens of hours of discussion on criteria for schizophrenia in which I participated during the work on DSM-IV where this subject was a major focus. In my training, the "praecox feeling" was mentioned once or twice as an example of the terrible and unscientific practices of an earlier generation that we best avoid at all costs. Do experienced clinicians develop a "sense" of a schizophrenic patient early in an interview? Certainly! Can I tell sometimes with the briefest contact that an unkempt homeless person who might be gesticulating peculiarly with that "odd look" in their eyes has a good chance of being schizophrenia? Yes. The task as I see it, which Dr Parnas is well positioned to pursue, is how to bring these important but hard to define impressions into a more scientific light and to show, if we can, that they can be reliably rated and have high sensitivity and specificity. He will, I suspect, have an uphill battle with American psychiatry here. But that does not mean it is not worth the effort.

In summary, I share many of Dr Parnas's values. We have impoverished our intellectual and clinical lives in American psychiatry by our lack of knowledge and appreciation for the rich descriptive psychiatric tradition that he represents. But I will still defend the DSM concept of schizophrenia. Much empirical data suggests that this definition does a lot of what we want. I do not claim is it perfect—or that it represents an optimal description of this deeply complex syndrome. But I would challenge Dr Parnas to prove that the construct which he defends performs in a superior fashion on these key validators. As might be expected given my background, I am not as pessimistic as Dr Parnas about the current status and future of psychiatric nosology. Should we teach and read classics of descriptive psychiatry more than we do? Absolutely! Is the current status of the DSM process hopelessly muddled and in need of an entire overhaul? I don't think so. It does have a number of problems. As outlined in my chapter in this volume (Chapter 15), the deepest concern is to ensure the cumulative nature of the nosologic enterprise. But do we have "basic epistemological issues haunting psychopathology" that need to be "addressed, discussed, and re-dressed" and which would thereby "entail a dramatic and massive re-learning of what psychiatry is about and how it should be exercised." I am not convinced that we are quite that badly off.

Comments References

Jaspers, K. (1963). *General Psychopathology*. Chicago, IL: University of Chicago Press.

Kendler, K. S. (1980). The nosologic validity of paranoia (simple delusional disorder). A review. *Archives of General Psychiatry*, **37**(6) 699–706.

Kendler, K. S., McGuire, M., Gruenberg, A. M. and Walsh, D. (1994). Outcome and family study of the subtypes of schizophrenia in the west of Ireland. *American Journal of Psychiatry*, **151**(6) 849–56.

Robins, E. and Guze, S. B. (1970). Establishment of diagnostic validity in psychiatric illness: its application to schizophrenia. *American Journal of Psychiatry*, **126**(7) 983–7.

Spitzer, R. L., Endicott, J., and Robins, E. (1975). *Research Diagnostic Criteria for a Selected Group of Functional Disorders* (2nd ed.). New York: New York Psychiatric Institute.

Spitzer, R.L., First, M. B., Kendler, K. S., and Stein, D. J.(1993). The reliability of three definitions of bizarre delusions. *American Journal of Psychiatry*, **150**(6) 880–4.

Part V

The way(s) forward

Chapter 13

Introduction

Josef Parnas

Dr McHugh offers the reader a concise critique of the DSM-III/IV and related psychiatric culture, a critique followed by quite concrete proposals of improvements of our classification. I believe that McHugh's recommendations will find a grateful echo in the hearts of the majority of clinical psychiatrists. In a certain sense, this is one of the most straightforward and pragmatically oriented chapters of the book (but see Ghaemi, Chapter 3, this volume, for related ideas).

McHugh's paper may be read in continuation of Andreasen's pessimistic assessment of the heritage of DSM-III's "operational revolution" (Andreasen 2007). McHugh recognizes stagnation and misdirections of the past 30 years that have passed since the DSM-III, then proclaimed as a so-called agnostic or atheoretical approach to classification. Thus classification became based on symptom likeness and diagnosis on "symptom counting," says McHugh, and classification was deprived of any overarching, guiding intelligibility principle. This official agnostic stance allowed for a steady proliferation of diagnostic entities, and may "have bred as many fallacies and misdirections (. . .) as did those explanatory 'theories' it replaced."

In the constructive part of his chapter, McHugh looks up to the *medical model* for help and outlines several steps adopted in such model for classificatory purposes. He advocates "a change based on fundamentals that render mental disorders intelligible and thus ultimately explicable." One issue that merits a special attention here is his recommendation of a return to a thorough clinical psychiatric interview, providing bottom-up information for diagnosis (including biographical data and mental status examination). McHugh sees consciousness as psychiatry's target domain and the concept of emergence as the best way of linking consciousness to the brain. I will leave to the reader the pleasure of suspense in following McHugh's steps through which he proposes to rework psychiatric nosology.

I will end this introduction with two remarks of partial dissent. First, DSM was never atheoretical because there is no such system. Rather, as McHugh himself remarks, the "bio-psycho-social" turned into "bio-bio-bio." Yes, consciousness is indeed the target domain of psychiatry. Yet, precisely for this very reason psychiatry needs other conceptual and methodological resources than those solely offered by the medical model. Consciousness is not a spatial object. To deal with consciousness, to address it without undue simplification, distortion or reification, we need some help from phenomenological psychopathology and philosophy of mind. Only such refinement of psychopathology can make our phenotypic descriptions and distinctions useful for linking the phenotypes to biological substrate of interest and to form an integrative bridge to neuroscience (Parnas and Bovet 1995; Parnas and Sass 2008).

Introduction References

Andreasen, N. C. (2007). DSM and the death of phenomenology in America: An example of unintended consequences. *Schizophrenia Bulletin*, **33/1**, 108–12.

Parnas, J., and Bovet, P. (1995) Research in psychopathology: Epistemological issues. *Comprehensive Psychiatry*, **36**, 167–181.

Parnas, J., and Sass, L.A. (2008). Varieties of "phenomenology": On description, understanding, and explanation in psychiatry. In K. Kendler and J. Parnas (eds.), *Philosophical Issues in Psychiatry: Explanation, Phenomenology, and Nosology*. Baltimore, MD: Johns Hopkins University Press), pp. 239–77.

Chapter 13

Rendering mental disorders intelligible: addressing psychiatry's urgent challenge

Paul R. McHugh

13.1 The issue

In contrast to most other medical specialties, psychiatry has yet to "come of age," i.e., matured as a clinical practice of applied science providing rational treatments directed at known causes of patients' disorders. A generation ago (1980) the profession's authorities, believing that the discipline was intractably divided into camps warring over the causes and treatments of mental disorders, proposed a consoling agnosticism about these matters and promoted a method for naming and distinguishing disorders based on those features all could recognize, namely the symptoms. In good faith they presented what amounted to an epistemological, "knowledge-theory" approach to diagnosis—"reliability first, validity second"—in the hope that eventually stability of diagnostic discourse would lead practitioners and investigators together to discern the true natures of mental illnesses and their best treatments.

In line with this approach the editors of the disciplinary manual (*Diagnostic and Statistical Manual of Mental Disorders* (DSM)) had it operate as a denotative classification abandoning any effort to "key" the mental disorders according to their natures. Rather in its third edition (DSM-III) they aggregated and defined the disorders by diagnostic "criteria" based on their clinical appearance. In this way they chose to use an "artificial" rather than a "natural" key to identify and distinguish disorders—not, it must be admitted, so different from Ptolemaic astronomers using motion in the sky to differentiate "fixed stars" from "planets."

Despite an introductory statement by the editors of DSM that clinical experience and judgment are essential for the proper use of the manual, it functions in identifying mental disorders just as does a naturalist's field guide for naming birds, wild flowers or trees with all the seductive ease and narrow purposes of that "artificial" classificatory method. The manual became a "best seller" outside of psychiatry and medicine— novelists are said to consult it for shaping their characters and trial lawyers keep it handy when defending or prosecuting clients.

At first several of its advantages—as in pacifying clinical argument and in providing consistency for cross-laboratory case identification and for population-wide census of mental disorders—obscured its weaknesses. But, they emerged with practice over time.

For example: as symptom counting blurred meaningful patient distinctions the use of diagnoses such as major depression and attention deficit disorder spread beyond credibility (Parker 2005). So many new mental disorders were "recognized" (but not explained) that the manual grew thicker edition after edition. Too often the use of the manual by advocates with political, ideological and even financial commitments for claims about the nature and treatment of disorders (such as dissociative identity disorder and post-traumatic stress disorder (PTSD)) embarrassed the profession and re-awakened some of the disciplinary conflict that DSM-III was intended to pacify (McHugh and Treisman 2007).

DSM's agnostic method, lacking any principle for denying its official recognition to any proposed entity conceived and vigorously advanced by a sizable group of advocates, may have bred as many fallacies and misdirections in psychiatry as did those explanatory "theories" it replaced (McHugh 2008).

The agnostic stance has not proven much more successful on the therapeutic side of the discipline. If mental disorders are identified by symptoms rather than by cause or nature, then treatments must be symptomatic and mostly "rule of thumb." This explains the haphazard outcomes (Fournier et al. 2010) with many medications (despite their promises as "anti-depressants," "anti-psychotics," "mood stabilizers," etc.). Horwitz and Wakefield in their aptly titled monograph, *The Loss of Sadness* (2007), identify the absence of coherence in assessment and treatment when normal grief is, as so often the case, mistaken to be major depression.

A stark, apt observation on these unintended consequences was voiced in his presidential address to a recent meeting of the American Psychiatric Association by Dr. Steven Sharfstein. "We have allowed the bio-psycho-social model to become the bio-bio-bio model" he announced with chagrin to an audience that responded with a standing ovation.

Recently and disconcertingly (Kupfer et al. 2010), the present DSM editors, many of the same people who encouraged the agnostic idea some 30 years ago, now say that despite the time and energies invested in practice and research under its umbrella, the practical results have been insufficient to propose for the new edition (DSM-5) an approach that even bows towards grouping disorders by their natures. They specifically say, "Psychiatry as a field and DSM users in general are not yet ready for a drastic overhaul of DSM's organization" (p. 90), confirming, for those interested in matters methodological, that the natural tendency of epistemology is to preserve a scientific status quo rather than encourage new thinking and action.

Surely, something better should be suggested and tried than a method used for over a generation and still so troubled. The adage holds: "nothing can be more dangerous than an idea when it's the only one you have."

What we have previously proposed (McHugh 2005; McHugh and Slavney 1998) (and I intend to reiterate here) is not so much a fundamental change but a change based on fundamentals that render mental disorders intelligible and thus ultimately explicable. It proposes a frame of reference, derived from an approach familiar to doctors, revealing what mental disorders exist and how. Being an ontologic (what exists?) rather than an epistemologic (how do you know?) approach it intends to free psychiatrists from the fading prospects of "reliability first, validity second" by proposing the challenging path of "intelligibility first, explanation second."

13.2 **The idea**

The method begins by addressing the question "From what comprehensible and empirically based explanatory principles do physicians and surgeons derive their systematic knowledge and rational therapies that might today be employed in psychiatry for mental disorders?" These principles—specifically propositions illuminating what disorders exist in nature and how—are not difficult to discern given that they configure the International Classification of Diseases (ICD) that DSM is intended to accompany.

Medical disorders are classified (as in ICD-10) according to two critical aspects of the nature of an affliction: (1) the organ or part affected (the "localization") and (2) its generation or pathogenesis (the "process").

Ever since William Harvey discerned the pump function of the heart and the circulation of the blood noting "the number of questions that can be settled, doubts resolved, and obscure places made clear given this illuminating truth, in every part of medicine" (Keele 1965), the concepts of "Localization" of pathology (as affecting the functioning of heart, lung, kidney etc.) and the pathogenic "Process" (as found in vascular, infectious, traumatic, neoplastic, etc. guises) have, in intelligible and progressive ways, directed coherent medical and surgical thought and practice. As became apparent to Harvey, "localization" could explain most of the signs and symptoms of an illness whereas "process" could make sense of its course and, by implication, its rational as against symptomatic treatment.

Psychiatrists can and should start employing such fundamental concepts in their discipline today. They can draw upon much implicit knowledge accrued by clinicians and upon investigative enterprises especially spurred during the last three decades by the diagnostic consistency of DSM. From these sources they can propose simple, intelligible hypotheses about the nature and causes of mental afflictions (making sense of what exists and how), describe what these proposals imply for patient assessment, treatment, and research, and eventually work with the results.

13.3 **The specific elements**

There are three steps in applying "medical" reasoning to psychiatry. Step 1: illustrate and explain how "localization" can be applied to features of consciousness. Step 2: identify "processes" that either damage or misdirect these features. Step 3: tie localization and process together for what they entail for treatment and research.

Each of these steps has a conceptual, empirical foundation particular to the discipline of psychiatry. They are fully compatible, though, with the methods that have advanced the understanding and treating of physical disorders.

Step 1: illustrate and explain how one can apply the concept of "localization" when referring to features of consciousness

Psychiatrists often hesitate over this issue asking how the psychological domain can offer a place or render support to a concept such as "localization" carrying as it does connotations of site and structure? In fact, some psychiatric authorities hold that only progress in neurology, with its material foundations in brain tissue and neuronal systems, can render mental disorders scientifically comprehensible. They imply and sometimes flatly state that psychiatrists must await the neurologists rather than command their own future.

We've long believed this problem should and can be confronted directly as it hinders the disciplinary discourse. Psychiatrists can join with neuroscientists (for example, Michael Gazzaniga in his 2009 Gifford Lectures) who note that consciousness (wherein mental and behavioral disorders have their expression) is an "emergent property" of the brain and not a "product" of the brain as bile is a product of the liver or urine a product of the kidney.

That is: the conscious mind is a functional biological domain that, although evoked by and contingent upon the integrative actions of brain elements, has features of its own (faculties, responses, drives, etc.) that, in dynamic, programmatic ways, assume roles and responsibilities in human life. These unique properties of consciousness justify separating psychology and psychiatry from neuroscience and neurology. They also imply that there will be different "kinds" of mental disorders—those that reflect damage to the neural systems supporting mental life and those that represent misdirection/misalignment of mind and behavior provoked by personal encounters and situational demands.

The concept of emergence is an empirical one spelled out thoroughly in the 19th century by such people as George Lewes and John Stuart Mill. Both T. H. Huxley and Niels Bohr, in explaining the concept of emergence to other scientists, used the analogy of water emerging from combining hydrogen and oxygen. They pointed out how water, with its features of liquidity and its powers as a solvent etc., was qualitatively unlike anything the most thorough knowledge of its elemental components predict and, as an emergent phenomenon, demanded its own scientific study (Mayr 2004).

This analogy should encourage psychiatric confidence in emergence as the best way of linking human consciousness and the brain. And, to continue the analogy, just as when one has trouble with water, one calls a plumber not an atomic physicist, so when one has trouble with mind, one should call a psychiatrist not a neuroanatomist. But, only the psychiatrist who can identify the mind's component features and how they are disrupted is prepared for the call.

Four interactive but conceptually separable functional "sets" (Marini and Singer 1988) comprise the emergent features of mind: (1) the "intrinsic" set that includes features such as consciousness itself and other staples of the mind such as perception, memory, language and affect. (2) The "self-differentiating" set that includes each individual's characteristic intelligence (IQ), temperament, and maturational stage. (3) The "teleological" set that encompasses those features of mind that organize and inform goal-directed behaviors such as appetites, drives, intentions, choices and habit conditioning. (4) The "extrinsic/experiential" set comprised of the features that, responding to life events, social networks, education and all the influences of family life, occupation and culture, bring about individuation, psychosocial development and character formation.

Normal mental life takes shape from the dynamic interaction of these four sets. Likewise they represent the psychological sites for "localizing" the pathogenic "processes" that beget mental unrest and disorder.

Step 2: identify "processes" that can damage or misdirect these features of mind

In making this step in delineating mental disorders according to their nature, my colleague Phillip Slavney and I proposed what we called "the Perspectives of Psychiatry" (1998). With this metaphor of "perspective" we suggested that one could, by "looking into" the personal history and mental state of a disturbed person, appreciate some "process" provoking his or her symptoms even while appreciating that other "ways of looking" would help one "see" other causal contributions to a disorder and note how, in the "whole person," psychological strengths and vulnerabilities contribute to the expressed condition.

We proposed four distinct "Perspectives": the Disease Perspective (what a patient "has"), the Dimensional Perspective (what a patient "is"), the Behavior Perspective (what a patient ("does") and the Life Story Perspective (what a patient "encountered"). These "perspectives" highlight "processes" generating mental disorders and tie them to the "localizations" within mind identified as the intrinsic factors, self-differentiating factors, teleological factors, and extrinsic/experiential factors.

Diseases of the brain primarily disrupt intrinsic features of mind. In fact each intrinsic feature can be separately and explicitly damaged giving rise to a specific mental disorder. For example delirium is the clinical manifestation of a disease process disrupting consciousness, dementia cognition, bipolar disorder affect, and schizophrenia the integrative and executive capacities built into conscious life. A conceptual triad frames the explanatory approach of the Disease Perspective and, familiar to internal medicine and neurology, renders these particular conditions clinically intelligible; etiology—pathology—clinical syndrome.

With some of these psychiatric diseases we know the specifics of etiology and pathology in detail, but for others, although rendered intelligible by the concept of disease, we await a full explanation. For example, the pathogenesis and pathophysiology of bipolar disorder and schizophrenia remain elusive, but identifying the nature of such conditions as diseases a patient "has" encourages research framed by the disease triad as David Lewis and his group in Pittsburgh describe with schizophrenia. (Lewis et al. 2005). Notice how their work exemplifies the ontological approach of "intelligibility first, explanation second."

Quite different in nature are the disorders tied to what a patient "is" that the Dimensional Perspective grasps. Here an encounter with personally challenging circumstances provokes symptoms and disorders dependent upon and explained by the self-differentiating factors. Again a framing triad of generative interrelations makes sense of this family of disorders (most encompassed in DSM on Axis II): personal vulnerability—provocative life circumstance—emotional/behavioral responses.

The key to the nature of these conditions comes from recognizing that graded measurable dispositional features such as intelligence and temperament are universal, constitutional, dimensional characteristics that characterize persons psychologically and individually in the same way that height and weight characterize them physically. Individuals, who by constitution stand at the extremes of these dimensions, are vulnerable to being disturbed and emotionally disrupted by circumstances others would manage successfully.

The particular dispositions most likely to represent potentials for distressful states of mind are suboptimal IQ (<80), high "neuroticism" combined with high extraversion or introversion (as measured by such psychological instruments as the NEO (Costa and McCrae 1990), and psychic immaturity. A good example of a mental disorder explained by such factors is social phobia—an affliction generated by the vulnerability to sustained and powerful "negative" conditioning found in people high in introversion and neuroticism (Brandes and Bienvenu 2006; Eysenck 1957).

Encompassed by the Behavior Perspective are those disorders tied to what a patient "does." They rest upon the "teleologic" features of mental life and appear in the form of deviant choices, habits, and intentions (Heyman 2009). They come in several distinct varieties.

Some represent problematic habitual choices tied to innate drives as in sexual paraphilias and certain eating disorders, others represent the disruptive effects of acquired drives as in alcoholism and drug addiction, others are patterns of choice provoked by social attitudes, purpose and meaning such as hysteria, anorexia nervosa and some examples of self-injury, still others develop because of the emotional arousal ("thrill") their choices provoke, such as pathological gambling and kleptomania.

Again, further research will specify more details generating particular behavioral disorders but a framing triad of interrelating factors familiar to behavioral and physiological psychologists: physiological drive—conditioned learning—problematic choice characterizes their nature and renders their study and treatment intelligible.

Finally those mental disorders grasped by the Life Story Perspective are states and symptomatic conditions that depend upon extrinsic/experiential factors of the mind and represent the emotional and behavioral reactions to life circumstances (the "encounters") that are humanly understandable and meaningful. States of mind such as grief, demoralization, homesickness, jealousy and post-traumatic stress disorder are the most common afflictions in this family. The concept of narrative or "the story" best grasps how they emerge with encounters. Again, a triad: setting—sequence—outcome frames their generative elements and renders intelligible the symptoms expressed.

These states of mind—essentially species-specific responses to distressful events—can certainly debilitate the afflicted. A recent study from Denmark (Bennedsen et al. 2008) demonstrated the loss of profitability in business enterprises led by executive officers who suffered a grief-inducing loss of a child or spouse. Also explicable under the Life Story Perspective are the distressful life outcomes of individuals exposed in childhood to crime, abuse, and parental divorce and who take on assumptions (what E.O. Laumann has referred to as "life scripts" (Browning and Laumann 1997)) that shape their decisions as adults and have sequential effects extending across lives and even generations.

Step 3: tie "localization" and "process" together for the various psychiatric disorders to identify what they entail for treatment and research

The final advantageous implication found with this method comes from deriving and identifying—and in the process de-mystifying—the therapeutic enterprises of psychiatrists.

Thus psychiatric patients suffering from diseases that disrupt the intrinsic faculties of their mind are in need of remedies that could correct the disease processes and cure the condition. When these are not available other treatments to alleviate the effects or slow the advance of the process can be sought. The place of medications and other physical treatments for disease is clear.

Individuals whose problematic dispositions render them vulnerable to exaggerated emotional reactions need guidance to help them anticipate and avoid threatening circumstances by teaching them about their special vulnerabilities and what to do about them. For example, a plan counseling abstinence from beverage alcohol for patients identified as neurotic extraverts (Axis II Cluster B patients in DSM-IV) will, if followed, do much to reduce their emotional travails.

Patients in the grip of habitual behavioral disorders need help first in interrupting their deviant choices but then, given that their behavior can both poison their minds and social circumstances (Heyman 2009), they need help in living without relapsing into their maladaptive habits. Therapeutic programs that include regular monitoring of intentions, rewarding good choices and burdening injurious ones, and structuring daily life such as does Alcoholics Anonymous are, for this reason, demonstrably successful.

Patients whose lives have been derailed by distressful encounters need therapeutic programs that offer them ways of attaching fitting meanings to their emotional reactions. Teaching patients that such states of mind as grief or post-traumatic stress disorder are normal, to be expected, and have natural courses of recovery hastens their healing.

Programs such as cognitive behavioral therapy specifically help such patients reframe or "rescript" their interpretations of their distressful life experiences and in the process change disruptive attitudes and points of view these experiences provoked. They encourage the patients to think and respond in coherent ways to what they've experienced.

As an aside to these matters of therapy (and mentioned only for completeness), a place always remains for using medications and other modes of symptomatic relief with all of these conditions—as in medications providing temporary relief for anxiety, discouragement, or demoralization or in satisfying, with a substitute, a pressing hunger for addictive substances such as heroin or nicotine. But the distinctions between what is symptomatic and temporary from what is essential and ultimately corrective can and should be made here in psychiatry as it is in general medicine.

13.4 **Making sense for today and tomorrow**

Figure 13.1 presents a graphic way of framing these concepts of "localization," "process," and "implication" hierarchically. Its intention is to support the "medical," ontologic stance about mental disorders that could come eventually to replace the "agnostic," epistemologic stance of DSM-III/IV. What psychiatrists, just like internists, need is not freedom *from* theory but freedom *within* theories that offer them an intelligible vision of scientific and clinical realities that can be studied and enlarged through experience.

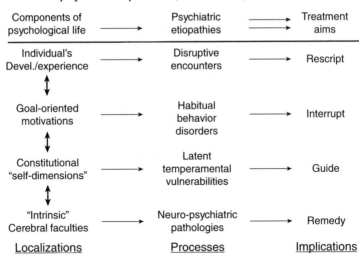

Bio-psych. Components, Processes, Treatments

Figure 13.1 A comprehensive hierarchical representation of the "perspectives of psychiatry."

What though can be done in practical terms to bring about this change for the profession? Psychiatrists are now so accustomed to the denotative diagnostic terms of DSM and so encouraged by the consistency it brought to their clinical discourse that they will be naturally reluctant to change radically. But psychiatrists need not abandon what they've gained with DSM-III/IV as they begin moving towards an intelligible sense of different mental disorders.

The simplest and easiest first step in that direction could come from DSM editors officially recognizing that Axis I disorders, despite the connotation of "Axis," are hardly of the same nature. The conditions could be organized and listed in a way that begins to speak to what naturally distinguishes them—the connotative implications of a diagnosis.

Without changing the present diagnostic criteria the Axis I disorders could easily be listed in DSM-5 so that, instead of being arranged according to "phenomenologic" features, they were organized by their presumed generative "families"—the diseases with the diseases, the behaviors with the behaviors, the encounters with the encounters. This would hardly call for "heavy lifting" given that DSM-III first gestured towards some distinctions amongst mental disorders by nature when separating the so-called Axis-II disorders from the others. Figure 13.2 displays how the several conditions could be separated into generative groups.

Such a simple classificatory rearrangement would at first hardly affect diagnostic practice as it would not alter the allocating of a diagnosis to a patient according to "criteria." It would, however, promote salutary practices in assessing patients before they were "given" a diagnosis.

In a subtle way, this simple classificatory notice of how mental disorders with similar symptoms can differ in fundamental natures—as with what a patient *has*, what a

Diseases	Behaviors	Dimensions	Life stories
Delirium	Alcohol-depend.	Subnormal IQ	Demoralization
Dementia	Drug-depend.	"neuroticism"	Grief
Frontal lobe	Sex. paraphilia	Personality dis.	Loneliness
syndrome	Anorexia/bulemia	(A,B,C clusters)	Homesickness
Schizophrenia	Sleep disorders	Immaturity	Adjustment dis.
Bipolar disorder	*Et cetera*	*Et cetera*	Jealousy
Panic disorder			PTSD
Et cetera			*Et cetera*

Figure 13.2 Arranging disorders by "perspectival" generation.

patient *is*, what a patient *does*, or what a patient *encountered*—would come to affect what psychiatrists in their assessment process strive to accomplish. Mere checklists for diagnostic "criteria"—habits of assessment that explain why conditions with similar symptoms are often confused—would soon become suspect. Just as fever or pain can be symptoms of different physical "processes" so symptoms such as depression or mood lability can occur with disease, dimensional, behavioral or life story processes and do not on their own determine the matter. Again, just as in medicine, only a full assessment of the patient will suffice.

This is why the assessment model that was standard to psychiatry before DSM-III shall soon again be viewed as professionally essential and clinically justified. All psychiatric textbooks published prior to DSM-III describe it (see, for example, Kolb (1977) and Mayer-Gross et al. (1963)). It called for a "bottom-up" study of the patient that included: (1) an extensive personal background history from birth to presentation, (2) a thorough description of the onset and progress of the presenting illness or disorder, (3) a complete mental status examination as the patient first appeared to the psychiatrist, and, whenever possible, (4) inquiry with "external informants" who knew the patient and could provide contexts and continuities enriching what the distressed patient could report.

Not only does this "bottom up" method of assessment provide information for more deliberate diagnostic formulations than any "top-down" checklist or "structured" interview, it restores to psychiatrists what was previously thought their greatest strength as physicians, namely that they "knew their patients as people," could differentiate their symptoms, and build treatment alliances accordingly.

In addition to encouraging this thorough way of assessment, the realignment of conditions would, as does moving any classificatory enterprise from an artificial towards a natural "key," enrich the daily discourse of psychiatrists and inspire their investigative energies. Science provokes research not by terminologic consistency but by presenting challenging proposals as to the nature of the objects of interest. Here is how the sequence "intelligibility first, explanation second" brings direction and energy to every enterprise of science.

For a clinical example, would it not be salutary for psychiatry to have the kind of stimulating debate and critical research that the challenging of the cause of peptic ulcer produced in internal medicine some decades ago (Marshall and Warren 1984)? Think of the helpful clamor that would break forth if the diagnostic manual even suggested that Axis I disorders such as schizophrenia, alcoholism and PTSD differ not only because their symptoms are different but because the first is a brain disease, the second a disorder of choice and the third an emotion of adjustment.

Even the editors of DSM would gain a modest but real advantage from rearranging Axis I in this fashion. It would encourage all advocates for new diagnostic entrees to specify their nature and cause rather than just provide a name and a list of "diagnostic criteria." This would hinder the overgrowth of the manual and further help to clarify which presentations are distinct "species" of disorder as against pathoplastic varieties, *formes frustes*, or some mixture of mental states.

This rearrangement need not disturb cross-laboratory research where the need for definite identifying criteria is clear. ICD-10 dealt with this issue by providing two psychiatric classificatory volumes. One labeled "clinical descriptions and diagnostic guidelines" functions to encourage the thoughtful and interpretive diagnostic formulations for individual patients such as are recommended here. The other labeled "diagnostic criteria for research" provides official sets of criteria permitting easy communication between investigators. Something of the same would relieve that hindrance to change felt and expressed by the editors of DSM as they strive to serve simultaneously the differing needs of clinicians and investigators.

13.5 **Summation**

This essay has argued that psychiatric practice needs a more intelligible grasp of mental disorders than that provided now by the DSM. Its "agnostic" strictly denotative approach to mental disorders, which may have served a pacifying purpose when proposed 30 years ago, is now at the root of a growing set of problems within the discipline that will not improve until the issues of cause and nature of mental disorders start to be resolved.

The time is right to propose that psychiatric disorders now be classified by DSM in a more connotative and intelligible way such that those with similar generative derivations (localization and process) are clustered together in a fashion analogous to that employed by medical classifiers.

Such an official act would encourage psychiatrists to elucidate, distinguish, formulate and treat patients not simply according to some recipe tied to the diagnosis assigned and the "criteria" those patients "meet," but according to what is the nature of the problems the diagnosis reveals and the therapies are aiming to correct. Psychiatrists would come to know and teach how fundamental natural differences amongst mental disorders make sense of who is a patient, what is psychopathology and ultimately what is meant by "normal" in human mental life and behavior. Then this clinical discipline will truly "come of age."

Chapter References

Bennedsen, M., Perez-Gonzalez, F. and Wolfenzon, D. (2008). *Do CEOs Matter? NYU Working Paper No. FIN-06–032* Available at SSRN: http://ssrn.com/abstract=1293659 posted November 2008.

Brandes, M. and Bienvenu, O. J. (2006). Personality and anxiety disorders. *Current Psychiatry Reports*, **8**, 263–9.

Browning C. R. and Laumann, E. O. (1997). Sexual contact between children and adults: A life course perspective. *American Sociological Review*, **62**, 540–60.

Costa, P. T. **Jr**. and McCrae, R. R (1990). Personality disorders and the five-factor model of personality. *Journal of Personality Disorders*, **4**, 362–71.

Eysenck, H. J. (1957). *The Dynamics of Anxiety and Hysteria*. New York: Frederick A. Praeger, Inc.

Fournier, J. C., DeRubeis, R. J., Hollon S. D., Hollon, S. D., Dimidjian, S., Amsterdam, J. D., *et al.* (2010). Antidepressant drug effects and depression severity: a patient-level meta-analysis. *Journal of the American Medical Association*, **303**, 47–53.

Heyman, G. M. (2009). *Addiction: A Disorder of Choice*. Cambridge, MA: Harvard University Press.

Horwitz, A. V. and Wakefield, J. C. (2007). *The Loss of Sadness: How Psychiatry Transformed Normal Sorrow into Depressive Disorder*. New York: Oxford University Press.

Keele, K. D. (1965). *William Harvey: The Man, the Physician, and the Scientist*. London: Nelson.

Kolb, L. C. (1977). *Modern Clinical Psychiatry* (9th ed.). Philadelphia, PA: W.B. Saunders Co, (chapter 8).

Kupfer, D. J., Kuhl, E. A., Narrow, W. E. and Regier, D. A. (2010). *On the Road to DSM-V. Cerebrum 2010*. New York: Dana Press, pp. 83–93.

Lewis, D. A., Hashimoto, T. and Volk, D. W. (2005). Cortical inhibitory neurons and schizophrenia. *Nature Reviews Neuroscience* **6**, 312–24.

Marini, M. M. and Singer, B. (1988). Causality in the social sciences, *Sociological Methodology*, **18**, 347–409.

Marshall, B. J. and Warren, J. R. (1984). Unidentified curved bacilli in the stomach of patients with gastritis and peptic ulceration. *Lancet*, **1**, 1311–15.

Mayer-Gross, W., Slater, E. and Roth, M. (1963). *Clinical Psychiatry* (3rd ed.) London: Cassell and Co, (chapter 2).

Mayr, E. (2004). *What Makes Biology Unique?* Cambridge: Cambridge University Press, pp. 74–7.

McHugh, P. R. (2005). Striving for coherence: Psychiatry's efforts over classification. *Journal of the American Medical Association*, **293**, 2526–8.

McHugh, P. R. (2008). *Try to Remember: Psychiatry's Clash over Meaning, Memory, and Mind*. New York: Dana Press.

McHugh P. R. and Slavney, P. R. (1998). *The Perspectives of Psychiatry* (2nd ed.). Baltimore MD: Johns Hopkins Press.

McHugh, P. R. and Treisman, G. (2007). PTSD: A problematic diagnostic category. *Journal of Anxiety Disorders* **21**, 211–22.

Parker, G. (2005). Beyond major depression. *Psychological Medicine*, **35**, 467–74.

A search for coherence

Assen Jablensky

With a characteristic eloquence, Dr McHugh presents a pithy critique of the DSM-III/ IV enterprise and of the gist of the current debate on DSM-5. To summarize his main points, the DSM system dominates the practice of psychiatry in the United States (and, to some extent worldwide). One of its positive effects is that it has brought consistency to the diagnostic discourse which, in the not too distant past, lacked a common language and was riddled with dissention. However, in Dr McHugh's "search for coherence," the top-down decision-tree process of DSM diagnosis neglects the "generative sources" of the disorders it claims to identify and ignores a century of clinical research and practice. Moreover, according to Dr McHugh, the DSM approach is predicated on the assumption that mental disorders are exclusively biologically based and that their ultimate understanding would be reducible to "as yet unattainable neurological foundations." His justified concern is that this approach ignores the accumulated and detailed knowledge and wisdom of psychiatrists and psychologists who have focused on "the essentials of mental life and its disorders." So, the unstated DSM philosophy (despite claims of it being "atheoretical") is implicitly reductionistic and ignorant of the complex issues arising in any serious discussion of the fundamental questions about the nature of mental disorders and their intrinsic relevance to the perennial question of brain and mind relationships. Dr McHugh's next argument refers precisely to this fundamental problem. He explicitly endorses a creative, though still controversial "emergentist" point of view, which can be distilled into a syllogism with two premises and a conclusion. First, "conscious mental life" is undeniably derived from neural organization and brain activity. Secondly, once "emerged" from the complex organization of the brain, it brings into existence a novel "level of capacities, properties and modes of action" which are not explicable or predictable from the properties of the underlying neural components. And finally, this novel level becomes a self-propelled domain that brings about causal determinants of mental events, in health and disease. Thus, "emergentism" postulates that an emergent system, such as conscious life, is in real life qualitatively more than the sum of properties of its underlying base components in brain structure and function. In this particular instance, the adoption of an "emergentist" position implies the acceptance of mental causation— something that cannot be directly tested by any imaginable empirical research design. Karl Jaspers wrote about two levels of interpretation of mental events—the intuitive grasping of "meaningful connections" in the stream of consciousness, and the search for objective conjunctions between brain function and psychological performance—

but he never thought that the two were reducible to one another (Jaspers 1946/1963). This is where we stand now—torn between "emergentist" thought experiments that are not amenable to empirical validation, and an implicit belief in the ultimate, future vindication of the reductionist approach. It is a particular merit of Dr McHugh's paper that it draws our attention and interest to deep and significant problems in our relationship with everyday clinical reality.

At this point we can turn to our current expectations and concerns about the future shape of psychiatric classifications, referring to the points so pertinently raised by Dr McHugh in his paper.

First, I have to bring up the comments of Dr Pincus, who had to leave the conference prior to Dr McHugh's presentation, and authorized me to convey his viewpoints. Dr Pincus points out Dr McHugh's enormous contributions to psychiatric education and his efforts to help students engage with the clinical phenomena to develop a coherent understanding of the person they are trying to help. However, Dr Pincus feels that Dr McHugh attributes to DSM-IV far too much power than it deserves, while agreeing that DSM-IV is often greatly misused. Furthermore, he disagrees with the statement that DSM-IV is locked into a purely biological interpretation of mental illness. Dr Pincus emphasizes the need for "understanding" the patient and believes that a purely descriptive nosology is not the way leading to this goal.

Concerning the issue of relevant criteria for the assessment of a classification in psychiatry, I should like to add to this discussion my own take on the problem. Can a classification of mental disorders be a biological classification? This is doubtful, at least in the foreseeable future. Psychiatric classifications and biological classifications are dissimilar in several key aspects:

- The objects classified in psychiatry are explanatory concepts, i.e., abstract entities rather than physical organisms.
- The taxonomic units of "disorders" DSM-IV and ICD-10 do not form hierarchies.
- The current psychiatric classifications contain no supraordinate, higher-level organizing concepts.

Leaving aside the vexing issue of validity of the categories, the criteria for assessing psychiatric classifications should at present focus pragmatically on their clinical relevance and utility (Kendell and Jablensky 2003), e.g.:

- Representative scope (coverage) of mental disorders that are of clinical concern.
- Capacity of discriminating between syndromes and between degrees of their expression in individual patients.
- Adaptability to different population and cultural settings.
- Reliability.
- Cognitive ease of use.
- Meeting the needs of various users.
- Reducing stigma.

In the foreseeable future, neuroscience and genetics are likely to play an increasingly important role in the understanding of the etiology and pathogenesis of psychiatric disorders. However, the extent of their impact on the diagnostic process is difficult to predict. A possible (but unlikely) scenario is the advent of an "eliminativist" or "mindless" psychiatry driven by biological models and jettisoning psychopathology. It is much more likely that clinical psychiatry will retain psychopathology as its core. The eventual outcome is less likely to depend on the knowledge base of psychiatry per se, than on the social, cultural and economic forces that shape the public perception of mental illness and determine the clinical practice of psychiatry.

In his chapter, Dr McHugh speaks from the point of view of great clinical experience and wisdom. His critique of the present state of psychiatric classification—be it DSM-IV or ICD-10—should be given considerable weight in the present debate.

Comments References

Jaspers, K. (1946/1963). *Allgemeine Psychopathologie* (7th ed.). Hoenig J. and Hamilton, M. W. (trans. and eds.) (1963). *General Psychopathology*. Manchester: Manchester University Press, pp. 302–13; 451–62.

Kendell, R. and Jablensky, A. (2003). Distinguishing between the validity and utility of psychiatric diagnoses. *American Journal of Psychiatry*, **160**, 4–12

Chapter 14

Introduction

Kenneth S. Kendler

Darrel Regier treats us to an autobiographic journey through his long and distinguished career in psychiatric epidemiology and psychiatric nosology. His broad goal is to provide us with a conceptual and historical framework for the current discussions leading up to DSM-5, a process in which he is a central player. His story indicates how closely intertwined has been the growth of psychiatric epidemiology in the US with the problems of the assessment and definition of psychiatric illness. In first-generation psychiatric epidemiology studies, assessment was by self-report symptom scales. Then, with the Feighner Criteria (Feighner et al. 1972), Research Diagnostic Criteria (Spitzer et al. 1975), and DSM-III (American Psychiatric Association 1980), operationalized diagnostic criteria became standard. This quickly led to the development of the new technology of structured interviews. As a psychiatric resident, I can still recall the thrill of watching my first structured interview with the SADS-L (Schedule for Affective Disorders and Schizophrenia-Lifetime) given to a depressed patient as part of the Collaborative Study of Depression by Gene Redmond, MD—then a young faculty member. We were very enthusiastic (and in retrospect rather full of hubris) that we had finally really solved the problem of measurement in psychiatry.

These interviews sought to produce dichotomous diagnoses as defined by the relevant criteria. One of the main problems with which Regier's essay struggles is that the criteria were, in almost all cases, created for clinical populations by psychiatrists who worked in clinical settings. It is no trivial thing to take such criteria—as instantiated in a diagnostic interview—and figure out how to calibrate it for subjects in an epidemiological study. In particular, how do measures of functioning inter-relate with clinical criteria in the definition of illness in community populations? Under what circumstances is it sensible to diagnose someone as suffering from a psychiatric disorder if he or she meets diagnostic criteria but has no evident impairment in daily life? This problem, largely rising initially in epidemiologic studies, came back to the fore with the ultimately successful debate in DSM-IV about the addition of a "clinically significant distress or impairment" criteria, on top of the other diagnostic criteria, with the goal of trying to establish a better way of distinguishing between "normal unhappiness" and psychopathology.

One useful way to think about the problem is the relative balance of false positives (well people improperly diagnosed as psychiatrically ill for whom a diagnosis and the subsequent therapy would probably be inappropriate) versus false negatives (ill individuals who miss a diagnostic cut-off but who presumably would benefit from care).

Those especially concerned about false-positives sometimes express this point by talking about the problems of the "medicalizing of normal human experience (or suffering)" or, a bit more stridently, of "unleashing waves of false epidemics." Regier outlines some of the controversies with Wakefield, Kessler, and others about this balance. Since we will never have prefect criteria, at some level we have to balance which of these problems is the greater and calibrate from there.

Let me comment briefly on one other issue in this rich essay. Regier discusses the problem of the reification of existing diagnostic criteria. Here too, there is a balance. As Regier points out, perhaps the DSM-III paradigm has major limitations. To carry those forward solely out of respect for "tradition" might be unwise. However, as I focus on in my essay in this volume ("Epistemic iteration as a historical model for psychiatric nosology: promises and limitations," Chapter 15), if you take this approach, how do you avoid a "random walk" in nosologic space? That is, what will occur if in each iteration of DSM (or ICD), folks just re-think the issues and decide they don't like the prior paradigm and change it? Is it fair to increase the empirical evidence necessary to make changes in a nosologic system? It increases the chances of an iterative process working, but only if the process is in the right ball-park. If the whole system needs a re-boot, tightening up the rigor of needed changes from the old system is a recipe for stasis and stultification. How do we get this balance right?

This thoughtful essay raises many of the current major issues in psychiatric nosology and provides an historical context for their development.

Introduction References

American Psychiatric Association (1980). *Diagnostic and Statistical Manual of Mental Disorders, Third* Edition Washington, DC, American Psychiatric Association.

Feighner, J. P., Robins, E., Guze, S. B., Woodruff, R. A., Jr., Winokur, G., and Munoz, R. (1972). Diagnostic criteria for use in psychiatric research. *Archives of General Psychiatry,* **26**(1), 57–63.

Spitzer, R. L., Endicott, J., and Robins, E. (1975). *Research Diagnostic Criteria for a Selected Group of Functional Disorders* (2nd ed.). New York: New York Psychiatric Institute.

Diagnostic threshold considerations for DSM-5

Darrel A. Regier

When I began my career in psychiatry as a resident in the early-to-mid 1970s, I had a major interest in the role of primary care physicians in providing mental health services in collaboration with community psychiatrists. My initial mentors in this area were Leon Eisenberg, MD, Chair of the Massachusetts General Hospital (MGH) Department of Psychiatry; Gerald Klerman, MD, who was Director of the MGH Lindemann Community Mental Health Center in Boston; and Alexander Leighton, MD, at the Harvard School of Public Health. Leighton had directed the community-based Stirling County Study (Leighton et al. 1960) and completed analyses and publication of the Midtown Manhattan Study (Srole 1962) when the director, Thomas Rennie, MD, died suddenly. Another critical mentor was Morton Kramer, ScD, at the National Institute of Mental Health (NIMH), who helped initiate and then support the US-UK study (Cooper et al. 1972), and who hired me in 1975 to start a primary care mental health research program at NIMH. He also introduced me to Michael Shepherd, MD, at the London Institute of Psychiatry, whose ground-breaking epidemiological studies of mental disorders in primary care settings had established the international standard for such research (Shepherd et al. 1966). His careful study of primary care physicians in England reliably found that only about 15% of the population could be identified as having significant mental disorders in a single year.

The lessons I learned from these mentors were often hard to reconcile. On the one hand, the Midtown Manhattan Study proclaimed that up to 84% of community residents had significant psychiatric symptoms that were widely interpreted as mental illness. The Stirling County Study of another community population found rates of mental disorders as high as 50%, with about 25% of the population in need of mental health services. The Stirling County and Midtown Manhattan Studies used psychiatrists to assess data obtained from survey staff, who collected data with standardized symptom questionnaires that had emerged from the US Army Neuropsychiatric Instrument (NPI) to screen World War II soldiers for mental disability. In that period, the clinical judgment of a psychiatrist was considered the gold standard of psychiatric diagnosis—even though the subsequent US/UK study showed that the reliability of mental disorder diagnoses by psychiatrists was very poor without an agreed-upon definition of terms and explicit diagnostic criteria.

After several years at NIMH, my colleagues and I produced a paper that summarized the available literature on epidemiological studies of mental disorders and mental health service use drawing on the earlier cited studies (Regier et al. 1978). However, we were most worried about false positives and the medicalization of normal human experiences and had much greater confidence in the clinical assessments of physicians with some longitudinal knowledge of all persons requesting care for identifying appropriate rates of mental disorders. The question then, as is now, is, if 84% of the population has active psychopathology, what is normal? We were not interested in the very transient mood or anxiety states that caused no impairment or need for care, and the prominent idea at the time that everyone could use a good psychoanalysis was not convincing for a good percentage of us coming out of Eisenberg's training program. The Baltimore morbidity study (Pasamanick et al. 1956) was the most prominent US example of a study that used all physicians in a community to identify the rates of all medical and mental illnesses in the community. They found a point-prevalence rate of 10% in the community, and from a well established case register, it was possible to estimate an annual incidence rate of 5% for an annual prevalence of 15%—about the same prevalence reported by Shepherd in his studies. This prevalence rate was then contrasted with available data on mental health service use that could be identified in specialty mental health, general medical, and other human services settings as well as a voluntary self-help sector—the totality of which my colleagues and I referred to as the DeFacto US Mental Health Services System (Regier et al. 1978).

At NIMH, I was asked to direct the research Division of Biometry and Epidemiology when Kramer retired to Johns Hopkins University. In the late 1970s, our NIMH primary care research unit was able to conduct under contract a very useful primary care study in the Marshfield Clinic (Regier et al. 1985) in Wisconsin that used the General Health Questionnaire (GHQ) from David Goldberg, DM (1972), as a first stage screening instrument and the Schedule for Affective Disorders and Schizophrenia (SADS-L) instrument prepared by Robert Spitzer, MD, and Jean Endicott, PhD (1977), as a second-stage instrument to assess Research Diagnostic Criteria (RDC) diagnoses (Spitzer et al. 1978) and disability status according to the Global Assessment Scale (GAS) (Endicott et al. 1976). Goldberg had been one of Shepherd's protégés, then in Manchester, who served as a consultant to this study. Although about 30% of primary care patients were identified with RDC mental disorders, only 15% of the population had a GAS score of less than 70, 9% a GAS score less than 60, and about 2% less than 50. We also found that the GAS was the best predictor of mental health service use in both the primary care and the specialty mental health sectors.

Under Kramer, the NIMH Division of Biometry and Epidemiology had historically supported the American Psychiatric Association's DSM-I (American Psychiatric Association (APA) 1952) and DSM-II (APA 1968) revisions in conjunction with the World Health Organization's (WHO) ICD-8 (WHO 1965) and ICD-9 (WHO 1977) revisions. Hence, my Research Division inherited the opportunity to support the DSM-III (APA 1980) field trials as well as to coordinate a new generation of epidemiological mental disorder studies that incorporated DSM-III criteria—supported by an endorsement from the President's Commission on Mental Health (1978) during the Carter Administration.

This Epidemiologic Catchment Area (ECA) study (Regier et al. 1984; Robins et al. 1991) was our opportunity to resolve the issue of true community prevalence rates of mental disorders defined by explicit DSM-III criteria. The case-identification instrument would be a new Diagnostic Interview Schedule (DIS) developed by Lee Robins, PhD, Spitzer, and colleagues (Robins et al. 1981) that would replace the symptom checklists of earlier surveys, which lacked diagnostic specificity. Although the Marshfield Clinic experience should have made us more cautious, we had great confidence that far lower rates of any mental disorder would be found than were identified in Midtown Manhattan and Stirling County, and that we would also identify the rates of specific mental disorders in community settings comparable to those seen in specialty mental health settings.

When 1-month point prevalence rates for mental and addictive disorders came in at about 16%, and prospective 1-year incidence rates at 12%, for a total 1-year rate of 28%, we realized it would have been very helpful to have had a measure like the GAS to assess global disability level (Regier et al. 1993). Of equal concern was that lifetime rates of any mental disorder identified in two interviews (1 year apart) were closer to 50% (Regier et al. 1998). Even higher rates in a single interview were found by Ronald Kessler, PhD, in the National Comorbidity Survey (Kessler et al. 1994), which was supported by a grant from our Division, using a somewhat different diagnostic instrument—the University of Michigan version of the Composite International Diagnostic Interview (UM-CIDI). The CIDI (Robins et al. 1988) was developed by NIMH and WHO as a slight revision of the DIS. In all of these studies, we failed to obtain information on global impairment from a scale like the GAS or the Global Assessment of Function (GAF). Clinical reappraisal studies comparing the diagnoses of subjects assessed by the lay-administered DIS and a clinician-administered DSM-III diagnostic checklist showed that clinicians often identified higher rates of some disorders among community residents.

We also noted the Robins and Guze expectations (Robins and Guze 1970) that valid diagnoses with explicit diagnostic criteria should delineate patients with separate disorders. We found, however, that strict application of the criteria could only separate disorders cleanly if there was an explicit hierarchy of disorders (e.g., a diagnosis of a higher level condition like schizophrenia would subsume symptoms associated with all lower level conditions, such as depressive or anxiety disorders). Incorporating such a hierarchy in the scoring algorithm resulted in the suppression of a great deal of useful clinical information, and its elimination provided a richer description of individual symptomatology while producing a high level of multiple DSM-III disorders or comorbidity (Boyd et al. 1984; Regier et al. 1990).

The lessons from the ECA for DSM-III-R (Regier 1987) were to drop the hierarchy and substitute the GAS for the previous rarely used DSM-III Axis V (highest level of adaptive functioning in the past year). The new Axis V became known as the GAF scale in DSM-III-R (APA 1987) and DSM-IV (APA 1994)—the latter gave full credit to Lester Luborsky, PhD, for his 1962 Health-Sickness Rating Scale (Luborsky 1962) from which the GAS and GAF were derived. However, the continued high rates of disorders found with DSM-III and DSM-III-R led the editors of DSM-IV to also add a "clinically significant distress or impairment" criteria on top of the other diagnostic criteria to help establish a better threshold for separating normality from psychopathology.

This "clinical significance" addition led me to work with colleagues William Narrow, MD, MPH; Lee Robins; and Donald Rae to re-evaluate our ECA and the NCS data to see if we could operationalize the clinical significance criteria of DSM-IV. The resulting paper showed that the 1-year prevalence rate of 28% would be reduced to about 18% if the same clinical significance criteria used to assess individual symptom thresholds was used in the scoring algorithm to establish composite diagnostic syndrome thresholds (Narrow et al. 2002).

To put it mildly, howls of protest arose from Spitzer at the presentation of that paper, first at the American Psychopathological Association (APPA) in 2000 (Regier et al. 2002) and later from Jerome Wakefield, PhD, Spitzer (1998), and others (Pincus et al. 1998) with its publication in the *Archives of General Psychiatry* (Narrow et al. 2002). Our objective was to address the probability of false positives and the risk of medicalizing normal human emotional experiences that concerned me with the Midtown Manhattan Study at the start of my career. Spitzer had been adamantly opposed to the addition of the "clinical significance criterion" in DSM-IV and used our APPA paper and the subsequent *Archives* publication as a vehicle to make his opposition public. He and Wakefield believed that diagnostic criteria alone should define disorders and that such disorders might also be recognized by better measures of their environmental context and by their association with some evolutionary or biological disadvantage. Interestingly enough, the strategy that Wakefield and his co-author Allan Horwitz, PhD, have recently taken is to assert that the way to reduce false positives is to eliminate any depression that can be associated with grief reactions and any other loss or adverse event—i.e., any adverse environmental context. Their book, *The Loss of Sadness: How Psychiatry Transformed Normal Sorrow into Depressive Disorder* (Horowitz and Wakefield 2007), was based on this theory and some rather selective analyses of the NCS (Wakefield et al. 2007). Lost completely in this conceptual approach is the reality of gene–environmental interactions for individuals exposed to adverse events with a genetic vulnerability to a major depressive disorder. It is safe to say that analyses of Avshalom Caspi, PhD (Caspi et al. 2003), Sidney Zisook, MD, and Kenneth Kendler, MD (Kendler et al. 2008), have likely convinced the DSM-5 Mood Disorders Work Group that this use of social context is unlikely to prove convincing to either clinicians or research investigators.

Lost to the general public was another concern of Spitzer, recently raised by a different psychiatrist in *Psychiatric Times* (Moffic 2010), which was a previous paper on "Are psychiatrists still needed for making a diagnosis?" (Spitzer 1983). The underlying scientific issue is the following: can diagnostic criteria be made sufficiently explicit that non-clinicians (using the DIS) can actually separate psychopathology from normal distributions of human emotional, behavioral and cognitive expressions? The rather blatant guild issue raised in the recent *Psychiatric Times* article was the following: should non-psychiatrists be allowed to make mental disorder diagnoses even with the explicit DSM-5 criteria, or are there so many additional inferential assessments needed to make such a diagnosis that, like the famous line from a Major League Baseball umpire about calling balls and strikes, psychiatrists could claim, "it ain't nothin' till I call it"?

What is striking about this debate is that it became even more personal in an *Archives of General Psychiatry* article written by Kessler and colleagues (2003), who became alarmed that Narrow and I might have some influence on the development of DSM-5. Their concern was that DSM-5 would enact additional measures to eliminate mild cases of mental disorders that they had found in multiple epidemiological surveys using the DIS, created for the ECA study, or its international version, the CIDI. Although our concern was that DSM-III and DSM-IV criteria were admitting too many people with little-to-no distress or impairment, their analysis showed that some of the "mild" cases had as much impairment as those meeting full diagnostic criteria. Please note that this concern is directly opposite to that of Wakefield, who thought DSM-IV was letting in too many false positives—which could be eliminated not by assessing the patient's distress or impairment but only by the environmental context in which the syndrome occurred.

In response to this scientific critique, we thought it would be helpful to highlight the central issue in DSM-5 revisions very clearly and chose the James Carville approach by responding with a letter to the editor in *Archives* entitled, "For DSM-5, It's the 'Disorder Threshold,' Stupid!" (Regier et al. 2004). The purpose of this letter was to point out that we did not intend to eliminate mild cases of any disorder; we simply needed to find a way of establishing a threshold for psychopathology that differed in some quantitative or qualitative manner from normal homeostatic variations of brain functions. We also noted that the DIS and CIDI method for determining that individual symptoms were associated with "clinically significant distress or impairment" were exactly the same that Narrow et al. (2002) used in assessing whether the syndromes (composed of aggregated symptoms) met the same distress or impairment criteria.

Lee Robins had carefully observed how the residents and staff conducted clinical interviews to assess the presence of Feighner criteria in patients at Washington University and replicated the cross-examination techniques that were incorporated into the DIS probe-flow chart (i.e., "Did the symptoms interfere with your life a lot?" "Did they bother you enough that you told someone about them?" "Did they ever occur in the absence of drugs or alcohol?" "Did you have to take anything to treat these symptoms?"). Although the critics claimed that there was a potential confounding of treatment seeking with diagnosis, we pointed out that if that was their true concern, the entire epidemiological enterprise of the last 30 years would collapse like a house of cards. If the method wasn't good for syndromes, it wasn't good for symptoms. We also noted that a relatively large percentage of people who met the clinically significant syndrome criteria did so on the basis of the interference it caused with their social roles rather than from telling a doctor or other mental health professional about their symptoms. A well-known fact from most epidemiological studies is that only about half of people who meet criteria for a DSM-IV disorder in Western countries actually receive any mental health services (Regier et al. 1993; Robins et al. 1988).

It is ironic that our epidemiological and nosological critics were most concerned that the DSM-5 criteria might become too strict and leave out major segments of the population who had significant psychopathology and needed treatment—thereby creating many false negatives. In contrast, the major concern that some of these same critics have voiced more recently is that all depression in the context of grief or any other adverse life experiences should not be considered mental disorders—the result of which has been many false positives. Certainly some of the loudest concerns in the blogs and print media are that we will unleash a wave of false epidemics—with the past editor of DSM-IV claiming credit for creating false epidemics of pediatric bipolar disorder, ADHD, and autism as a result of insufficient attention to making the criteria sufficiently clear (Frances 2009). He also proclaims little confidence that the current editors can fix his problems or do better for the next edition. As Zachar (Chapter 2, this volume) documents in his historical summary of progress in the calibration and validation of scientific constructs in astronomy, biology, and psychiatry, defenders of the current construct do not yield easily to suggested changes in paradigms.

What has become abundantly clear in the epidemiological testing and attempt to validate DSM-III, DSM-III-R and DSM-IV diagnostic criteria "hypotheses" is that current hierarchically based, categorical diagnostic criteria, created to separate patient groups in specialty psychiatric settings, were never validated in primary care or community population settings. In retrospect, the US/UK study demonstrated that the ICD-7 through ICD-9 criteria were insufficient for clinical research, and the ECA and subsequent epidemiological studies have demonstrated that DSM-III to DSM-IV criteria are insufficient for epidemiological, genetic, and more advanced neurocircuitry and clinical research. What is most remarkable is that the simple advance of having some more reliable, explicit diagnostic criteria, regardless of their validity, has made it possible for our research enterprise to advance as far as it has (Regier 2003).

The practical aspects of building on past experience and the emerging research base have occupied much of our thinking for DSM-5 (Regier et al. 2009). It is clear that some explicit diagnostic criteria will be needed if reliability is to be maintained. However, the reification of our existing criteria has resulted in a failure to adequately test alternative or more encompassing criteria that could better capture the clinical syndromes that present in nature—not only in tertiary care psychiatric settings, but also in primary care and community settings. There are obviously missing criteria in the current classification system that could be associated with persons in the community with similar conditions who never come into primary care or specialty care settings.

The DSM criteria themselves are attempts to capture essential components of an underlying pathophysiology and psychopathological process. Even the aggregation of these components allows us to see only the tip of the iceberg that represents a complex neurophysiological mechanism, which exceeds the range of normal homeostatic brain functioning (Hyman 2007). The range of the processes underlying these "disorders" can extend from those that cross a continuum of normal physiological functioning, like blood pressure, glucose metabolism, cholesterol levels, depressed mood, elevated anxiety, compulsive behavior, or cognitive acuity. There may also be more abrupt discontinuities of major genetic or structural defects that are incompatible with normal organ tissue function, such as neoplasms, stroke, acute psychoses and Alzheimer's disease.

One of the clearest limitations of our current diagnostic criteria has been the lack of quantitative measures in routine diagnostic practice and in epidemiologic studies to help set diagnostic thresholds for disorders that fall on the extreme end of a continuum of normal emotional, behavioral and cognitive functions. The reliance on a few symptomatic criteria, which are then used to render a "yes/no" diagnostic answer, has not been used to assess effectiveness of new treatments for such disorders in clinical trials and should not be considered sufficient for either setting thresholds for diagnosis in primary care and community studies or to establishing severity levels for clear communication with colleagues and monitoring of treatment response (Kraemer 2008).

As detailed in previous publications, our plans for DSM-5 are to provide a range of cross-cutting measures that will identify continuous measures of emotional, cognitive, addictive and other domains that are expressed in both mental and other medical/surgical disorders (Kupfer et al. 2009). These domains will be used somewhat like a mental status examination to make sure that major functional areas are probed and to facilitate the characterization of all mental disorders beyond established criteria. Diagnoses will require the use of specific criteria, and a diagnostic checklist will be suggested to assist clinicians in a systematic assessment of the relevant symptom domains. A measure of severity will be developed for all disorders that may be patient-reported or clinician-assessed with reliable quantitative anchors for ongoing monitoring of treatment response.

The overall organization of the manual has yet to be determined but will give priority to clinical utility and prepare the groundwork for adding more biological and continuous psychosocial criteria in the future. The DSM-5 approach to accomplishing this as well as increasing validity can be summarized in the following steps:

1. Identify the benefits of blending categorical and dimensional approaches to psychiatric diagnosis (Kraemer 2008).

2. Propose a blend of bottom-up latent class analysis with evidence-based dimensional constructs for grouping related disorders and expert top-down proposals for categorical criteria revisions based on literature reviews (Helzer et al. 2008).

3. Identify 11 validators to go beyond Robins and Guze (Hyman 2010a; Kupfer et al. 2009).

4. Encourage application of these to developing a new organization (metastructure) for mental disorders chapter in DSM-5 and for ICD-11 (Kupfer and Regier, 2008). This specific effort resulted in publication of six papers on "metastructure" in *Psychological Medicine* (Andrews et al. 2009).

5. Establish guidelines for inclusion and exclusion of disorders in DSM-5 (Kendler et al. 2010).

6. Prioritize the inclusion of cross-cutting dimensional measures and dimensional severity measures in DSM-5 Field Trial testing.

7. Assess the degree to which "pure" cross-cutting psychological domains are eventually linked to temperament, personality traits, and biological variables, including "neurocircuitry" and genetic vulnerability as vulnerability factors for psychopathology (Hyman 2010b).

8. Evaluate how core concepts of disorders with specified traits/symptom profiles can be used clinically in field trials (Kraemer et al. 2010).

9. Evaluate models for displaying integrated categorical/dimensional descriptions to permit better characterization of psychopathology (Kraemer et al. 2010).

Now that our 13 DSM-5 diagnostic work groups have developed proposed revisions of diagnostic criteria over the past 3 years, posted them on the public http://www.dsm5.org website for a thorough public and professional vetting, and revised the criteria based on this extensive feedback, we are ready to test them out in a series of field trials in large academic settings as well as in routine individual practice settings (Kraemer et al. 2010). Revisions of the proposed criteria will be made based on the field trials, and additional field trials will be conducted on selected disorders that appear in need of additional substantial change. All of these proposed changes will need to be reviewed by the entire DSM-5 Task Force before recommendations are made to the APA Board of Trustees for their approval. It has also been recommended that we have a scientific review of proposed changes to see if they follow the inclusion/exclusion guidelines that have been in place for the past year. Some of our colleagues have also devoted some time to reviewing the DSM-IV "definition of a mental disorder" to see if the past two decades have given us any additional epistemological wisdom for providing an encompassing definition for all mental disorders (Stein et al. 2010).

The challenge for this enterprise has been illustrated recently as the DSM-5 and ICD-11 groups have attempted to harmonize an overall organizational structure of the mental disorder classification into large groups of disorders. A new Neurodevelopmental Disorders section has been proposed to replace the "Disorders Usually First Diagnosed in Infancy, Childhood, or Adolescence." When David Shaffer, MD, chair of the ADHD and Disruptive Behavior Disorders Work Group, initiated an effort to describe this section, he provided the following definition:

> A disorder that is presumed to reflect an abnormality of CNS development in which the appearance and subsequent refinement and elaboration of a physical and/or psychological capability is delayed beyond a specified period. The emergence of normal function may continue at either a delayed pace or normal pace and may or may not reach a level that would be broadly regarded as within normal limits.

This definition is quite different than that found in DSM-IV, which is as follows:

> A clinically significant behavioral or psychological syndrome or pattern that occurs in an individual and that is associated with present distress (e.g., a painful symptom) or disability (i.e., impairment in one or more important areas of functioning) or with a significantly increased risk of suffering death, pain, disability, or an important loss of freedom. In addition, this syndrome or pattern must not be merely an expectable and culturally sanctioned response to a particular event, for example, the death of a loved one. Whatever its original cause, it must currently be considered a manifestation of a behavioral, psychological, or biological dysfunction in the individual. Neither deviant behavior (e.g., political, religious, or sexual) nor conflicts that are primarily between the individual and society are mental disorders unless the deviance or conflict is a symptom of a dysfunction in the individual, as described above (APA 1994, pp. xxi–xxii).

It may be of interest to this audience that almost none of the DSM-5 Task Force or Work Group meetings struggled with these definitional issues as they evaluated the research literature to determine the evidentiary basis for revisions. One notable exception would be the group that addressed the proposal for including Parental Alienation Syndrome. The issue here is one of determining whether this is a parent-child relational problem or "a dysfunction in an individual."

Moving forward, I believe the more critical issue for work group members is how to avoid mind–body dualism in which mental disorders are moved in neurological classifications as more precise pathophysiological, neuroimaging, genetic, nutritional, infectious, traumatic or other etiological characteristics are discovered. The implicit belief that there is an underlying, incompletely understood brain-based dysfunction for the behavioral, cognitive, emotional and physical symptom syndromes is the de facto definition of mental disorders used by most members of the DSM-5 Task Force and Work Groups. Certainly, there is a substantial appreciation that the biologically based temperament and personality traits from infancy to adulthood constitute protective or vulnerability factors for "gene–environmental interactions" that may lead to mental disorders.

In summary, members of the DSM-5 Task Force are acutely aware of the broader social impact of mental disorder definitions—beyond their use for clinical decision-making and for facilitating research studies. However, we are also aware that advances in our understanding of these disorders will only occur if the definitions and diagnostic criteria for these disorders are constructed to facilitate their testing as scientific hypotheses. Since the broad definition in DSM-IV and in the Stein revision (Stein et al. 2010) are almost impossible to test, most of our efforts will focus on the individual diagnostic criteria and dimensional measurements that permit better assessments of the thresholds between normal and pathological states. As Jablensky has so aptly pointed out in his remarkable history of "the nosological entity in psychiatry," even Kraepelin in his later publications moved decisively from a strict categorical to a dimensional approach to comprehend the essential nature of psychopathology (Jablensky, Chapter 5, this volume). Although we are guided by current diagnostic boundaries, we are deliberately collecting information from 12 psychological domains that will allow us to characterize patient presentations better than the current criteria—where "Not Otherwise Specified" is often the norm. In collecting such information, we will see if new syndromes emerge from this "bottom-up" empirical approach. Hence, both the syndrome categories and more quantitative thresholds can be tested to determine whether they can differentiate between normal and pathological functioning, thereby suggesting revisions for DSM-5.1.

Chapter References

American Psychiatric Association. (1952). *Diagnostic and Statistical Manual of Mental Disorders*. Washington, D.C.: American Psychiatric Association.

American Psychiatric Association. (1968). *Diagnostic and Statistical Manual of Mental Disorders*, *2nd* Edition. Washington, DC: American Psychiatric Association.

American Psychiatric Association. (1980). *Diagnostic and Statistical Manual of Mental Disorders*, *3rd* Edition. Washington, DC: American Psychiatric Association.

American Psychiatric Association. (1987). *Diagnostic and Statistical Manual of Mental Disorders*, *3rd* Edition, Revised. Washington, DC: American Psychiatric Association.

American Psychiatric Association. (1994). *Diagnostic and Statistical Manual of Mental Disorders, 4th* Edition. Washington, DC: American Psychiatric Association.

Andrews, G., Goldberg, D. P., Krueger, R. F., Carpenter, W. T., Hyman, S. E., Sachdev, P., *et al.* (2009). Exploring the feasibility of a meta-structure for DSM-V and ICD-11: Could it improve utility and validity? *Psychological Medicine,* **39**, 1993–2000.

Boyd, J. H., Burke, J. D., Gruenberg, E., Holzer, C. E., 3rd, Rae, D. S., George, L. K., *et al.* (1984). Exclusion criteria of DSM-III: A study of co-occurrence of hierarchy-free syndromes. *Archives of General Psychiatry,* **41**, 983–9.

Caspi, A., Sugden, K., Moffitt, T. E., Taylor, A., Craig, I. W., Harrington, H., *et al.* (2003). Influence of life stress on depression: moderation by a polymorphism in the 5-HTT gene. *Science,* **301**, 386–9.

Cooper, J. E., Kendell, R. E., Gurland, B. J., Sharpe, L., Copeland, J. R. M. and Simon, R. (1972). *Psychiatric Diagnosis in New York and London.* London: Oxford.

Endicott, J., Spitzer, R. L., Fleiss, J. L. and Cohen, J. (1976). The Global Assessment Scale: A procedure for measuring overall severity of psychiatric disturbance. *Archives of General Psychiatry,* **33**, 766–71.

Frances, A. (2009). A warning sign on the road to DSM-V: Beware of its unintended consequences. *Psychiatric Times,* 26 June. Available at: http://www.psychiatrictimes.com/dsm-5/content/article/10168/1425378?pageNumber=2 (accessed 26 October, 2010).

Goldberg, D. P. (1972). *The Detection of Psychiatric Illness by Questionnaire.* London: Oxford.

Helzer, J. E., Wittchen, H. U., Krueger, R. F. and Kramer, H. C. (2008). Dimensional options for DSM-V: The way forward. In J. E. Helzer, H. C. Kraemer and R. F. Krueger (eds.) *Dimensional Approaches in Diagnostic Classification: Refining the Research Agenda for DSM-V.* Arlington, VA: American Psychiatric Association, pp. 115–27.

Horwitz, A. V. and Wakefield, J. C. (2007). *The Loss of Sadness: How Psychiatry Transformed Normal Sorrow into Depressive Disorder.* New York: Oxford.

Hyman, S. E. (2007). Can neuroscience be integrated into the DSM-V? *Nature Reviews Neuroscience,* **8**, 725–32.

Hyman, S. E. (2010a). Diagnosis of mental disorders in light of modern genetics. In D.A. Regier, W. Narrow, E. Kuhl and D. Kupfer (eds.) *The Conceptual Evolution of DSM-5.* Arlington, VA: American Psychiatric Association, pp. 3–18.

Hyman, S. E. (2010b). The diagnosis of mental disorders: The problem of reification. *Annual Reviews in Clinical Psychology,* **6**, 155–79.

Kendler, K. S., Myers, J. and Zisook, S. (2008). Does bereavement-related major depression differ from major depression associated with other stressful life events? *American Journal of Psychiatry,* **165**, 1449–55.

Kendler, K. S., Kupfer, D. J., Narrow, W. E., Phillips, K. A. and Fawcett, J. (2010). *Guidelines for making change to DSM-5.* Memorandum to DSM-5 Task Force and Work Groups. Available at: http://www.dsm5.org/about/Pages/faq.aspx#7 (accessed 8 November, 2010).

Kessler, R. C., McGonagle, K. A., Zhao, S., Nelson, C. B., Hughes, M., Eshleman, S., *et al.* (1994). Lifetime and 12-month prevalence of DSM-III-R psychiatric disorders in the United States: results from the National Comorbidity Survey. *Archives of General Psychiatry,* **51**, 8–19.

Kessler, R. C., Merikangas, K. R., Berglund, P., Eaton, W. W., Kortez, D. S. and Walters, M. S. (2003). Mild disorders should not be eliminated from the DSM-V. *Archives of General Psychiatry,* **60**, 1117–22.

Kraemer, H. C. (2008). DSM categories and dimensions in clinical and research contexts. In J. E. Helzer, H. C. Kraemer, R. F. Krueger, H. U. Wittchen, P. J. Sirovatka and D. A. Regier (eds.) *Dimensional Approaches in Diagnostic Classification: Refining the Research Agenda for DSM-V*. Arlington, VA: American Psychiatric Association, pp. 5–18.

Kraemer, H. C., Kupfer, D. J., Narrow, W. E., Clarke, D. E. and Regier, D. A. (2010). Moving toward DSM-5: The field trials. *American Journal of Psychiatry*, **167**, 1158–60.

Kupfer, D. J., Kuhl, E. A., Narrow, W. E. and Regier, D. A. (2009). On the road to DSM-5. *Cerebrum*, 13 October, 2009 Available at: http://www.dana.org/news/cerebrum/detail. aspx?id=2356

Kupfer, D. J. and Regier, D. A. (2008). *DSM-5 Task Force and Work Group Update: APA Division of Research Report to the APA Board of Trustees*. Available at: http://www.dsm5.org/ ProgressReports/Pages/CurrentActivitiesReportoftheDSM-VTaskForce(November2008). aspx (8 November, 2010).

Leighton, D. C., Harding, J. S., Macklin, D. B., Macmillan, A. M. and Leighton, A. H. (1960). *The Character of Danger*. New York: Basic Books Inc.

Luborsky, L. (1962). Clinician's judgments of mental health. *Archives of General Psychiatry*, **7**, 407–17.

Moffic, H. S. (2010) Caution! Who should be the DSM-V diagnostician? *Psychiatric Times*, 3 February. Available at: http://www.psychiatrictimes.com/dsm-5/content/ article/10168/1518607 (accessed 26 October, 2010).

Narrow, W. E., Rae, D. S., Robins, L. N. and Regier, D. A. (2002). Revised prevalence estimates of mental disorders in the United States: Using a clinical significance criterion to reconcile 2 surveys' estimates. *Archives of General Psychiatry*, **59**, 115–23.

Pasamanick, B., Roberts, D. W., Lemkau, P. V. and Krueger, D. E. (1956). A survey of mental disease in an urban population. *American Journal of Public Health*, **47**, 923–9.

Pincus, H., Ustun, T. B., Millman, E. J. and Regier, D. A. (1998). [Letters to the Editor]. *Archives of General Psychiatry*, **55**, 1145–48.

The President's Commission on Mental Health. (1978). *Report to the President From the President's Commission on Mental Health*. Washington, D.C., stock No. 040–000-00390–8, vol. 1.

Regier, D. A. (1987). Introduction, Part VII Nosologic principles and diagnostic criteria. In G. L. Tischler (ed.) *Diagnosis and Classification in Psychiatry: A Critical Appraisal of DSM-III*. New York: Cambridge University Press, pp. 399–401.

Regier, D. A. (2003). Mental disorder diagnostic theory and practical reality: an evolutionary perspective. *Health Affairs (Millwood)*, **22**, 21–7.

Regier, D. A., Burke, J. D., Manderscheid, R. W. and Burns, B. J. (1985). The chronically mentally ill in primary care. *Psychological Medicine*, **15**, 265–73.

Regier, D. A., Farmer, M. E., Rae, D. S., Locke, B. Z., Keith, S. J., Judd, L. L., *et al.* (1990). Comorbidity of mental disorders with alcohol and other drug abuse: Results from the epidemiologic catchment area (ECA) study. *Journal of the American Medical Association*, **264**, 2511–18.

Regier, D. A., Goldberg, I. D. and Taube, C. A. (1978). The de facto U.S. mental health services system: A public health perspective. *Archives of General Psychiatry*, **35**, 685–93.

Regier, D. A., Kaelber, C. T., Rae, D. S., Farmer, M. E., Knauper, B., Kessler, R. C., *et al.* (1998). Limitations of diagnostic criteria and assessment instruments for mental disorders: Implications for research and policy. *Archives of General Psychiatry*, **55**, 109–15.

Regier, D. A., Myers, J. K., Kramer, M., Robins, L. N., Blazer, D. G., Hough, R. L., *et al.* (1984). The NIMH epidemiological catchment area (ECA) program: Historical context, major objectives, and study population characteristics. *Archives of General Psychiatry*, **41**, 934–41.

Regier, D. A. and Narrow, W. E. (2002). Defining clinically significant psychopathology with epidemiologic data. In J. E. Helzer and J. J. Hudziak (eds.) *Defining Psychopathology in the 21st Century: DSM-V and Beyond.* Washington, DC: American Psychiatric Association, pp. 19–30.

Regier, D. A., Narrow, W. E., Kuhl, E. A. and Kupfer, D. J. (2009). The conceptual development of DSM-V. *American Journal of Psychiatry*, **166**, 645–50.

Regier, D. A., Narrow, W. E. and Rae, D. S. (2004). For DSM-V, it's the "disorder threshold," stupid. *Archives of General Psychiatry*, **61**, 1051–52.

Regier, D. A., Narrow, W. E., Rae, D. S., Manderscheid, R. W., Locke, B. Z. and Goodwin, F. K. (1993). The de facto U.S. mental and addictive disorders service system: Epidemiological catchment area prospective 1-year prevalence rates of disorders and services. *Archives of General Psychiatry*, **50**, 85–94.

Robins, E. and Guze, S. B. (1970). Establishment of diagnostic validity in psychiatric illness: Its application to schizophrenia. *American Journal of Psychiatry*, **126**, 983–87.

Robins, L. N. and Regier, D. A. (eds.) (1991). *Psychiatric Disorders in America: The Epidemiologic Catchment Area Study.* New York: The Free Press.

Robins, L. N., Helzer, J. E., Croughan, J., Williams, J. B. W. and Spitzer, R. L. (1981). *NIMH Diagnostic Interview Schedule: Version III (May 1981).* Rockville, MD: NIMH.

Robins, L. N., Wing, J., Wittchen, H. U., Helzer, J. E., Babor, T. F., Burke, J., *et al.* (1988). The composite international diagnostic interview: An epidemiologic instrument suitable for use in conjunction with difference diagnostic systems and in different cultures. *Archives of General Psychiatry*, **45**, 1069–77.

Shepherd, M., Cooper, B., Brown, A. C. and Kalton, G. W. (1966). *Psychiatric Illness in General Practice.* London: Oxford.

Spitzer, R. L. (1983). Psychiatric diagnosis: are clinicians still necessary? *Comprehensive Psychiatry*, **24**, 399–411.

Spitzer, R. L. (1998). Diagnosis and need for treatment are not the same. *Archives of General Psychiatry*, **55**, 120.

Spitzer, R. L. and Endicott, J. (1977). *Schedule for Affective Disorders and Schizophrenia: Life-Time Version (SADS-L)*, ed 3. New York: New York State Psychiatric Institute.

Spitzer, R. L., Endicott, J. and Robins, E. (1978). Research Diagnostic Criteria. *Archives of General Psychiatry*, **35**, 773–85.

Srole, L. (1962). *Mental Health in the Metropolis: The Midtown Manhattan Study.* New York: McGraw-Hill Book Co Inc.

Stein, D., Phillips, K. A., Bolton, D., Fulford, K., Sadler, J. and Kendler, K. (2010). What is a mental/psychiatric disorder? From DSM-IV to DSM-V. *Psychological Medicine*, **40**, 1759–65.

Wakefield, J. C., Schmitz, M. F., First, M. B. and Horwitz, A. V. (2007). Extending the bereavement exclusion for major depression to other losses: evidence from the National Comorbidity Survey. *Archives of General Psychiatry*, **64**, 433–40.

Wang, P. S., Lane, M., Olfson, M., Pincus, H. A., Wells, K. B. and Kessler, R. C. (2005). Twelve-month use of mental health services in the United States. *Archives of General Psychiatry*, **62**, 629–40.

World Health Organization. (1965). *Manual of the International Statistical Classification of Diseases, Injuries, and Causes of Death. Eighth Revision of the International Classification of Diseases.* Geneva: World Health Organization.

World Health Organization. (1977). *Manual of the International Statistical Classification of Diseases, Injuries, and Causes of Death. Ninth Revision of the International Classification of Diseases.* Geneva: World Health Organization.

The tangible burden of mental disorder in the absence of mental disorder categories in nature: some reflections on Regier's contribution

Robert F. Krueger

Darrel Regier has been a pioneer in the closely related areas of psychiatric nosology and epidemiology. For example, Regier was a leader of the Epidemiologic Catchment Area Study, a landmark effort in psychiatric epidemiology (Regier et al. 1984), and he is currently the co-chair of the DSM-5 task force. Regier's paper provides a personal account of his intellectual journey to date in these areas, and makes clear how his thinking has evolved over the years, leading to his current, forward-thinking perspectives. My goal here will be to amplify some themes that emerge in Regier's paper by providing my own perspective on those themes, with particular emphasis on the importance of constructing an empirically-based dimensional model of mental disorders.

14.1 Most mental disorders are probably dimensional in nature

One key issue Regier touches on pertains to the nature of mental disorder variation. For example, he discusses the challenges of estimating precise prevalence rates for specific disorders, and the myriad factors that influence these rates. Obviously, knowing the prevalence rate for a mental disorder is a critical consideration in distributing scarce resources effectively. For example, one often encounters the idea that the prevalence of a mental disorder justifies its place in a nosology, and thereby, in research and clinical thinking (see, e.g., Miller and Campbell 2010; writing about narcissistic personality disorder and corresponding commentary by Krueger 2010). Why, then, is it so challenging to accurately estimate the prevalence of mental disorders? One reason is likely that most mental disorders are probably not categories in nature, as revealed by recent research.

Recent years have seen key developments in statistical modeling techniques that can distinguish among forms of human variation (e.g., mental disorders) that are dimensions, categories, or have both dimensional and categorical (mixed) aspects. These developments are important because they place deep questions about the nature of mental disorder variation on an empirical playing field. Historically, the conceptualization of mental disorders has been driven by a priori assumptions. For example, the DSM-IV-TR renders all mental disorders as binary dichotomies (i.e., a person either meets criteria for a specific mental disorder or does not meet those criteria)—not because of evidence that this is an accurate model of mental disorder variation, but because this is how mental disorders are traditionally conceived of in official nosologies.

Recent modeling developments take the problem of modeling mental disorder variation out of the realm of tradition and assumptions and into the realm of empirical inquiry. Models can be compared that render mental disorder variation in terms of degree (e.g., the extent to which a specific person has none, some, or all of the symptoms of major depression) as opposed to rendering it in terms of kind (e.g., people tend to have all or most of the symptoms of major depression or none or few of the symptoms).

The relevant literature is growing and is too voluminous to review thoroughly in this brief commentary, but a number of psychopathological phenomena have been formally modeled and have been found to be better fit by dimensional as opposed to categorical models. For example, specific externalizing syndromes (e.g., Walton et al. 2011) as well as the overall extent of comorbidity among externalizing (substance use and antisocial behavior) disorders (e.g., Markon and Krueger 2005) are better conceptualized using dimensional as opposed to categorical models. Importantly, the apparent dimensionality of psychopathology is not limited only to the more "common" mental disorders. For example, Prisciandaro and Roberts (2011) provided three independent lines of support for conceptualizing mania as a dimension of psychopathological variation. Two lines of evidence were more "internal" (i.e., latent structural analyses) whereas the third line of evidence was more "external" (i.e., the relative ability of discrete and continuous models to predict outcomes such as suicidal behavior and health service utilization). This combined strategy of both internal and external modeling is important because the conjunction of both provides evidence that a specific mental disorder is structured dimensionally, as well as evidence regarding why a dimensional conceptualization is important for validity. For example, dimensional models tend to be more replicable than categorical models across different samples (e.g., Eaton et al. in press), and tend to have improved validity in predicting important external criteria (Prisicarando and Roberts 2011), as well as enhanced temporal stability (Watson 2003). In addition, a recent meta-analysis by Markon et al. (2011), involving 58 studies and 59,575 research participants, showed that continuous measures of psychopathology are associated with a 15% increase in reliability and 37% increase in validity, relative to discrete measures.

14.2 The social costs of mental disorders are probably a continuous function of psychopathology dimensions

Mounting evidence indicates that most forms of psychopathology are probably dimensional in nature, with little evidence for distinguishable groups of persons or "zones of rarity" (Kendell and Jablensky 2003) in the distributions of psychopathological signs and symptoms. We anticipate that this literature will continue to grow as additional investigators begin working to compare dimensional, categorical and hybrid models, and we also hypothesize that dimensional models (or hybrid models with continuous latent variables that capture key aspects of psychopathological variation) will provide a better fit to data than models with only categorical latent variables. Importantly, this hypothesis could be wrong, and data can be used to test it. These hypotheses are more than a matter of opinion and preference; we are past the age where authority is all we can rely on in constructing a nosology.

A key question this raises, vis a vis Regier's chapter, is: if psychopathology is dimensional, how shall we determine its prevalence and social costs? A major theme of psychiatric epidemiology, and Regier's seminal contributions, lie in using the tools of epidemiology to document both the prevalence and social costs of mental disorders. If mental disorders are continuous, however, what is their "prevalence" and how do we document their costs?

This question is critical, and fortunately, also tractable. I will highlight here a recent contribution from Markon (2010) because it nicely illustrates this point. Markon (2010) studied the relationship between internalizing (overall extent of mood, anxiety and somatization symptoms) and impairment (impairment in activities of daily living and work, social relationships, and other activities) using a sophisticated series of formal models. He concluded that the relationship between internalizing psychopathology and impairment was linear and constant throughout the range of both constructs, and that the data did not reveal a "natural dividing line" beyond which impairment accelerated dramatically.

More model-based research of this type is needed, but our prediction is that this kind of finding will be the norm rather than the exception. That is, psychopathology per se and its consequences (impairment) are probably linked in a monotonic, continuous fashion in nature. This situation is not unusual in medicine, so perhaps it is unsurprising with regard to psychopathology. However, it does suggest a need to recognize the continuity of psychopathology and impairment in official classification systems, and the need to move away from the empirically inaccurate conceptualization of mental disorders as polythetic dichotomies.

14.3 **Toward a dimensional nosology of mental disorders**

Our reading of the literature is that mental disorders are likely more dimensional than categorical in nature, and that their relationships with external consequences are likely monotonic and linear. This emerging empirical understanding does run counter to the model of mental disorders in the DSM, which remains the dominant model of mental disorders in both research and clinical settings.

Regier has been heroic in his efforts to promote more dimensional thinking about mental disorders. For example, I had the distinct pleasure of working with him to organize a meeting on "Dimensional Approaches in Diagnostic Classification," as part of the process leading up to DSM-5 (Helzer et al. 2008). Nevertheless, the DSM is accompanied by a fair degree of tradition and inherency; changing the DSM in a dramatic way is challenging at best. As Regier notes in his chapter, "defenders of the current construct do not yield easily to suggested changes in paradigms."

Because of Regier's tireless advocacy, it seems likely that DSM-5 will feature more dimensional elements, such as the cross-cutting measures he describes in his chapter and "evidence-based dimensional constructs for grouping related disorders." However, in spite of this, some have argued that the magnitude of change possible within the DSM paradigm may be insufficient for the needs of contemporary researchers. For example, the United States National Institute of Mental Health (NIMH) has initiated the "Research Domain Criteria" (RDoC) effort in an attempt to circumvent the limitations of the DSM paradigm, e.g., through a focus on genetics and neurobiology.

Unfortunately, scientifically viable models of psychopathological variation are unlikely to simply "bootstrap" themselves from research in genetics and neurobiology. Clearly, biological factors are important contributors to mental disorder, and that is not in question. Instead, my concern is that pathways from genetic polymorphisms through central nervous systems to psychopathological outcomes are circuitous and are also influenced by factors external to the organism per se. As a result, it seems unlikely that there will be some major breakthrough where a specific biological variant is suddenly discovered to be "the cause" of a mental disorder.

Nevertheless, the structure of manifest signs and symptoms of psychopathology is a highly tractable problem. A critical next step in psychopathology research is the continued formal delineation of a comprehensive dimensional model of psychopathology. This step is tractable and can be placed on solid scientific footing. It can proceed in a way that is interwoven with research on biological factors. Indeed, biometrical genetic research suggests close parallels between the genetic and phenotypic dimensional structure of psychopathology (e.g., Kendler et al 2003). It seems likely that there are important parallels between manifest structure and neurobiology as well (e.g., Gilmore et al. 2010).

In sum, our hope is that empirical research on the dimensional structure of mental disorder signs and symptoms becomes a major focus of research, and that infrastructures relevant to this (e.g., testable dimensional hypotheses in DSM-5, relevant funding streams) will emerge. Regier's openness to these kinds of new ideas bodes well for the role DSM-5 can play in facilitating and encouraging novel work on classification from a dimensional perspective.

Comments References

Eaton, N. R., Krueger, R. F., South, S. C., Simms, L. J. and Clark, L. A. (2011). Contrasting prototypes and dimensions in the classification of personality pathology: Evidence that dimensions but not prototypes are robust. *Psychological Medicine*, **41**(6): 1151–1163.

Gilmore, C. S., Malone, S. M. and Iacono, W. G. (2010). Brain electrophysiological endophenotypes for externalizing psychopathology: A multivariate approach. *Behavior Genetics*, **40**, 186–200.

Helzer, J. E., Kraemer, H. C., Krueger, R. F., Wittchen, H.-U., Sirovatka, P. J. and Regier, D. A. (eds.) (2008). *Dimensional Approaches in Diagnostic Classification: Refining the Research Agenda for DSM-V*. Arlington, VA: American Psychiatric Association.

Kendell, R. and Jablensky, A. (2003). Distinguishing between the validity and utility of psychiatric diagnoses. *American Journal of Psychiatry*, **160**, 4–12.

Kendler, K. S., Prescott, C. A., Myers, J. and Neale, M. C. (2003). The structure of genetic and environmental risk factors for common psychiatric and substance use disorders in men and women. *Archives of General Psychiatry*, **60**, 929–37.

Krueger, R. F. (2010). Personality pathology is dimensional, so what shall we do with the DSM-IV personality disorder categories? The case of narcissistic personality disorder: Comment on Miller and Campbell (2010). *Personality Disorders: Theory, Research, and Treatment*, **1**, 195–6.

Krueger, R. F. and Markon, K. E. (2005). Categorical and continuous models of liability to externalizing disorders: A direct comparison in NESARC. *Archives of General Psychiatry*, **62**, 1352–9.

Markon, K. E. (2010). How things fall apart: Understanding the nature of internalizing through its relationship with impairment. *Journal of Abnormal Psychology*, **119**, 447–58.

Markon, K. E., Chmielewski, M. and Miller, C. J. (2011). The reliability and validity of discrete and continuous measures of psychopathology: A quantitative review. *Psychological Bulletin*, **137**(5), 856–79.

Miller, J. D. and Campbell, W. K. (2010). The case for using research on trait narcissism as a building block for understanding narcissistic personality disorder. *Personality Disorders: Theory, Research, and Treatment*, **1**, 180–91.

Prisciandaro, J. J. and Roberts, J. E. (2011). Evidence for the continuous latent structure of mania in the Epidemiologic Catchment Area from multiple latent structure and construct validation methodologies. *Psychological Medicine*, **41**, 575–88.

Regier, D. A., Meyer, J. K., Kramer, M., Robins, L. N., Blazer, D. G., Hough, R. L., *et al.* (1984). The NIMH Epidemiologic Catchment Area program: Historical context, major objectives, and study population characteristics. *Archives of General Psychiatry*, **41**, 934–41.

Walton, K. E., Ormel, J. and Krueger, R. F. (2011). The dimensional nature of externalizing behaviors in adolescence: Evidence from a direct comparison of categorical, dimensional and hybrid models. *Journal of Abnormal Child Psychology*, **39**(4), 553–61.

Watson, D. (2003). Investigating the construct validity of the dissociative taxon: Stability analyses of normal and pathological dissociation. *Journal of Abnormal Psychology*, **112**, 298–305.

Chapter 15

Introduction

Josef Parnas

In this chapter we find a realist proposal of scientific progress, modeled upon mathematics, applied to psychiatric nosology, and illustrated through the permutations of the DSM, from its III-rd edition, over III-R, to DSM-IV. The chapter is *descriptive*, describing scientific progress, and *prescriptive*, outlining certain law-like conditions that science must obey, in order to reach its goal, which is truth.

We have all witnessed spectacular transformations in science and, especially, in technology and the idea of progress is deeply entrenched in the Western mind (in the East there are more cyclical views), and that despite our allegedly "post-modernist" condition (see Ghaemi, Chapter 3, this volume). Evolution, though most likely working in a proscriptive rather than prescriptive way, is seen in its vulgar, anthropocentric version as an engine of biological improvement. The idea of progress has conceptual affinities to the notions of purpose (telos), final cause, vital force (entelechy), teleology, and self-organization (spontaneous transition from indeterminate, disorganized homogeneity to determinate, patterned heterogeneity ((structure))). The general idea of progress can be defined as a process of gradual, cumulative, incremental, linear-chronological "improvement" or refinement of humanity. This idea, quite vague in Antiquity, became clearly articulated in the Christian theology of Middle Age, to achieve its more contemporary form in the rationalism of the Enlightenment, early championed by Leibniz. More recent and famous versions of theories of progress comprise Hegel's dialectic of Spirit and Marx's claim of historical laws (on analogy with laws of nature), asymptotically leading to a totally emancipated free society. Yet, the credentials of the *historicism* (a belief in historical laws and their inevitable causal sequences) have diminished dramatically in our time (Popper 1957). Progress in science is both a parcel of more overarching ontological and epistemological debates, including issues such as realism, pragmatism, etc. (see Chapter 1 by Bolton, Chapter 2 by Zachar and Chapter 9 by Schaffner, this volume), and, at the same time, a specific field of philosophy of science, with the names of Karl Popper and Thomas Kuhn in the foreground.

Kendler proposes the concept of "epistemic iteration" (EI): the progress in (science of) nosology works in analogy with a computational method which, using available information, generates a series of "*increasingly accurate estimations of a desired parameter.*" Optimal iterative system, "improves each estimate on its predecessor so that, with a sufficient number of iterations, the process asymptotes to a stable and accurate parameter estimate" (solution). Transposed into nosology, epistemic iterations (i.e., successive stages of research ensuing from each, scientifically based, DSM modification) yield typologies which are increasingly consistent with the really existing nosological categories. As a contrast to the EI process, Kendler describes the horror of "random walk," where parameter estimates change in unpredictable manner, making the computer to "walk" randomly, producing inconsistent results, and failing to reach the endpoint of truth. As concrete or incarnated example of a "random walk" situation in the domain of schizophrenia, "Great German Professors" (GGP) are invoked: Kraepelin, Bleuler, Langfeldt and Schneider, each one with a specific (presumably dogmatic) view on what constitutes the essential feature of schizophrenia. Kendler notes the following, successive, defining emphases ("nothing like a progressive process"): course →symptoms→course→symptoms. This random walk scenario seems to betray a subtle transatlantic perspectivism, however. First, two (50%) of the GGP were in fact non-German: Bleuler was Swiss and Langfeldt was Norwegian. Second, it would be quite possible (but out of place) to convincingly argue that GGP *did not disagree* on the typical outcome of schizophrenia, and were in a substantial agreement on the essentials of the *clinical core* of schizophrenia (see Chapter 12 by Parnas, this volume, for a detailed assessment of Schneider's views), a core that was *raison d'être* of the category "schizophrenia" (and which, through its important "trait"-component, was necessarily linked to course). Langfeldt, for example, tried to differentiate between the typical clinical picture of "true," poor outcome, schizophrenia, and clinical patterns of paranoid-hallucinatory syndromes with apparently benign course (affective turbulence, clouding of consciousness, etc).

Kendler presents us with an intriguing account of scientific progress, perhaps applicable to psychiatric nosology. This proposal invites to certain conservatism in our attitude to changes in the specifications of diagnostic categories. Kendler's proposal deserves a further fleshing out in terms of practical options for improving our nosological categories.

Introduction Reference

Popper, K. (1957). *The Poverty of Historicism*. London: Routledge.

Chapter 15

Epistemic iteration as a historical model for psychiatric nosology: promises and limitations

Kenneth S. Kendler

As evident from the history of Science, a mature science's progress may be interpreted as asymptotic, i.e., coming closer and closer to the way the world really is.
Marcum (2010, p. 44)

In this essay, I want to expand upon my earlier discussion of epistemic iteration (EI) as a historical framework within which to understand the development of psychiatric nosology (Kendler 2009). I mean this discussion to be both descriptive and prescriptive. That is, I think that the concept of EI captures an important part of what has been implicit in what we might call "the DSM-III model." That is, the initial revisions of DSM-III—DSM-III-R and DSM-IV—implicitly assumed an EI model. I also see EI as serving a prescriptive function. Given a certain set of assumptions that I will review, I want to argue that EI is a good method for psychiatric nosology to use at this point in its historical development. I will try to show under what conditions EI might work in future generations of the DSM effort and when it may not work.

15.1 Iteration

Let us begin by reviewing the concept of iteration. It originates in mathematics as a computational method which, using available data, generates a series of increasingly accurate estimations of a desired parameter. In a properly working iterative system, each estimate improves on its predecessor so that, with a sufficient number of iterations, the process asymptotes to a stable and accurate parameter estimate. Iteration is robust in that, given some key features of the likelihood surface over which it "crawls," it can begin with widely divergent starting values and reliably converge to the same correct solution.

Figure 15.1a represents a vertical slice through a very simple and idealized likelihood surface. The current solution is depicted at point A. The ideal solution—which represents the lowest possible point on the surface—is depicted by point X. In this case, the fit function has an easy task of it. It must simply crawl "downhill" a little bit at a time, until it arrives at point X. This process is depicted in Figures 15.1b–e.

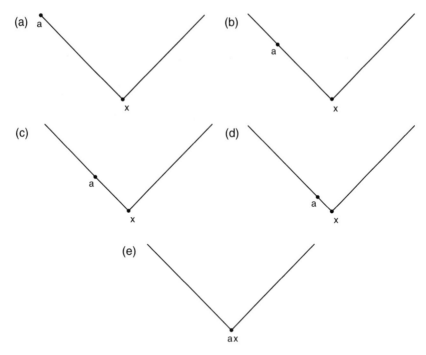

Figure 15.1 A simple model of iteration seen from the side. The current solution is depicted at point A. The ideal solution—which represents the lowest possible point on the surface—is depicted by point X.

Three key assumptions, each of which will be explored, are required for iteration to work. First, an un-ambiguous solution is required. There needs to be something out there—a solution with a roughly stable place in the world—toward which the iteration is aiming. By definition, iteration won't work if there is no target toward which to aim. Second, the process of iteration needs to have some stability over time. This can be thought of in two ways that are roughly equivalent. Either the "aim" of the iterative machinery has to be roughly stable at each stage, or, alternatively, the location of the "solution"—the target of the iterative process—cannot shift about wildly between iterations. Third, the likelihood surface needs to be reasonably smooth. Ideally, it should be "all downhill" from the initial location of the estimate to the final destination. As we will discuss below at length, bumpy likelihood surfaces, especially with local minima that can capture and trap an iterative solution—pose major problems.

15.2 **Epistemic iteration**

In a thoughtful book published in 2004, Chang expands this concept of iteration to develop the concept of EI and applies it to the history of the measurement of temperature specifically and the history of science more generally (Chang 2004). In agreement with the introductory quote, Chang defines EI (where "epistemic" refers to the acquisition of knowledge) as a historical process in which successive stages of knowledge in a given area build in a sequential manner upon each other. Directly analogous to its original mathematical meaning, when correctly applied, the process of EI should lead through successive stages of scientific research toward a better and better approximation of reality in "a spiral of improvement." Of note, before the development of thermometers, there was no external referent for temperature—simply the human perception of cold and warmth. Over time, a series of different "measures" were proposed—especially the expansion of air, water, mercury, and even pottery. Importantly, these measures worked given assumptions that were not at first known—especially about the degree to which changes in volume with temperature were linear. We now know that the nature of the expansion of these different substances was not the same. So, the early thermometers didn't agree. In the language with which psychiatry is familiar, they were using "validators" that were—although correlated—not exactly the same.

Another important part of the story told by Chang is that the search for a good thermometer had to begin with somebody designing what was a very crude thermometer. Start somewhere. At that point, EI could get started. That is, for EI to work "you've got to start somewhere."

15.3 **Modified random walk**

The main alternative to iteration that I want to consider is a modified "random walk." While a central feature of iteration is the progressive approach of the model toward a solution, this is lacking in a random walk. While the model is changing, there is no trend over time for the model to approach the goal.

I call it "modified" because it is probably not quite random. In affairs of human opinion, there are often detectable historical cycles. One viewpoint dominates and holds sway for a period of time. Then, a new viewpoint arises, the bearers of which often look with derision at those of their predecessors, concluding that they now surely have the "correct" view of things. This is illustrated beautifully in Figure 15.2 which depicts the average skirt length in women's dresses from 1605–1936 (Richardson and Kroeber 1940). There are a series of irregular cycles, with periods of maximum length seen in 1641–1660, 1794, 1860, 1902–1905, and 1934–1936. There are also times of shorter skirts, by far the most striking of which is seen in 1927 (think "flappers"). I here have to quote the original authors, "At this time [1927], skirts nearly reached their upper limit of possibility, and probably our less definable limits of decency." (Richardson and Kroeber 1940, p. 129).

Of course, there is no "true" skirt length out there toward which skirts should be approximating over time. Rather, we have changes of style and taste, with a tendency for irregular historical cycles. That is, one style becomes dominant—let us say long dresses—then, there is a reaction against that style and short dresses come into fashion. But then that becomes the dominant style and that is reacted against, and longer dresses come back into fashion. And on it goes.

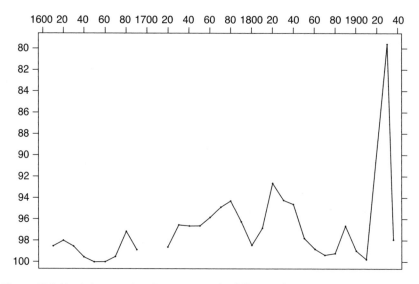

Figure 15.2 X-axis in years. Y axis represents the following fraction multiplied by 100: the distance from the mouth of the female figure to the hem of her dress divided by the distance from the mouth of the female figure to the bottom of her feet.

15.4 **Epistemic iteration and psychiatric illness**

So, is EI a viable model for psychiatric illness? Let us first ask under what conditions would it clearly not work? Let us illustrate how the three problems with iteration outlined earlier would play out for psychiatry.

First, it would make some sense to argue that EI has to assume a realist model for psychiatric illness—that is, if psychiatric disorders don't exist out there in the world in any real way, then EI will have to fail. It would be like iterating toward a target which isn't there. In considering this issue further, I am less convinced of the absoluteness of this position. While it might seem odd to iterate toward a target that you were not firmly convinced was real, EI could be used given certain weaker pragmatic models for psychiatric illness. I expand on this later. Putting this point a bit differently, I do not think it would be correct to assume that in the absence of a strong realistic model for psychiatric disorders we would inevitably be doomed to a random walk across DSM editions.

Second, EI clearly won't work if the method used to move the process forward differs dramatically over time. In the temperature story, some scientists were trying to improve the design of mercury thermometers and others with air thermometers. These approaches were not the same, but were, pretty highly correlated. But what would happen if the validating methods—the empirical methods used to try to move the iterative process forward—differed dramatically over time? I have used the term "wobbly iteration" to describe this process (Kendler 2009). Why will it wobble? It will wobble because, as we will outline in a moment, the "aim" in the iterative process would not be exactly the same at each step. This would occur if, for example, different diagnostic validators were emphasized at each iteration. Or, we can express this same point in a roughly analogous way by saying that the target of the iteration—the true nature of the psychiatric disorder—itself, changes over iterations. As we will try to show, the process can tolerate some degree of wobble of the aim of EI or the location of its target. However, if this becomes too great, the system will spin out of control and lose its cumulative character.

Third, EI won't work if the clinical historical concepts of psychiatric illness with which this process began in DSM-III are not even "in the right ball-park." EI requires that "you can get there from here." This problem might arise if some scientific break-through, the nature of which we cannot currently conceive, is required to truly under-stand the nature of psychiatric illness. For EI to work, some proximity in multivariate space is required between our current clinical-historical constructs and the true typol-ogy of psychiatric illnesses. If that true typology differs dramatically from our current conceptions of psychiatric illness, we are likely in deep trouble.

15.5 Graphical approach

So now, in the meat of this essay, I utilize a simple-minded graphical approach to explore the applicability of the EI model to psychiatric nosology over historical time. Let's start with assumptions. Turning again to Figure 15.1, we start out in a large likeli-hood surface. This surface now represents the degree to which a current diagnostic construct represents "roughly" the true or real form of the psychiatric disorder under consideration. So the bottom of this function, spot X, is the true place we want our syndrome definition to be. It is the spot for which a psychiatric nosologist should yearn. That is where he or she wants to get—so that the diagnostic criteria well capture the true nature of the illness.

But instead of being at X, we are actually at point A. In psychiatry, we can, for the sake of the current argument, assume that this point reflects the clinical-historical constructs that were articulated in DSM-III.

How would we get from A to X? In the simple model of EI, researchers would revise the criteria describing the syndrome under consideration using a range of validators each of which reflects to some limited degree the true disorder. That is, to be explicit, we expect that the true disorder will perform better on our key validators—have a more homogeneous outcome, be more diagnostically stable, have a distinct pattern of comorbidity, a clearer pathophysiology, and be more familial—than any approxima-tion of the disorder. So if we change criteria of syndrome A to improve its perform-ance on these validators, we will of necessity move syndrome A closer to position X. So this is the process that I am trying to capture in Figure 15.1.

Now, for reasons that hopefully will become clear, I want to look at this process from the top looking down and will ask you to imagine the three-dimensional compo-nent. Figures 15.3a–e show you the same process as Figure 15.1, but top-down. This is what progressive, simple EI should look like. If only life were this simple.

Let us now depict the opposite extreme. Figures 15.4a–e illustrate what would I will call the "modified random walk." Here, over time, the position of A is changed but there is no systematic use of empirical methods to more closely approximate X. While this may seem cynical (and possibly incorrect), I would suggest this is how a lot of traditional clinical psychiatry worked. We had the "great German Professors"—a few

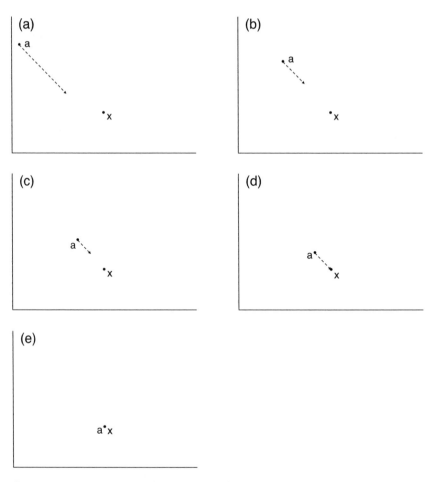

Figure 15.3 A simple model of iteration seen from the top. The current solution is depicted to be stably located at point A. The ideal solution—which represents the lowest possible point on the surface—is depicted by point X.

great individuals who articulated visions of individual disorders. The impact of these visions had to do with persuasiveness of the description and the prestige of the author.

An illustration might help. If we have a concept of what true schizophrenia might be, then think of where we would represent on this graph the position of—in rough historical order—E. Kraepelin (Kraepelin 1899), E. Bleuler (Bleuler 1950), G. Langfeldt (Langfeldt 1939), and K. Schneider (Schneider 1959). Each of them wrote cogent monographs that were internally consistent and rather clinically convincing describing a concept of schizophrenia. But, was there anything like a progressive process—a greater proximity to a true concept of schizophrenia? Or was there a cycle? Kraepelin focused largely on a deteriorative course of illness in defining dementia praecox. Bleuler focused largely on symptoms in his approach to schizophrenia—e.g. his "four As."

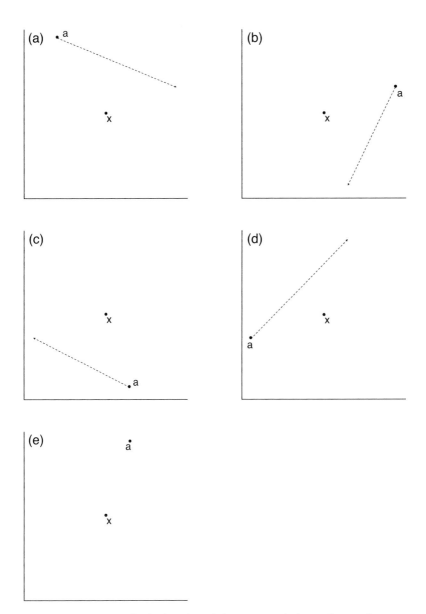

Figure 15.4 A random walk. The location of the current solution X changes from iteration to iteration but with no tendency to approach the solution at point A. The true position of the syndrome in multivariate space is stable at point A. This produces no evidence for a cumulative process as A does not get closer to X over time.

Langfeldt distinguished his true schizophrenic disorders from schizophreniform cases largely on the basis of course of illness. Schneider, as we all know, defined schizophrenia solely on the basis of specific psychotic symptoms. Although quite oversimplified, we might have had something a bit like a "course →symptoms→course →symptoms" progression in this little historical sequence in the defining features of schizophrenia.

If there were a true illness out there, it was not clear that subsequent great professors were inherently getting closer. Berrios reaches the same conclusion from a more thorough examination of the historical record (Berrios et al. 2003). He concludes that the idea that the diagnosis of schizophrenia has been steadily improving up to the DSM-IV is a "myth." He goes on to say, "The history of schizophrenia can best be described as the history of a set of research programs running in parallel rather than serialism and each based on a different concept of disease, of mental symptom and of mind."

So, in our language, the resulting process for schizophrenia is probably closer to a modified random walk than to EI. (This may be too harsh a verdict in that even "great professors" are likely to incorporate works of current science in their thinking. But if you were to look at the history of more traditional psychiatric nosology prior to DSM-III, it would be hard, I suspect, to defend rigorously a model of progressive scientific progress.)

Now I want to examine the space between simple EI and the modified random walk. First, what might happen if the criterion for detecting the solution is stable but slightly off? That is, it is subtly inaccurate across iterations—such as might occur if we didn't model quite accurately the non-linear expansion of mercury in our thermometer. A psychiatric example might be that our validating measures do not exactly point toward the true diagnosis but they do so approximately. Figures 15.5a–e show that generally this will still iterate, albeit more slowly. This informal modeling suggests, consistent with common sense, that our "validating" criteria do not need to have perfect aim for the basic iterative process to work.

Second, what would happen if the true nature of the psychiatric disorder shifted over time? Most of us working in psychiatric nosology hope that the syndromes we describe are broadly stable over time, space and culture. But what if this is not true? In his provocative book, *Mad Travelers* (Hacking 1998), Ian Hacking described a historically and spatially constrained mini-epidemic of "wandering fugue" states largely in France over a few decades toward the end of the 19th century. He makes a strong case that for some psychiatric syndromes, social and historical influences can be critical.

A more contemporary model may be that the war-induced "post-traumatic stress disorder" (PTSD) syndrome might be contextually influenced (e.g. by the nature of the war, the quality of medical care, the population support of the war effort, etc.). Therefore, the "PTSD-like" syndrome that has arisen in World War I, World War II, Korea, Vietnam, Iraq and Afghanistan is not exactly the same syndrome. Another example might be the influence of technological developments on patterns of psychopathology. A proportion of people who used to suffer from traditional voyeurism (for males—"Peeping Toms") may now find these urges more easily satisfied on the Web (Metzl 2004).

Figures 15.6a–e illustrate what might happen if the nature of the syndrome shifted short distances in multidimensional space. As one might suspect, the iterative system

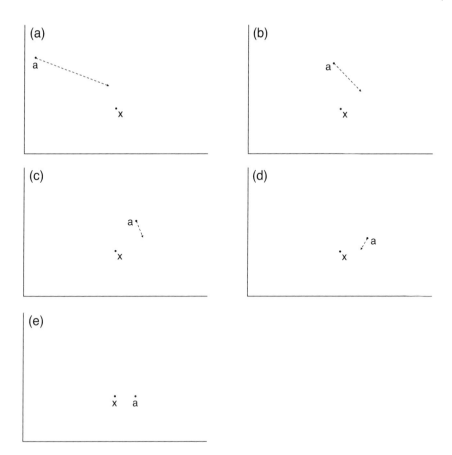

Figure 15.5 A model of epistemic iteration in which the "aim" of the iterative process is a bit off. The true position of the syndrome in multivariate space is stable at point A. Compared to Figures 15.3a–e, the model is less efficient and takes longer to approach the target. However, a cumulative process is evidence as A tends to approach X.

would still work, albeit more slowly and inaccurately. Figures 15.7a–e illustrate what would happen if the nature of the syndrome shifted dramatically over time. In this case, a cumulative process is unlikely to unfold. The target is shifting too far and too rapidly. One might think of this as a "random chase." Like the story of Achilles and the hare, the nosologic construct (point A) will never catch up to the "true" disease location in multivariate space.

Third, what would happen if the validators that were used at each iteration to assess the construct shifted dramatically? This would be one way to tell the brief story of diagnostic approaches to schizophrenia articulated earlier. Looking forward, this might be expected if, in one DSM edition, all disorders were evaluated on the basis of

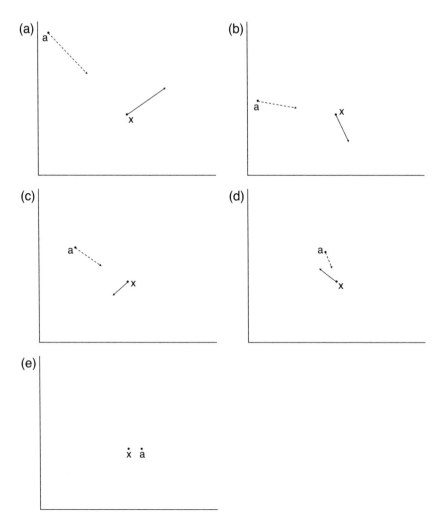

Figure 15.6 A model of epistemic iteration in which the target of the iterative process—point A—shifts modestly from iteration to iteration. Like Figure 15.5a–e, compared to Figures 15.3a–e, the model is less efficient and takes longer to approach the target. However, a cumulative process is evidence as A tends to approach X.

patterns of familial aggregation. By the next edition, opinion had shifted dramatically and drug responsiveness was considered the sole critical validating criterion. Then in the next edition, brain imaging was seen as the be-all and end-all of nosology.

What happens under this circumstance depends critically on the correlation between the true nature of psychiatric disorders defined by different validators (Kendler 1990). For example, how similar would a "schizophrenic" or a "major depressive" syndrome be if that syndrome were designed to maximize familial aggregation, treatment response or magnetic resonance imaging patterns? An optimistic response would be

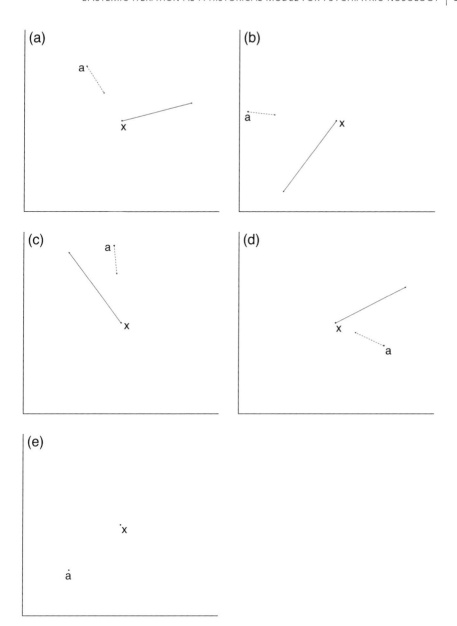

Figure 15.7 A model of epistemic iteration in which the target of the iterative process shifts substantially from iteration to iteration. Unlike Figures 15.3a–e and 15.5a–e, but like Figures 15.4a–e, the model spins out of control and approaches a "random chase." No cumulative process is evident and A does not tend to approach X over time.

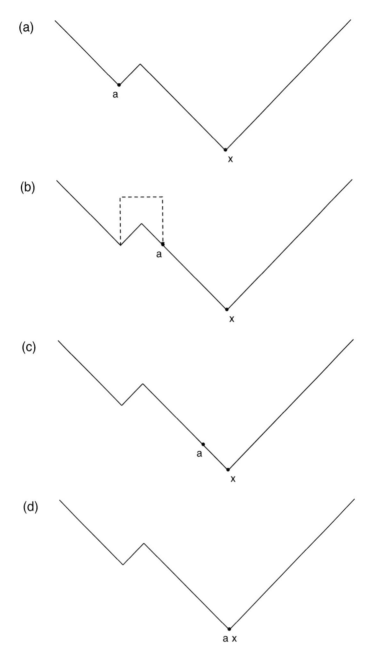

Figure 15.8 A model in which the process of epistemic iteration gets stuck in a local minimum in Figure15.8a. The process needs to be "re-booted" so that the iterative process gets over the local minimum as depicted in Figure 15.8b. With this done, the iterative process can again get back to work and find the target X which it reaches in Figure 15.8d.

"close enough"—meaning that the shifting of the true nature of syndrome would resemble that seen in Figures 15.5a–e and EI could still be expected to work. A pessimistic assumption is that these syndromes would actually differ a lot and the expected pattern would be closer to Figures 15.6a–e in which cases the nosologic systems would be more of a "random chase" than a cumulative iterative process.

I doubt that anyone can reach a definitive global conclusion about whether the optimistic or pessimistic scenario is closer to the truth here. The answer is likely to vary substantially across disorders and the exact nature of the shifts of the validating criteria. There are some examples where the shifts will be large (Kendler 1990) but these results may not generalize. This is, in part, an empirical question.

Fourth, up until now, I have unrealistically assumed that psychiatric disorders represent a "point" in likelihood space. While convenient, this approach assumes an essentialist model for psychiatric illness to which I do not ascribe. There is not one central feature (like the number of protons in an atomic nucleus) that defines a psychiatric disorder and sets it apart from all other disorders. Rather, it is more realistic to think of psychiatric disorders as closer to biological species. They exist as "blobs" in multidimensional space with more central and more peripheral cases (Kendler et al. 2011). This is what we would find for any multifactorial syndrome in medicine. This reality just adds a further degree of "wobble" to the process but is not, in my view, a crippling problem and I won't further explore its implications here.

Finally, what happens if the iterative process gets stuck in a local minimum? Let me go back and modify our original Figure 15.1 to demonstrate this in Figure 15.8a. Local minima are the bane of statistical modelers. If a lot of them exist, you cannot start from any point in the iterative process and always get to the true solution. Rather, you get stuck in these local minima. We see this state in Figure 15.8a. Little changes won't get you out. Instead, we have to "re-boot" the system and get over the hump as seen in Figure 15.8b. This "deux ex machina" mechanism lifts our point A over the obstacles and then EI takes over and the target is reached in Figure 15.8d.

(For readers familiar with population genetics, it might be helpful to understand this problem as analogous to a population being in a trough in an evolutionary landscape. You have to flip over top to bottom, but otherwise the picture is the same. To get to where you need to go, you have to get over an adaptive valley to reach the "hill" of maximal fitness. Small mutations (which equal our tiny iterative steps) cannot do it. You need a big one.)

Why might our disorders get stuck in a local minimum? While there might be several small "technical" reasons for this, the most interesting (and worrying) possibility is that the clinical-historical syndromes that we have started this process with are not close enough to the truth about psychiatric illness for us to get there from here. This is the "not even in the ball-park" metaphor I used previously.

Here the population genetics example is helpful. Generally, our approach to modifying psychiatric diagnoses is like a small mutation. We consider adding a criterion (like "craving" to substance dependence or "hopelessness" to major depression), simplifying criteria (as we did with generalized anxiety disorder from DSM-III-R to DSM-IV) or changing duration. These small changes are like the small steps of an iterative evolutionary process.

But maybe the place we started with a diagnosis is like an evolutionary box canyon. Small changes cannot fix it. We need a big re-design. According to some experts, this is the position in which personality disorders in DSM-IV finds itself.

The problem of local minima is a deep one. In particular, how will you know when you are in one? When do you decide that a diagnostic category is so broken that small fixes are not going to work? I cannot now provide any satisfactory answers for these questions.

15.6 **Implications**

I want to start by contrasting starkly and melodramatically two different historical models for psychiatric nosology. Do we want our nosology to be progressive and cumulative as seen in most examples of Western science and captured by the concept of EI, or do we want it to reflect a modified random walk though time as seen in a variety of social trends and values and exemplified here by dress length?

I want to suggest that if DSM and ICD iterations do not require empirical evidence that the changes made in psychiatric disorders are an improvement over the previous version (that is—in our language—are moving closer to point X), then a modified random walk is likely to result. It is human nature to feel that your predecessors (those who worked on the prior manual) were not as smart or insightful as you. You can do it better. Especially given the prestige within psychiatry that arises from having your imprint on DSM, this process will guarantee that diagnostic changes will occur but this alone will not necessarily produce progression.

However, it is also clear that merely saying we will "rely on data to produce change" is no guarantee of success. If in leading one revision we focus on one sort of validating data, and our predecessors and successors focus on completely different kinds of data, this is unlikely to work either. Fortunately, I don't think we have to (and don't think we could if we wanted to) get it "exactly right" each time. Our science is just not up to that. However, we can probably tolerate some wobble and still get pretty close to where we want to go.

Is EI a fool-safe method to solve the problems of psychiatric nosology? No. It is the best alternative I can see but there are reasons to be skeptical. Of the various problems, an obvious one is the possibility that psychiatric disorders as even semi-discrete entities do not really exist in nature. That is, there is no "there there" toward which to aim. While this might at first seem a fatal objection to the whole idea of EI, the reality may be more subtle. If we took a more instrumentalist rather than realistic approach to psychiatric disorders (similar to the practical kinds model of Peter Zachar (2003)), it still might be possible to develop an iterative approach. But here it would be toward some agreed upon set of tasks at which we wanted our diagnoses to optimally perform, rather than toward some external reality out there.

I am quite worried about whether we can sustain the level of historical discipline to keep the iterative process on track. We are still a young and rather immature science. We are prone to trends and, dare I say, fashions. Can we keep the EI machinery on target for a few more iterations of DSM and ICD by focusing on a common set of key validators? That is not at all clear to me.

The deepest issue, and the one that is most worrisome, is whether we are even "in the right ball park?" Imagine transporting ourselves 100 years in the future and looking back on the DSM-IV manual. Is it possible that we will be laughed at for the backwardness of our approaches to psychiatric illnesses the way we might regard the Hippocratic humoral theory of disease today? A closely related issue is the question: "How would we know if we were not?" Here we get into speculations about the future of psychiatric research. I do not think that our future genetics and neuroscience are going to discover single simple causes of our psychiatric disorders—true essences. Rather, I think that our disorders are, with rare exceptions, inherently multifactorial. That is, we have not found the cause for schizophrenia or depression, not because we are stupid or because our science is so crude, but because there is no one cause.

However, perhaps we will someday be able to describe psychiatric disorders at a systems level—as disturbances in specific psychobiological pathways that have an anatomy and a physiology. If we are to make a move toward an etiologically-based diagnostic system, this seems to me as the most likely direction we will take. All kinds of questions will arise—especially about the idea level at which to describe our systems—psychological, systems neuroscience and molecular neuroscience.

But if such a shift toward etiologically based diagnoses does occur, how will we make the shift from our current historical-clinical syndromes? Is this the "re-booting" that we depict in Figure 15.8b? How will we know when we need the boot—when it is time to stop making small incremental advances and go in for a major overhaul? If we make major overhauls when small steps are likely to work, then we are at risk for ending up further from the target. However, if we are stuck in an iterative box canyon, we could go on for a long time making no real progress.

There is a long tradition in the philosophy of science of trying to illustrate and potentially validate a philosophical claim from historical analysis. While beyond my charge here, it is worth sketching out what we might find if we considered some of the modest "successes" we have had in psychiatric nosology over the last century. Kraepelin conceptualized manic-depressive illness as a broad category including what we now would consider unipolar and bipolar illness (BPI) (and perhaps a few other conditions) (Kraepelin 1990). By contrast, Leonhard saw it something differently—and suggested that bipolar disorder should be separated from the other mood syndromes (Leonhard et al. 1999). Leonhard's concept of BPI was later robustly supported by its differential treatment response to lithium. This heightened awareness of the importance of a history of mania led a range of new studies focused on BPI, and the rise of focused operationalized diagnostic criteria. A new generation of research then showed that it was meaningful to divide bipolar from non-bipolar cases of mood disorder as a function of age at onset, course, risk of illness in relatives, heritability and patterns of comorbidity. Would this story represent a success for the process of EI?

Another case to consider would be Donald Klein's separation of panic disorder from other anxiety states on the basis of pharmacologic response to low-dose imipramine (Klein 1964). This work was followed by a generation of studies showing that panic disorder, now diagnosed using operationalized diagnostic criteria, had a distinct set of precipitants (lactate, carbon dioxide) and patterns of illness in relatives. Or going back into the 19th century, what could we learn about the role of EI in the history of general paralysis of the insane, from the first proposals based only on gross anatomy and limited follow-up that it represented a distinct form of insanity, to the detailed pathology and clinical studies documented in Kraepelin, to the eventual clarification of the specific etiology by Nogouchi and Moore (Noguchi and Moore 1913)? Might it be useful to look at a less successful story? For example, atypical depression attracted a lot of attention in the 1980s and 1990s in part because of evidence suggesting that this syndrome was particularly responsive to a particular type of antidepressant drugs—the monoamine oxidase inhibitors (Quitkin et al. 1988; Stewart et al. 2007). Several epidemiological studies using latent class analysis identified it as a distinct subtype of depression (e.g. Horwath et al. 1992; Sullivan et al. 2002). However, although there remains an "atypical features specifier" for major depression in DSM-IV, the disorder has not "caught on" and is rarely a subject of clinical or research interest. Or, finally, would it be useful to review whether the operationalized DSM-III concept of schizophrenia really was more valid than the descriptive DSM-II diagnosis that it replaced?

Further scholarly work on these and other potential psychiatric disorders might shed important light on the construct of EI as I have here articulated it. One potential lesson that these case examples might already illustrate is that my focus on single disorders is naïve. What may happen more for psychiatric disorders is that single syndromes split up over time into two or more conditions each with greater validity (and greater resemblance to the way things really are) than the parent diagnosis from which they sprang. This progression is schematically shown in Figures 15.9a–c. Nosologists would begin with one diagnosis (a) that they are trying to improve (Figure 15.9a). However, as seen in Figure 15.9b, further studies show that syndrome A really consists of two syndromes, B and C, which have different targets toward which EI will bring them (x and y). So we end up with two validated disorders by two independent processes of EI (Figure 15.9c). Such a process is probably quite common in the history of medicine (e.g. the division of diabetes into type I and type II).

15.7 **Conclusions**

Psychiatric nosology is part of a time line. We are in the middle of a long historical process. We have to situate ourselves in that context. The EI model is one way to do that. We should admire our predecessors—both the great descriptive psychiatrics of past days like Kraepelin and those who launched us on our current trajectory (personally, I would here emphasize Eli Robins and Robert Spitzer). However, we can do something more important than admiration. We need to regard our nosologic systems as structures of substantial value to our young field. We should seek to pass them on to our successors in yet better shape than we found them. This is the essence of EI. However, EI is no panacea. There are situations where we can expect it to work and others where it will fail. It may be appropriate during some historical periods in the evolution of the science of psychiatry and not in others. How sensitive is it to the underlying external reality of psychiatric disorders? How would it respond to major scientific developments the nature of which we cannot now even accurately picture? The future holds many challenges for psychiatric nosology. Whether the concept of EI will provide any guidance through these difficulties remains to be seen.

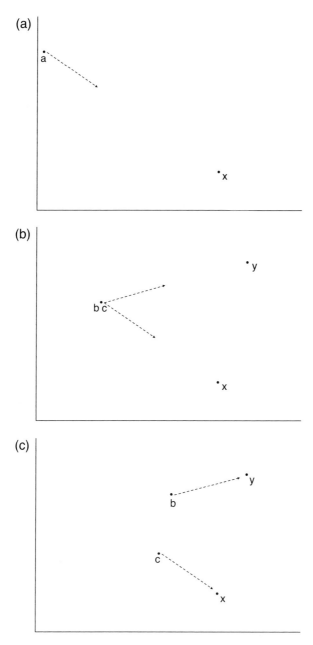

Figure 15.9 A model of epistemic iteration in which the initial syndrome A actually consists of two different syndromes B and C. When this division is discovered, it becomes possible to further improve each disorder (toward goals y and x) via two separate EI processes.

Chapter References

Berrios, G. E., Luque, R. and Villagran, J. M. (2003). Schizophrenia: A conceptual history. *International Journal of Psychology and Psychological Therapy*, 3(2), 111–40.

Bleuler, E. (1950). *Dementia Praecox, or The Group of Schizophrenias*. New York: International Universities Press.

Chang, H. (2004). *Inventing Temperature: Measurement and Scientific Progress*. New York: Oxford University Press.

Hacking, I. (1998). *Mad Travelers: Reflections on the Reality of Transient Mental Illnesses*. Charlottesville, VA: University Press of Virginia.

Horwath, E., Johnson, J., Weissman, M. M. and Hornig, C. D. (1992). The validity of major depression with atypical features based on a community study. *Journal of Affective Disorders*, 26(2), 117–25.

Kendler, K. S. (1990). Toward a scientific psychiatric nosology. Strengths and limitations. *Archives of General Psychiatry*, 47(10), 969–73.

Kendler, K. S. (2009). An historical framework for psychiatric nosology. *Psychological Medicine*, 39(12), 1935–41.

Kendler, K. S., Zachar, P. and Craver, C. (2011). What kinds of things are psychiatric disorders? *Psychological Medicine*, 41, 1143–50.

Klein, D. F. (1964). Delineation of two drug-responsive anxiety syndromes. *Psychpharmacologia*, 5, 397–408.

Kraepelin, E. (1899). *Psychiatrie: Ein Lehrbuch fur Studierende und Aerzte* (6th ed. 2 vols.). Leipzig: von Barth Verlag.

Kraepelin, E. (1990). *Psychiatry: A Textbook for Students and Physicians* (Metoui, trans., J. Quen, ed.). Canton, MA: Science History Publications.

Langfeldt, G. (1939). *The Schizophreniform States*. London: Oxford University Press.

Leonhard, K., Beckmann, H. E. and Cahn, C. H. T. (1999). *Classification of Endogenous Psychoses and their Differentiated Etiology*, (2nd revision, enlarged ed.). New York: Springer.

Marcum, J. A. (2010). *An Introductory Philosophy of Medicine: Humanizing Modern Medicine* (1st ed.). Netherlands: Springer.

Metzl, J. M. (2004). Voyeur nation? Changing definitions of voyeurism, 1950–2004. *Harvard Review of Psychiatry*, 12(2), 127–31.

Noguchi, H. and Moore, J. W. (1913). A demonstration of Treponema pallidum in the brain in cases of general paralysis. *Journal of Experimental Medicine*, 17, 232–9.

Quitkin, F. M., Stewart, J.W., McGrath, P.J., Liebowitz, M. R., Harrison, W. M., Tricamo, E., *et al.* (1988). Phenelzine versus imipramine in the treatment of probable atypical depression: defining syndrome boundaries of selective MAOI responders. *American Journal of Psychiatry*, 145(3), 306–11.

Richardson, J. and Kroeber, A. L. (1940). Three centuries of women's dress fashions A quantitative analysis. *Anthropological Records*, 5(2), 111–54.

Schneider, K. (1959). *Clinical Psychopathology*. New York: Grune & Stratton.

Stewart, J. W., McGrath, P. J., Quitkin, F. M. and Klein, D. F. (2007). Atypical depression: current status and relevance to melancholia. *Acta Psychiatrica Scandinavica*, 115, 58–71.

Sullivan, P. F., Prescott, C. A. and Kendler, K. S. (2002). The subtypes of major depression in a twin registry. *Journal of Affective Disorders*, 68(2–3), 273–84.

Zachar, P. (2003). The practical kinds model as a pragmatist theory of classification. *Philosophy, Psychology and Psychiatry*, 9(9), 219–27.

Chapter 15: Comments

Coherentist approaches to scientific progress in psychiatry: comments on Kendler

Kenneth F. Schaffner[1]

15.8 Introduction

It is a pleasure to provide comments on Kenneth S. Kendler's essay on "Epistemic iteration as a historical model for psychiatric nosology." The article is a stimulating inquiry into the way that psychiatry may profitably progress as it confronts both the scientific advances in genetics and neuroscience, and the intense discussions taking place around the DSM and ICD revisions.

Kendler offers modifications and extensions of an "epistemic iteration" model that was partially, at least, inspired by Hasok Chang's 2004 book on *Inventing Temperature* (Chang 2004). The present essay by Kendler builds on an earlier 2009 publication of his that also addressed epistemic iteration in psychiatry, as well as on an additional recent paper (Kendler 2009; Kendler and First 2010). In what Kendler terms "the meat of the essay," he explores several contrasting scenarios that vary depending on how far away the "true" state of the psychiatric disorder is from the point at which it is being considered, as well as what the impediments might be in moving from the state under consideration (roughly the current situation in psychiatry for any specific disorder). Such impediments might be that the current state is too far away from reality, or that it is "stuck" at a wrong but difficult to modify state, calling for a major "reboot" of the system to rectify this type of problem. Alternatively, the validators might change so radically that real progress will not occur, only a kind of "wobbly change." Kendler's more abstract analyses are also enriched by several historical examples, one discussing the apparent non-progressive cycle that four "great professors," Kraepelin, Bleuler, Langfeldt and Schneider exhibited in their influential monographs on schizophrenia. Other examples refer to the social aspects of psychiatry, including Hacking's account of the "mad travelers" of the 19th century and the explosion of PTSD today (Hacking 2002).

However, Kendler's main concern, and main alternative to progress, is with what he calls a "modified random walk." Kendler defines this as follows: "While a central feature of iteration is the progressive approach of the model toward a solution, this is lacking in a random walk. While the model is changing, there is no trend over time for the model to approach the goal." This is the kind of change we might see in fashion change, and here Kendler refers to changing women's skirt lengths, though he could as easily noted the width of men's neck ties. He writes: "Of course, there is no 'true' skirt length out there toward which skirts should be approximating over time. Rather, we have changes of style and taste, with a tendency for irregular historical cycles."

15.9 **Another more Chang-like EI alternative**

It is curious that while Kendler cites Chang's approach in *Inventing Temperature* as a major inspiration for his (Kendler's) extensions to psychiatry, he takes an *opposite* epistemic direction than does Chang on the nature of truth, reality and the nature of scientific progress. In his 2004 book, Chang adopts what philosophers call a "coherentist" or anti-realist approach to truth, whereas Kendler's analysis in this and his other EI articles, is robustly realist, or in line with a "correspondence" notion of truth. It is worth reiterating Kendler's key assumption underlining his view of EI, and then contrasting Chang's account. This will not of itself tell us who has the better overall general view, nor which approach—coherence or correspondence—might be more suitable for psychiatry. But I will then explore what might be the implications of turning (this aspect of) Kendler on its head, and speculate on how a more Chang-like coherentist account might be developed in contemporary psychiatry to characterize "progress."

Kendler proposes there are "three key assumptions" that "are required for [epistemic] iteration to work." The first of these, and the one directly related to the points in the previous paragraph, is that "an un-ambiguous solution is required. There needs to be *something out there*—a solution with at least a roughly stable place *in the world*— toward which the iteration is aiming. Iteration won't work if there is no target toward which to aim." [my emphasis] (Kendler's other two assumptions require a "stable 'process of iteration, and that the process needs to travel a 'relatively smooth' journey, but I will not dwell on these other two assumptions in these comments).

As a backdrop issue, it is important to note that Chang saw some important differences between iteration as practiced in mathematics, and the expanded notion of EI that he (Chang) developed in application to the physics of the temperature concept. Chang writes that EI "differs crucially from mathematical iteration in that the latter is used to approach the correct answer that is known, or at least in principle knowable, by other means. In epistemic iteration that is not so clearly the case"[2] (Chang 2004, p. 45).

As a prelude to further more specific comparison of Kendler and Chang, consider the following additional quotations from Chang's book. These contrast sharply with the Kendler notion of EI that targets (though it may well miss) the "truth," and the Chang notion that eschews the notion of "truth" as a goal for EI:

> How about truth? Can we ever say whether we have obtained the true values of an abstract concept like absolute temperature? The question of truth only makes sense if there is an objectively determinate value of the concept in each physical situation. In case we have a convergent operationalization, we could consider the limits of convergence as the "real" values; then we can use these values as the criteria by which we judge whether other proposed operationalizations produce true values. But we must keep firmly in mind that the

existence of such "real values" hinges on the success of the iterative procedure, and the successful operationalization is constitutive of the "reality." If we want to please ourselves by saying that we can approach true values by iterative operationalization, we also have to remember that this truth is a destination that is only created by the approach itself (Chang 2004, p. 217).

This *will* sound obscure, and perhaps suspiciously circular, especially the comment that "this truth is a destination that is only created by the approach itself."[3] To situate the points that I want to develop to clarify Chang's approach, it will be most useful to summarize the general theme of his chapter 6 on justification and progress, which is more philosophically reflective than his earlier more historical chapters. He writes, addressing a circularity he finds in the realist or foundationalist approach, that:

> The only productive way of dealing with that circularity is to accept and admit that justi-fication in empirical science has to be coherentist. Within such coherentism, epistemic iteration provides an effective method of scientific progress, resulting in the enrichment and self-correction of the initially affirmed system. This mode of scientific progress embraces both conservatism and pluralism at once (Chang 2004, p. 220).

We can perhaps find some further clarity in the use of two suggestive analogies that Chang develops, though these are not original analogies due to Chang. They arise out of the perennial debate among philosophers about realism (and the related correspondence theory of truth), and non-realism and its "coherence" theory of truth. Here non-realism, for our purposes, can be roughly read as equivalent to instrumen-talism. These analogies are the "turtles" and the "building" analogies, or, if you will, images, that may help situate the distinction between Kendler and Chang more intui-tively. The gist of the turtle analogy is the ancient mythology where the flat earth rested on the back of very large elephants and the elephants stood on the back of a giant turtle, raising the question on what did the turtle stand—i.e., the beginning of an infinite regress for any type of "foundationalism." As an alternative analogy, Chang suggests we think of the earth as round, and as our structures, including scientific concepts, as being built outward. The earth Chang adds is not "grounded," but it can serve as a foundation "simply because it is a large solid and dense body that coheres within itself and attracts other objects to it. In science to, too, we build structures around what we are first given, and that does not require the starting points to be absolutely secure." This analogy is perhaps a bit obscure as regards this surrogate for a foundation, but it does resonate with another analogy Chang also uses of Neurath's boat which must be rebuilt at sea on a journey to an unknown land (see Chang 2004, pp. 156–157).

The question for us, now, is whether giving up on a foundationalist or correspond-ence notion of truth and accepting, at least provisionally, a coherentist notion, can make any sense when applied to the area of psychiatric disorders. Furthermore, can a coherentist notion of EI suggest certain directions regarding progress that can side-step the inaccessible notion of something "out there"—a notion that might be a meta-physically sound idea, but seems epistemically (and practically) empty? (More detailed arguments related to the meaning and roles of realism in psychiatry are developed in my paper in this volume.)

15.10 **Progress in science within a coherentist framework**

Chang's coherentist perspective recalls a similar view urged by Kuhn in the last chapter of his influential *Structure of Scientific Revolutions*. In that chapter, Kuhn (finally) turned to the notion of "truth" as well as the notion of drawing closer to it, and noted that truth at best enters only "as a source for the scientist's conviction that incompatible rules for doing science cannot coexist except during revolutions when the profession's main task is to eliminate all sets but one." Kuhn adds:

> The developmental process described in this essay has been a process of evolution from primitive beginnings-a process whose successive stages are characterized by an increasingly detailed and refined understanding of nature. But nothing that has been or will be said makes it a process of evolution *toward* anything. Inevitably that lacuna will have disturbed many readers. We are all deeply accustomed to seeing science as the one enterprise that draws constantly nearer to some goal set by nature in advance. (Kuhn 1970, p. 170).

Kuhn then suggested an important alternative:

> But need there be any such goal? Can we not account for both science's existence and its success in terms of evolution from the community's state of knowledge at any given time? Does it really help to imagine that there is some one full, objective, true account of nature and that the proper measure of scientific achievement is the extent to which it brings us closer to that ultimate goal? If we can learn to substitute evolution from-what-we-do-know for evolution-toward-what-we-wish-to-know, a number of vexing problems may vanish in the process. Somewhere in this maze, for example, must lie the problem of induction (Kuhn 1970, p. 171).

Kuhn then noted he "cannot yet specify in any detail the consequences of this alternate view of scientific advance" (p. 170). He does say that this is a "Darwinian" position and contrasts with earlier "teleological" approaches to evolutions. In his 1970 Postscript to his *Structure . . .*, Kuhn amplified on his views concerning truth, realism, and progress. In his Postscript he wrote, noting that his view of progress would not satisfy the typical "philosopher," (e.g., Popper), since for such a philosopher:

> A scientific theory is usually felt to be better than its predecessors not only in the sense that it is a better instrument for discovering and solving puzzles but also because it is somehow a better representation of what nature is really like. One often hears that successive theories grow ever closer to, or approximate more and more closely to, the truth. Apparently generalizations like that refer not to the puzzle-solutions and the concrete predictions derived from a theory but rather to its ontology, to the match, that is, between the entities with which the theory populates nature and what is "really there."
>
> Perhaps there is some other way of salvaging the notion of 'truth' for application to whole theories, but this one will not do. There is, I think, no theory-independent way to reconstruct phrases like 'really there'; the notion of a match between the ontology of a theory and its "real" counterpart in nature now seems to me illusive in principle (Kuhn, 1970, p. 206).

So far as I am aware, Kuhn never developed this "evolution from what we know" view further, though towards the end of my comments, I will point out a rough way Kuhn thinks one might compare paradigms and account for his kind of "progress."

And, Kuhn once stated (to me) that he felt that Darwinian progress notion was one of his least clear and least successful aspects of his *Structure* book (personal conversation, 1983).

There seem to be two ways that scientific progress might be assessed from a coherentist perspective. One was stated by Kuhn himself, and interestingly Chang seems to agree with this what I will call a "comparative" approach. The other approach, original to Chang, I believe, is to build up a concept—for him temperature and for us a psychiatric disorder—from basic elements, albeit not "foundationalist" elements. First a few words on the comparative approach. Elaborating on his Darwinian metaphor in his Postscript, Kuhn imagines a tree of theory descent where one could compare an earlier theory with a later theory, or paradigm. (Note that in even imaging this scenario, Kuhn has tempered his more radical claim that such a comparison is possible, and that these successive theories or paradigms are not incommensurable.) Envisioning such a comparison, Kuhn writes that "it should be easy to design a list of criteria that would enable an uncommitted observer to distinguish the earlier from the more recent theory time after time" (p. 205). Kuhn then provides a list of such criteria, suggesting that the most useful might be "accuracy of prediction, especially quantitative prediction; the balance between esoteric and everyday subject matter; and the number of different problems solved" (p. 206). Kuhn also indicated what he saw as "less useful though still important criteria, suggesting 'simplicity, scope, and compatibility with other specialties'" (p. 206). This is not yet a complete list, but Kuhn thought the project was doable and might provide a sense of irreversible direction to the scientific process of development.

What Kuhn is listing here then are prima facie trans-paradigmatic "values" or better epistemic "criteria" in terms of which one might judge a later theory better than a previous one. Kuhn was especially skeptical of the *application* of such criteria, particularly during periods of paradigm conflict. In another earlier part of his Postscript, Kuhn notes that these values are quite variable in application, citing the difference between Einstein on what seemed to be "an insupportable inconsistency in the old quantum theory," and Bohr, who saw that so-called inconsistency as a mere puzzle—"a difficulty that could be expected to work itself out by normal means." (p. 185) Kuhn continued to be skeptical of the application of such criteria, and reiterated that skepticism, even after refining a list of criteria of theory choice in chapter 13 of his later book *The Essential Tension* (Kuhn 1977).

I've argued elsewhere they can and do work to change paradigms quite extensively in the scientific community (but not necessarily in recalcitrant individuals) given enough time. How long a period? Actually usually only about 5–10 years in those examples I've looked at closely. (These examples include Einstein special relativity versus Lorentzian aether theory (Schaffner 1970, 1972) and the clonal selection theory versus an instructive theory of immunology (Schaffner 1993), esp. chapter 5). In a sense, more specific forms of these criteria would be the validators that Kendler has discussed in his paper.

It is of interest that Chang generally agrees with the use of these epistemic criteria, noting that though "historically contingent to a degree. . . they have considerable force in directing our judgments" (2004, p. 227).

The second way that progress might be achieved in a coherentist framework is suggested by Chang when he discusses the important role of "sensations" as a basis for our temperature concept. The proposal assumes what Chang calls a "principle of respect," which roughly means that one gives some prima facie credence to a pre-existing analysis, and does not dismiss it out of hand. (Bayesians might describe this as not attributing a zero probability to a hypothesis.) The approach is introduced fairly early in the book (p. 43) by describing the relation between human sensations and measuring instruments. Here sensation, such as our subjective feelings of hot and cold, are treated with *respect* and utilized, even as we initially "correct" them with instruments such as crude thermometers. Chang refers here to an experiment in which we put "one hand in a bucket of hot water and the other one in cold water." Here we at least initially respect the sensations not because they have a "stronger justification," but primarily because they are *prior* in time to the development of more sophisticated instruments, and, as Chang writes we really "do not have any plausible alternative" (p. 43.)

15.11 **Progress in psychiatry within a coherentist framework**

I now want to turn from a coherentist approach within science generally to how some of these proposals in the preceding section might be applied to progress in psychiatry. Here I will concentrate on the second approach just outlined, the one which proceeded from a "sensation" base. This is more complex in psychiatry, in part because many of the standard psychiatric disorders are not commonly subjectively experienced by most humans, even though all have likely been in kinds of "formes frustes" of major depressive disorder and various compulsion states, and perhaps even in mild psychoses. But there is no clear virtually universal intersubjective analogue of "putting one hand in a bucket of hot water and the other one in cold water." Thus it will be necessary to generalize from a "first-person" account of a sensory base, to a "second-" or "third-person" account of the psychiatric symptoms reported by those afflicted with these disorders. This is a kind of "heterophenomenology" to use Dennett's term, but it can be quite reliable and can be used as a starting point in this account. (Dennett 1991) (I should mention here that I am not averse to also exploring in this regard the classical philosophical phenomenological approach of the type one can find, for example, in the writings of Husserl and Merleau-Ponty.)

But more is needed, and for the next step I want to draw on a 1998 study by Kendler that develops a "numerical taxonomy" approach to generating psychiatric disorders (Kendler et al. 1998). The specific method is to use what is called "latent class analysis" (LCA) to seek categories underlying clusters of reported symptoms, signs and history items in a large group of psychiatric patients (in this case, probands in the well-known Roscommon Family Study Irish psychiatric registry). LCA (and other statistical clustering approaches) has been used before for similar psychiatric classification purposes, and Kendler et al. (1998) provide nine additional citations to other similar studies. In general, LCA creates non-observational, higher level or "latent" classes based on a collection of observable symptoms and signs in the population of interest.

This 1998 LCA analysis based the resultant latent classes on 21 signs and symptoms, of which 19 came from the standard list in the OPCRIT instrument (see website at: http://sgdp.iop.kcl.ac.uk/opcrit/). Representative OPCRIT items included "persecutory delusions" and "pressured speech." An additional seven items were constructed to increase coverage and limit computational demands. Examples of these composite symptoms are the merging of OPCRIT's "third-person auditory hallucinations" and "running commentary voices" into *Schneiderian hallucinations*; and compiling "abuse/accusatory/persecutory voices" and "other (nonaffective) auditory hallucination" into *other auditory hallucinations.*

The LCA generated six classes of psychiatric disorders, of which two fit well: class 1 with the classic schizophrenia of Kraepelin and Bleuler, and a class 2 that closely resembled the classical and current picture of major depression. Other classes fit somewhat less well, or did not replicate on a further validation study. A class 6, termed "hebephrenia," appeared to have loose relations to a syndrome that had once been identified by Kraepelin and Heckler. See Kendler et al.'s (1998) table 1 summarizing the classes and their item percentages.

Kendler et al. made no claims that this LCA analysis represented "a definitive nosology" (Kendler and Walsh 1998). In addition, there are some significant limitations, noted in the conclusion of this Kendler et al. (1998) article. But it does appear to be a significant "bottom-up" analysis that is in the spirit of Chang's suggestion that we can *build up and out* via a kind of epistemic iteration, and also re-examine other earlier traditions that are granted a modicum of "respect." I would also argue it is in this comparative re-examination that the *other* dimension of theory (or disorder) evaluation might be explored, i.e., developing and applying the "values" for assessing a better set of disorder definitions and classifications. Actually conducting such a comparative evaluation, for example here comparing the Kendler classes with DSM-IV-TR, would require a major effort, including historical inquiry and empirical reanalysis. This is a task that is well beyond this commentary, but perhaps may be a project for the future.

Endnotes

1 These comments have profited from extensive e-mails with Kenneth Kendler, Michael First and Robert Krueger, some earlier e-mails with Kyle Stanford, and also discussions with Kathryn C. Tabb on these topics, as well as from her unpublished paper "Progress Beyond Realism in Psychiatric Nosology."
2 I owe this citation to Kathryn C. Tabb.
3 I thank Kyle Stanford for first bringing to my attention this notion of Chang's that "truth is a destination that is only created by the approach itself."

Comments References

Chang, H. (2004). *Inventing temperature measurement and scientific progress.* New York: Oxford University Press.

Dennett, D. C. (1991). *Consciousness explained.* Boston, MA: Little, Brown and Co.

Hacking, I. (2002). *Mad travelers: reflections on the reality of transient mental illnesses.* Cambridge, MA: Harvard University Press.

Kendler, K. S. (2009). An historical framework for psychiatric nosology. *Psychological Medicine,* **39**(12), 1935–41.

Kendler, K. S. and First, M. B. (2010). Alternative futures for the DSM revision process: iteration v. paradigm shift. *British Journal of Psychiatry,* **197**(4), 263–5.

Kendler, K. S., Karkowski, L. M. and Walsh, D. (1998). The structure of psychosis: latent class analysis of probands from the Roscommon Family Study. *Archives of General Psychiatry,* **55**(6), 492–9.

Kendler, K. S. and Walsh, D. (1998). The structure of psychosis: syndromes and dimensions. *Archives of General Psychiatry,* **55**(6), 508–9.

Kuhn, T. S. (1970). *The structure of scientific revolutions* (2nd edn.). Chicago, IL: University of Chicago Press.

Kuhn, T. S. (1977). *The essential tension: selected studies in scientific tradition and change.* Chicago, IL: University of Chicago Press.

Schaffner, K. F. (1970). Outlines of a logic of comparative theory evaluation with special attention to pre- and post-relative electrodynamics. In: R. Stuewer (ed.), *Minnesota Studies in Philosophy of Science (V).* Minneapolis, MN: University of Minnesota Press, pp. 311–54 and 65–73.

Schaffner, K. F. (1972). *Nineteenth Century Aether Theories.* Oxford: Pergamon Press.

Schaffner, K. F. (1993). *Discovery and Explanation in Biology and Medicine.* Chicago, IL: University of Chicago Press.

Index

abnormality of the body 44, 54–5
absolute validity 19
acceptance of hypotheses and theories 178–9
Achenbach, T. M. 208
affective illness, schizophrenia and 75, 82, 84,
    229–30, 245–6
aggregation 184
alienists 29, 101, 106–7, 108, 109–10
Alzheimer's disease 79
anatomo-clinical model 110
Andreasen, N. C. 88, 170
antecedent validators 88
antidepressant induced mania 46
antisocial personality disorder 65–6, 153
anxiety
    comorbidity with mood disorder 203–4
    schizophrenia 245
Archambault, T. 109
artificial classifications 102
art of medicine 42
Ash, P. 128
assessment model 277
astronomy 24, 25
atheoretical approach 43, 44, 125, 132–4
atomic chemistry 24
atypical depression 320
atypical schizophrenic illnesses 84
audible thoughts 242–3, 244
Austin, J. L. 39

Bacon, F. 108
Baltimore morbidity study 286
baptismal event 28
basic realism 26
behavior perspective 273, 274
Berrios, G. E. 312
bio-bio-bio model 270
biological signal 118–19
biomarkers 4, 9–10, 48, 206
biomedical disease model 4, 9, 10, 13, 41
biopsychosocial model 44, 54
bipolar illness 319
bizarre delusions 242, 262
Bleuler, E. 249
BOGSAT process 141, 149
bold validation 30
Bolton, D. 38
bootstrapping 25
borderline disorders 83, 84
bottom-up study 277
Bouillaud, J. 105

Boyle, R. 23–4
broadcasting 243–4
Buchez, P. 106–7, 109

Caenorhabditis elegans 172, 174
calibration 20, 23–6, 36, 37
Cantor, N. 173
categorical classifications 89–91, 97, 102,
    131–2
categories 86
    real vs socially constructed 99–100
causes of psychiatric conditions 7, 13
cautious progressivism 30–1
Chang, H. 306–7, 324–5, 327
change paradigms 327
claim-making 26–7
Clarke, D. M. 224
classes 103
classification
    artificial 102
    benefits of 61–4, 104
    categorical 89–91, 97, 102, 131–2
    changing 181–5
    concept 101
    dangers of 64–6
    data-driven 205–6
    diagnosis and 78
    dimensional 27, 89–91, 97, 102, 137, 172,
        173–4, 203, 298–9, 300
    exhaustive 103
    folk classifications 86
    goals of 12–13, 145–7
    hierarchical 103
    historical definitions 105–6
    importance of in medicine 8–9
    modesty and caution towards 66–7
    natural 102
    partial 103
    prediction 104
    psychiatric vs biological 281
    scientific 77–8
    structural issues 89–91
    structured 103
    unit of classification in psychiatry 78–9
class-quantitative models 91
clinical care, research link 47–8
clinical-historical approach 197–8
clinically significant distress or
        impairment 287–8, 289
clinical observation 49–50, 56
clinical reality 171

clinical utility 97, 132, 142, 157, 159, 175–6, 181
clinical validity 171–2, 175–6, 183–4, 195
clustering of symptoms/traits 96, 183
cognitive behavioral therapy 275
coherence
  depression 231–2
  epistemic iteration 325
  progress in psychiatry 328–9
  progress in science 326–8
communication 12, 159, 163–4
community prevalence of mental
    disorders 285–8
comorbidity 198, 203–4, 208
  true and spurious 87
comparative approach 327
comparative validity 22, 25–6
Composite International Diagnostic
    Interview 287
concepts 8, 103
concurrent validators 88
conditionalized realism 167, 177–8, 193
consciousness 120, 267
  localization 271–2
consensus 51, 149
conservative science 121
conservative validation 29
construct validity 169–70, 176
context
  depressive symptoms 221–3, 225
  post-traumatic stress disorder 312
contrastive validity 19
convergences 101
Copernican model 25
core position 177, 193
course of disease, prediction 12–13
criterion counting 206–7
criterion variance 128–9
Cronbach, L. J. 169
culture-bound syndromes 200
curability 79, 80, 83
cycloid psychosis 84–5, 246

data-driven classification 205–6
deflationary approach 3, 7, 13
déjà lu 243
Delasiauve, L. J. F. 107
delusions 241–2, 262
demonstration 23–4
demoralization 224
dependent events 222
depression
  atypical 320
  coherence 231–2
  contextual issues 221–3, 225
  continuum of depressive states 226
  dependent events 222
  different concepts 155
  interviews 231
  life events 222
  polysemic nature 230–1

sadness and 221, 223–4, 225–6
schizophrenia 229–30, 245
temporal instability across relapses 230
descriptive approach 132–4
descriptive validity 170
despair 231
Desruelles, M. 106
Dewey, J. 179
diagnosis
  are psychiatrists necessary? 288
  classification and 78
  enlarging diagnostic categories 8
  keeping from patients 67
  latent variable modeling 206
  multiple 47, 205
  narratives 65–6
  new diagnostic categories 68
  possible harmful effects 65–6
  pragmatic view of diagnostic criteria 3
  process 78
  reliability 127–9, 199
  research 129–31
  sources of variation (unreliability) 125,
    128–9
Diagnostic and Statistical Manual of
    Mental Disorders, *see DSM headings*
diagnostic definitions 12
diagnostic entity, evolving changes 174–5
Diagnostic Interview Schedule 287
diagnostic pie 163
diagnostic validity 170, 176
dichotomous entities 203
Dick, D. M. 204
differential item functioning 207
dimensional classifications 27, 89–91, 97, 102,
    137, 172, 173–4, 203, 298–9, 300
dimensional perspective 273–4
direct evidence 178–9
disaggregation 184
discordance 250
discrete entity 90
disease
  as abnormality of the body 44, 54–5
  concept of 78–9
  definition of 44, 54–5
  implications of use of term 95
disease entity 78, 79–80
disease model 4, 9, 10, 13, 41
disease perspective 273
disorder
  ambiguous status 87
  implications of use of term 95
  replacing with disease/condition/
    syndrome 51
disorganized symptoms 246
dispositional features 273–4
distress 208–9, 274
domains 96, 102
Donabedian, A. 141
Down syndrome 39–40

drapetomania 28
DSM
  broadening research appendix 14–15
  history of classifications 147
  modesty of the system 66–7
  research role 14
  success in meeting goals of
    classification 13–14
DSM-I 147
DSM-II 147
DSM-III
  advantages 148
  atheoretical approach 43, 44, 125, 132–4
  disadvantages 148
  field trials 131
  multiaxial system 134–5, 136–7
  operationalized criteria 125, 127–31
  paradigm shift 147–8
  processes 149
  rejection of distinct diagnostic
    boundaries 132
  reliability 27
  structure–process–outcomes model 141
  success of 136, 141–2
DSM-III-R 148, 149
DSM-IV
  addition and deletion of disorders 151–2
  clinical goals 145
  communication role 159, 163–4
  controversies/disasters 155
  Craft Criteria 154
  educational goal 146
  false pragmatism 45–6
  first-rank symptoms 245
  folk classifications 86
  generalizability 152, 155
  goals 145–7
  information management 146–7, 158, 163–4
  introduction 156
  operationalization 153
  oversimplification of psychopathology 162–3
  placement issues 153–4
  pragmatic test for DSM-IV pragmatism 48–9
  principles and process 149–54
  reification problem 14
  research appendix 152
  research goals 146
  revising diagnostic criteria 153
  subtyping disorders 152
  tribes of users 158–9, 163–4
DSM-IV-TR, criteria for schizophrenia 238–9
DSM-5 289, 290, 291–2, 300–1
Dupré, J. 63

Edelbrock, C. S. 208
eliminativism 119, 168
Elkin, I. 225
Elliott, C. 64
emergence 272, 280
empiricists 178, 182

Endicott, J. 130
endophenotypes 91, 119, 171, 206
environmental factors 88
epidemiological studies 285–7, 300
Epidemiologic Catchment Area study 287
epistemic iteration 25, 303–4, 306–7, 324–5
  graphical approach 309–17
  psychiatric illness 308–9
epistemology 167, 168, 251–3
essence of disorders 163
Essen-Möller, E. 87–8
essential characteristics of mental disorder 47
essentialist view of disease 78
etiologically-based systems 126
etiology 6, 13
etiopathogenic validity 170–1
evidence
  direct 178–9
  DSM process 51
evidence-based approach 145, 154–5, 156–7
evidence-based medicine 145, 149–50
evolution 26, 172, 191
exhaustive classifications 103
experiment 23–4
experts 46, 51, 141, 149, 203
externalizing 183, 198, 208, 209, 210, 213–14
external validators 176–7
external validity 197, 200
extrinsic/experiential set 272
Ey, H. 85, 250

face validity 170
Falret, J. 107–8
false positives and false negatives 283–4, 288,
  289–90
false pragmatism 45–6
family resemblance 102
Faraday, M. 191
fear 208–9
Feighner criteria 13, 129–30
Fine, A. 177–8, 193
First, M. B. 176
first-rank symptoms 239, 240–5
folk classifications 86
Foucault, M. 104, 120
fuzzy sets 172

GAF scale 287
Galileo 25
Gardner, C.O. 224
Garnier, A. 108–9
Gedankenausspreitung 243–4
Gedankenlautwerden 242–3, 244
genetic issues 48, 83, 182, 195
genetic predisposition 88
gestalt
  prototype 246–7, 263
  schizophrenia 236, 248–9
g factor 201
Global Assessment Scale 286

glossary definitions 129
goals
   of classification 12–13, 145–7
   of nosology 47–8
good stories about life 65, 66, 67
grade of membership 172, 173
great German Professors 304, 310
Guze, S. B. 88, 170

Hacking, I. 64, 312
Hampton, J. 104
Healy, D. 223
hebephrenia 249–51, 262–3
Hecker, E. 249
Hempel, C. 89
heterophenomenology 328
hierarchical classifications 103
hierarchy of symptoms 47
Hippocratic tradition 42–3
Hobbes, T. 23, 24
hopelessness 231
Horwitz, A. V. 221, 288
Huntington's disease 67
hwa-byung 200
hybrid conditions 82
Hyman, S. E. 14, 170, 184
hypotheses 178–9
hypothetico-deductive spiral of
   reasoning 197, 202

ICD
   categorical approach 131–2
   research role 14
   success in meeting goals of
      classification 13–14
ICD-8 147
ICD-9, compatibility with DSM-IV 146
ICD-10
   compatibility with DSM-IV 146
   folk classifications 86
   processes 149
idealism 168
ideal types 104
identification 78
idiographic 103
implication 275
incredible insecurity of psychiatric nosology 29
incremental validation 29–30
incurability 79, 83
individual differences 182
information management 146–7, 158, 163–4
information variance 128
inner speech 242–3
insight 60
instrumentalism 169, 192, 193
interforms 171, 172
internalizing 198, 208–9, 210, 213–14
internal medicine approach 49–50
International Classification of Diseases, *see ICD*
   headings

International Pilot Study of Schizophrenia 81
interpretation variance 128
intrinsic set 272
inventing disorders 28–9, 36
IQ test performance 201
item response theory 174, 206–7
iteration 305–6; *see also* epistemic iteration

Jablensky, A. 171, 175, 191, 224
Jaspers, K. 85, 92

Kahlbaum, K. 249
kappa statistic 27
Kendell, R. 128, 171, 175, 191, 224
Kendler, K. S. 25, 63, 88, 154, 222, 224, 328–9
Kessler, R. L. 289
Kety, S. 253
Kirk, S. A. 26–7
Kissane, D. W. 224
Klein, D. F. 319
Klein, D. N. 225
Kotov, R. 209
Kraepelin, E. 79, 85–6, 133, 235
Kuhn, T. S. 36–7, 326–7
Kutchins, H. 26–7

labeling 28, 36, 64, 71
latent class analysis 174, 328–9
latent schizophrenia 82–3
latent trait analysis 174
latent variable modeling 206
   diagnosis 206
   symptoms 207
Laudan, L. 192
Lawrie, M. S. 230
l'echo de la lecture 243
l'echo de l'ecriture 243
l'echo de pensée 242–3, 244
Leonhard, K. 80, 319
Lewis, A. 222
life events 222
life scripts 274
life story perspective 273, 274
listings 103
lithium treatment 46
lived experience 104
localization 271–2, 274–5
local minimum 315–17
Loevinger, J. 201

MacIntyre, A. 64
major depressive disorder
   prevalence 221
   threshold for diagnosis 224–5, 226
making-up disorders 28–9, 36
man-made 102
Markon, K. E. 300
masochistic personality disorder 28
materialism 168
Maury, A. 108

McHugh, P. R. 273
Mead, M. 141
mechanistic models 194–5
medical humanism 44
medical model 22
medical taxonomy, dichotomies 102–3
medicine, Hippocratic school 42
Meehl, P. E. 89, 169
melancholia 226
mental disorder
  concept 6
  definition 47
mental illness, defining 43–4
meta-language 102–3
metaphysics 167–8
meta-structure 144, 209
Midtown Manhattan Study 285
mindless psychiatry 92
mineness 240
mirror-phenomenon 244
mixed models 91
model-based perspectives 194–5
modified random walk 307, 309–11, 323–4
molecular genetics 172, 174, 181–2, 184, 204–5
monothetic definitions 102
mood
  comorbidity of mood and anxiety
     disorders 203–4
  concept 231
  schizophrenia 245–6
Morel, B. A. 108
multiaxial system 134–5, 136–7
Multidimensional Personality
    Questionnaire 202
multilayered classifications 103
multiple diagnoses 47, 205
multiple levels of reality 167, 168, 171, 181
multiple personality disorder 28
multiple standards 20, 23, 25, 35–6

naming 28
narratives 64–6, 67
National Comorbidity Survey 287
natural classifications 102
natural kinds 59, 62, 102
natural ontological attitude 167, 177–8
natural selection 26
negative symptoms 246
Neptune 24
neuregulin gene 183
neuroscience 181–2, 184
neurosis 29, 133–4
new diagnostic categories 68
nomenclature 78
nomothetic 103
non-Hippocratic traditions 43
non-paranoid schizophrenia 249–51
non-realism 20, 26; *see also* scientific non-
    realism
normal science 36–7

norms 23–4, 28–9
nosography 78
nosological entity 79–80
nosology 78
  goal 47–8

observation
  clinical 49–50, 56
  units of 206
omega-sign 231
ontology 167, 168, 182
operationalized criteria 125, 127–31, 153
Osler, W. 49
outcome
  defining 79
  predictors 81–2
  schizophrenia 80–1
overlapping syndromes 46–7

panic disorder 319
panoply of operons 172
partial classifications 103
partial representations 195
passivity phenomena 244–5
pathologically defined disorders 79
Paykel, E. S. 225
Peirce, C. S. 177, 180
perfect language 104–5
periodic table 8–9, 24, 99
personality disorders
  dimensional approach 173–4, 183, 203
  internalizing–externalizing structure 183, 210
  symptom domains 96
perspectives of psychiatry 273–4, 276–7
pessimistic induction 38, 179, 192
philosophical realism 55
physicalism 168
Pinel, Ph. 105
plain old empirical confirmation 182
pluralism 194–5
  validity 19, 22
political campaigns 26–7
polythetic definitions 102
post-modernism 41, 43, 44–5
post-traumatic stress disorder, contextual
    issues 312
practical consequences 180–1
practical kinds 25
pragmatism
  diagnosis 3
  false pragmatism of DSM-IV 45–6
  pragmatic test for DSM-IV pragmatism 48–9
  reality 192–4
  truth 179–80
  utility 190–1
prediction
  classification 104
  course and treatment response 12–13
  outcome 81–2
  syndrome approach 8

predictive validators 88
predictive validity 170, 175
prevalence of mental disorders 286–8, 300
primary delusions 241–2
principle of respect 328
Prisciandaro, J. J. 299
private prototypes 252
privileged features 105
privileged perspective 120
probabilistic knowledge 50–1
procedures, validity-enhancing 88
process
  diagnosis 78
  pathogenic 271, 273–5
prognosis 81–2, 83
progress
  coherentist framework 326–9
  definition 303
  philosophical view of scientific progress 25–6
  scientific 326–8
  validity 22
promiscuous realists 63
proportionality 222
prototypes 104, 167, 172–4, 195
  gestalt 246–7, 263
  private ones 252
  role in teaching and training 252
proxy variables 102–3, 119
pseudoprecise diagnostic criteria 148
psychiatric object 102, 108, 110, 111, 118–20, 121, 122, 252
psychoanalysts 133
psychological test development 197, 201–2
psychometric model 22
psychosis risk syndrome 68
Ptolemaic model 25
Putnam, H. 100

random chase 315
random walk 304, 307, 309–11, 323–4
reading and writing echo 243
real 39, 40
realism 20, 168
  basic realism 26
  conditionalized 169, 177–8, 193
  promiscuous realists 63
  scientific 25–6, 38–40, 51, 99, 100, 169, 192, 193
  structural 38–9, 182–3
realistic attitude 167
reality
  clinical 171
  multilevel view 167, 168, 171, 181
  pragmatism 192–4
  realism 168
  scientific hypotheses/theories 178–9, 192
  scientific realists and non-realists 26, 39
  utility and 176, 190–1
recovery 80–1, 83
registers of psychopathology 86

reification of diagnostic categories 14, 30, 86–7, 121, 200, 284, 290
reliability 56, 199
  claim-making role 27
  diagnostic 127–9, 199
  diagnostic pie 163
  validity and 49, 190
repeatables 59, 62–4
representation 104
  partial 195
research
  classification in 14–15
  clinical care link 47–8
  clinical definitions 48
  diagnoses 129–31
  funding changes 149
  research goal of DSM-IV 146, 152
Research Domain Criteria (RDoC) project 15–16, 130, 131, 184, 206
respect 328
risks of psychiatric conditions 7
Roberts, J. E. 299
Robins, E. 88, 130, 170
Robins, L. N. 289
Rosch, E. 173

Sackett, D. L. 149
sadness, depression and 221, 223–4, 225–6
sampling 180
Scadding, J. G. 78
scale calibration 23
Schiller, F. C. S. 181
schizoaffective disorder 46–7, 246
schizophrenia
  affective illness and 75, 82, 84, 229–30, 245–6
  anxiety 245
  audible thoughts 242–3, 244
  core gestalt 248–9
  depressive symptoms and syndromes 229–30, 245
  dimensional approach 173
  disorganized symptoms 246
  DSM-IV 153
  DSM-IV-TR criteria 238–9
  entity of 79–80
  epistemic iteration 310–11
  first-rank symptoms 239, 240–5
  genetics 83
  gestalt approach 236, 248–9
  latent 82–3
  mineness 240
  mirror-phenomenon 244
  mixed (class-quantitative) models 91
  molecular complexity 184
  mood 245–6
  narratives 67
  negative symptoms 246
  non-paranoid 249–51
  outcomes 80–1
  oversimplification in DSM-IV 162–3

passivity phenomena 244–5
pre-Kraepelinian nosology 253–4
primary delusions 241–2
prognosis 81–2
recovery from 80–1
Schneider on 239–40
self-awareness 240, 241, 249
sub-threshold conditions in
    relatives 82–3
syndrome 79
third person perspective 236
thought block 244–5
thought diffusion 243–4
whatness of 248
schizophrenic autism 249
schizophrenic spectrum 89
Schneider, K. 239–40
Schwartz, M. A. 247
science
conservative nature 121
cynicism about 50
meaning of 50–1
of medicine 42
normal science 36–7
selling 26–7
scientific classification 77–8
scientific hypotheses/theories 178–9, 192
scientific non-realism 25–6, 38–40
scientific progress
coherentist framework 326–8
philosophical view 25–6
scientific realism 25–6, 38–40, 51, 99, 100, 169,
    192, 193
secondary delusions 242
second person perspective 253
secretive psychiatry 67
self-consciousness 240, 241, 249
self-differentiating set 272
self-perpetuating feedback loops 198, 202, 203,
    204
selling science 26–7
sensations 328
sets 272
Shaffer, D. 292
Sharfstein, S. 270
Shepherd, M. 78
signe du mirroir 244
signs
clusters 183
differentiating from symptoms 10
third person data 252
Slavney, P. R. 273
social constructionist theory 43, 45
socially constructed categories 99–100
social phobia 274
Société Médico Psychologique debate 106–10
somatoform disorder 153
spectrum disorders 83
Spiegelphänomen 244
Spitzer, R. 129, 130, 135, 261, 288

spurious comorbidity 87
standards 20, 23, 25, 35–6
states of mind 274
stereotypes 173
Stirling County Study 285
structural knowledge 207–10
structural realism 38–9, 182–3
structural validity 182–3, 197, 201, 203–4
consequences 204–5
nosology development 205–7
structural realism 182–3
structured classifications 103
structure–process–outcomes model 141
structures 89–91, 182
substances 78
sub-threshold conditions 82–3
subtyping 3, 7–8, 152
surface characteristics 6
symptoms
bimodal distribution 203
clusters 96, 183
differentiating from signs 10
domains 96
hierarchies 47
latent variable modeling 207
leading to other symptoms 47
severity scales 90
third person data 252
treatment 42, 43
syndrome approach 13–14, 79, 87–8, 95
epistemic iteration 312–15
overlapping syndromes 46–7
prediction 8
single syndromes splitting over time 319
susceptibility to classification 100
syphilis 9, 50, 55
system 102

taxa 86
taxonomy 78, 103, 105–6
technology 7
teleological set 272
Ten-country Study on Determinants of
    Outcome of Severe Mental
    Disorders 81
Thase, M. E. 225
'the homely line' 177, 194
theories 178–9, 192
therapy, localization and process 274–5
thinking 242–3
third major psychosis 82, 84–5, 246
third person data 252
third person perspective 236
thought block 244–5
thought diffusion 243–4
thought disorder 210
thought experiments 198
trait domains 96
transmission 243–4
treatment effects 46

treatment of symptoms 42, 43
treatment response
    prediction 12–13
    specificity 46
tribal classifications 122
tribes of users 158–9, 163–4
true comorbidity 87
truth of things 104
truth, validity and utility 179–81

unitary psychosis 230
units
    of classification 78–9
    of observation 206
unobserved entities 24
un-understandable 242, 262
Uranus 24
US-UK Study 128, 285
utilitarian approach 71–2
utility
    clinical 97, 132, 142, 157, 159, 175–6, 181
    pragmatism 190–1
    reality and 176, 190–1
    truth and 179–81
    validity and 75–6, 89, 97, 175–6, 190

vacuum 23–4
validation
    approaches 29–31
    bold strategy 30
    calibration and 23–6
    cautious progressivism 30–1
    conceptual norms 28–9
    conservative strategy 29
    determining valid disorders 37–8
    incremental strategy 29–30
validators
    additional 88
    antecedent 88
    concurrent 88
    epistemic iteration 315

external 176–7
predictive 88
validity
    absence of gold standard 176
    absolute 19
    big V, little v distinction 19, 22, 190
    clinical 171–2, 175–6, 183–4, 195
    comparative 22, 25–6
    concepts 169–71
    construct 169–70, 176
    contrastive 19
    descriptive 170
    diagnostic 170, 176
    diagnostic concepts 88
    etiopathogenic 170–1
    external 197, 200
    face 170
    indictors 35
    pluralism 19, 22
    predictive 170, 175
    procedures to enhance 88
    progress and 22
    reliability and 49, 190
    structural, see structural validity
    truth and 179–81
    utility and 75–6, 89, 97, 175–6, 190
value judgments 170
Venus 25
von Trostorff, S. 80
voyeurism 312

Wakefield, J. C. 221–2, 288
Ward, C. 129
weeds, classifying 38
Widiger, T. A. 183
Wiggins, O. P. 247
wild diagnosis 28
Williams, J. 134
Windelband, W. 103
wobbly iteration 308–9
Worrall, J. 38–9, 182